Competency Based

BD Chaurasia's

Human Anatomy

Tenth Edition

Volume 4

Regional and Applied | **Dissection and Clinical**

As per the latest NMC Guidelines | Competency Based Medical Education (CBME) Curriculum under Graduate Medical Education Regulation

Brain–Neuroanatomy

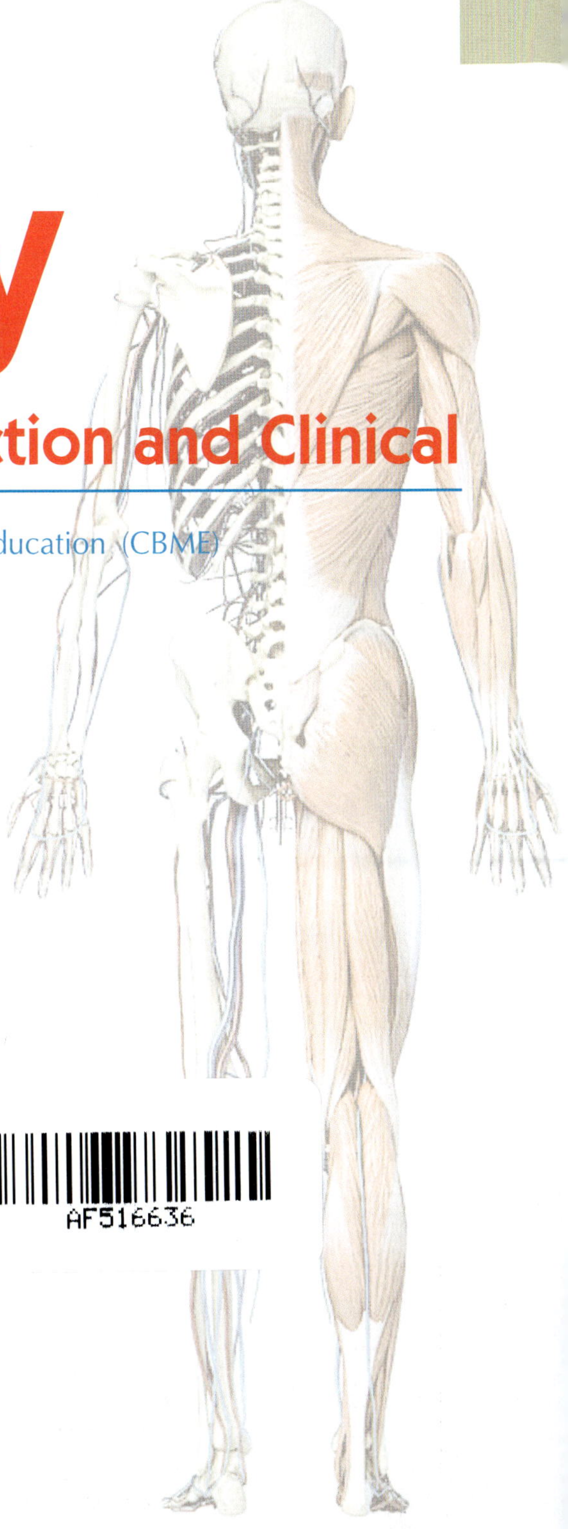

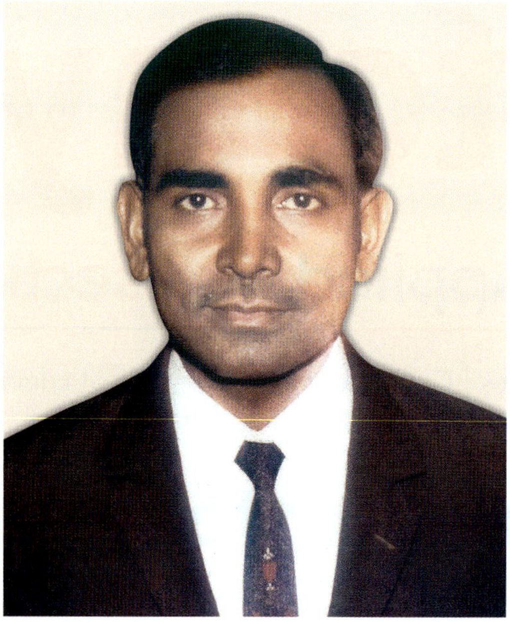

Dr BD Chaurasia (1937–1985)

was Reader in Anatomy at GR Medical College, Gwalior.
He received his MBBS in 1960, MS in 1965 and PhD in 1975.
He was elected fellow of National Academy of Medical Sciences (India) in 1982.
He was a member of the Advisory Board of the *Acta Anatomica* since 1981,
member of the editorial board of *Bionature*, and in addition
member of a number of scientific societies.
He had a large number of research papers to his credit.

Competency Based

BD Chaurasia's

Human Anatomy

Tenth Edition

Volume 4

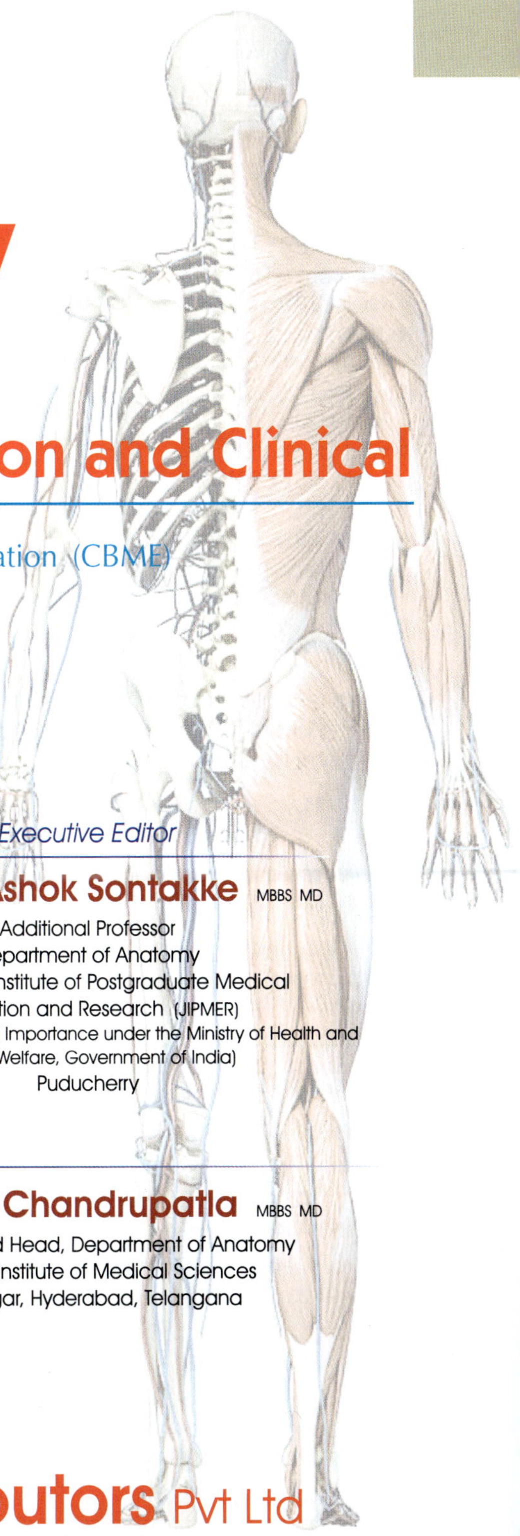

Regional and Applied **Dissection and Clinical**

As per the latest NMC Guidelines | Competency Based Medical Education (CBME) Curriculum under Graduate Medical Education Regulation

Brain–Neuroanatomy

Chief Editor

Krishna Garg
MBBS MS PhD FIMSA FIAMS FAMS FASI
Legend of Anatomy; Nation's Who's Who
Fellow, Anatomical Society of India
Lifetime Achievement Awardee
DMA Distinguished Service Awardee
Ex-Professor and Head, Department of Anatomy
Lady Hardinge Medical College, New Delhi

Executive Editor

Yogesh Ashok Sontakke MBBS MD
Additional Professor
Department of Anatomy
Jawaharlal Institute of Postgraduate Medical Education and Research (JIPMER)
(An Institute of National Importance under the Ministry of Health and Family Welfare, Government of India)
Puducherry

Editors

Pragati Sheel Mittal MBBS MS
Professor, Department of Anatomy
Government Institute of Medical Sciences
Greater Noida, Uttar Pradesh

Mrudula Chandrupatla MBBS MD
Professor and Head, Department of Anatomy
All India Institute of Medical Sciences
Bibinagar, Hyderabad, Telangana

CBS Publishers & Distributors Pvt Ltd

New Delhi • Bengaluru • Chennai • Kochi • Kolkata • Lucknow • Mumbai
Gujarat • Hyderabad • Jharkhand • Nagpur • Patna • Pune • Uttarakhand

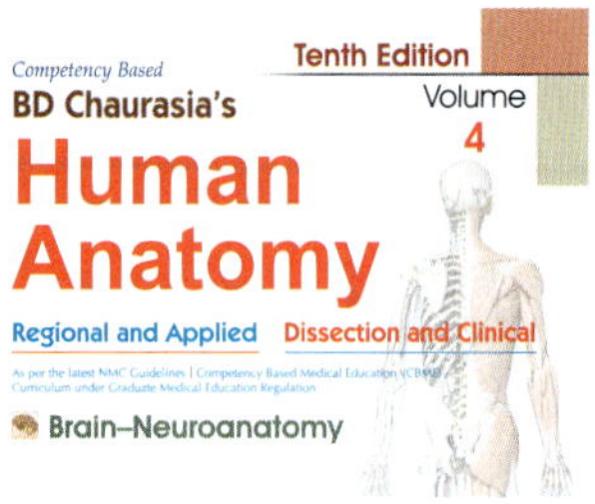

Disclaimer

Science and technology are constantly changing fields. New research and experience broaden the scope of information and knowledge. The editors have tried their best in giving information available to them while preparing the material for this book. Although, all efforts have been made to ensure optimum accuracy of the material, yet it is quite possible some errors might have been left uncorrected. The publisher, the printer and the editors will not be held responsible for any inadvertent errors, omissions or inaccuracies.

ISBN: 978-93-5466-943-9

Tenth Edition: 2025[1]
Reprint: 2026

First Edition: 1979
Reprint: 1980, 1981, 1982, 1983, 1984, 1985, 1986, 1987, 1988
Second Edition: 1989
Reprint: 1990, 1991, 1992, 1993, 1994
Third Edition: 1995
Reprint: 1996, 1997, 1998, 1999, 2000, 2001, 2002, 2003, 2004
Fourth Edition: 2004
Reprint: 2005, 2006, 2007, 2008, 2009
Fifth Edition: 2010
Reprint: 2011, 2012
Sixth Edition: 2013
Reprint: 2014, 2015
Seventh Edition: 2016
Reprint: 2017, 2018, 2019
Eighth Edition: 2020
Reprint: 2021, 2022
Ninth Edition: 2023
Reprint: 2024

Published by Satish Kumar Jain and produced by Varun Jain for

CBS Publishers & Distributors Pvt Ltd
4819/XI Prahlad Street, 24 Ansari Road, Daryaganj, New Delhi 110 002, India
Ph: 011-23289259, 23266838 Website: www.cbspd.com
e-mail: delhi@cbspd.com

Corporate Office: 204 FIE, Industrial Area, Patparganj, Delhi 110 092, India
Ph: 011-4934 4934 Fax: 011-4934 4935 e-mail: publishing@cbspd.com; publicity@cbspd.com

Branches

- **Bengaluru:** Seema House 2975, 17th Cross, K.R. Road, Banasankari 2nd Stage, Bengaluru 560 070, Karnataka, India
  Ph: +91-80-26771678/79 Fax: +91-80-26771680 e-mail: bangalore@cbspd.com
- **Chennai:** 18/8B, Subbarayan Street, Shenoy Nagar, Chennai 600 030, Tamil Nadu, India
  Ph: +91-44-42032115, 26681266 e-mail: chennai@cbspd.com
- **Kochi:** 42/1325, 1326, Power House Road, Opposite KSEB, Power House, Ernakulum 682 018, Kochi, Kerala, India
  Ph: +91-484-4059061–65, 67 Fax: +91-484-4059065 e-mail: kochi@cbspd.com
- **Kolkata:** 147, Hind Ceramics Compound, 1st Floor, Nilgunj Road, Belghoria, Kolkata 700 056, West Bengal, India
  Ph: +91-33-25633055/56 e-mail: kolkata@cbspd.com
- **Lucknow:** Basement, Khushnuma Complex, 7 Meerabai Marg (behind Jawahar Bhawan), Lucknow 226 001, UP, India
  Ph: +91-522-4000032 e-mail: tiwari.lucknow@cbspd.com
- **Mumbai:** PWD Shed, Gala No. 25/26, Ramchandra Bhatt Marg, Next JJ Hospital Gate No. 2, Opp. Union Bank of India, Noorbaug, Mumbai 400 009, Maharashtra, India
  Ph: +91-22-66661880/89 e-mail: mumbai@cbspd.com

Representatives

• **Gujarat**	0-9879558667	• **Hyderabad**	0-9885175004	• **Jharkhand**	0-9811541605	• **Nagpur**	0-8692091830
• **Patna**	0-9334159340	• **Pune**	0-9664372571	• **Uttarakhand**	0-9716462459		

Printed at: Thomson Press (India) Ltd., Faridabad, Haryana, India

to

my teacher
Shri Uma Shankar Nagayach

— BD Chaurasia

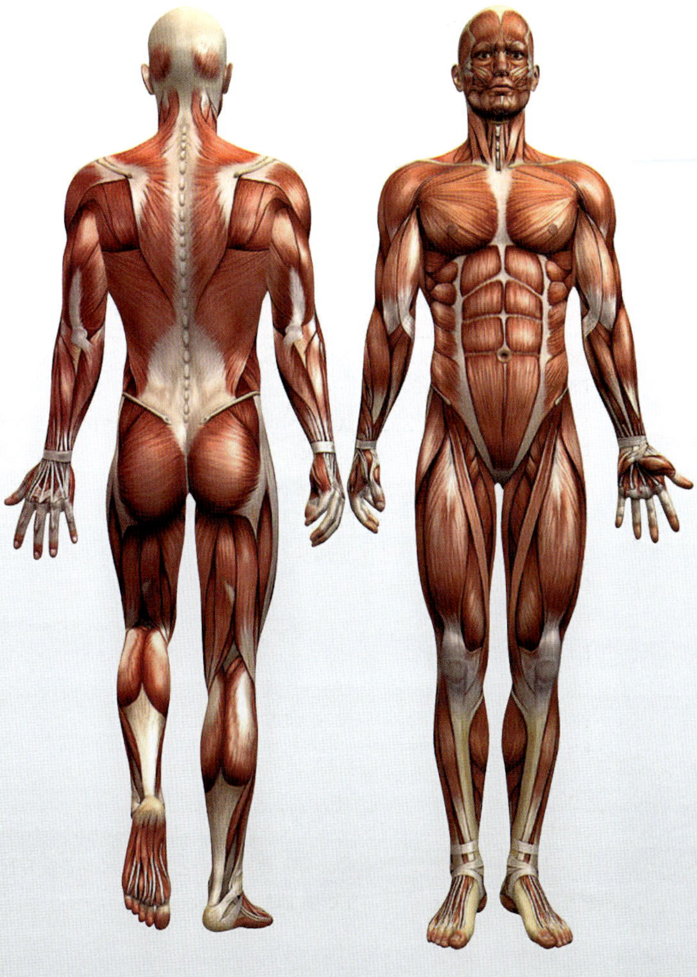

Volume 1 UPPER LIMB and THORAX

Volume 2 LOWER LIMB, ABDOMEN and PELVIS

Volume 3 HEAD and NECK

Volume 4 BRAIN–NEUROANATOMY

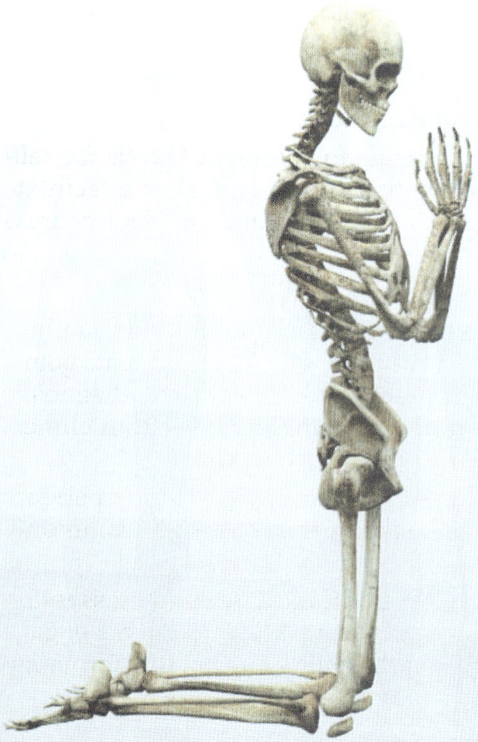

Preface to the Tenth Edition

With the change in time, the needs of the students and curriculum are continuously changing. The science is continuously evolving. To integrate the solutions to common problems faced by the students and to follow the latest NMC guidelines for the CBME curriculum, the most widely accepted and read book has been revised thoroughly to maintain the standards of the last half-century. The primary goal of this book is to help the students for easy understanding and rapid grasping of knowledge for their higher academic achievements, to prepare them for all academic formative, summative and entrance examinations and to make it extremely student-friendly.

Anatomy forms the foundation of the clinical knowledge. This book has been made more clinically oriented with the following salient features:

- **Complete** and **time-tested textbook** boasting unparalleled **quality content** designed to enrich both fundamental and clinical understanding for students.
- **Simple text** is the main feature of the book. It will facilitate easier understanding for students. Small sentences minimize effort, enhancing readability and accessibility. This approach ensures clarity of information, aiding students in grasping complex concepts effortlessly.
- **Updated text and images:** The text and images updated as per the updates in the field of medicine, in the terms updates the facts and the data from the authenticated reference books. All the deviations from the traditional concepts, have been duly sourced and referenced to the standard international publications. It make the book suitable for all the academic university and entrance examinations need the updated information.
- **3D colour illustrated plates** will aid the students in comprehending anatomical structures and their relationships with clarity. These visual aids offer a dynamic perspective, enhancing spatial understanding and facilitating the identification of anatomical features.
- **Simple line diagrams** are incorporated. These diagrams will allow students to easily redraw them during examinations. These diagrams are designed for clarity and simplicity, ensuring that students can accurately reproduce anatomical structures in assessments and examinations efficiently.
- **Flowcharts** will facilitate rapid revision and memorizing of facts, alleviating students' concerns about time constraints during the subject review. These visuals will enhance comprehension and retention. Students can quickly navigate through key concepts, optimizing study time and effectively addressing time limitations in their revision process.
- **Clinical anatomy** sections are integrated at the end of each topic to maintain the purpose towards **early clinical exposure (ECE)**. By seamlessly merging theoretical knowledge with practical application, this approach ensures students gain valuable insights into clinical contexts, enhancing their understanding and readiness for real-world clinical scenarios.
- **Dissection boxes** will guide the students in the step-wise dissection of the human cadaver.
- **Tables** are used to summarise essential facts for clear understanding and retention.
- ***QR codes*** for ***eSmartQuiz*** are embedded in the text, which will grant access to online MCQ tests for self-assessment at the end of each chapter. This interactive feature will enhance engagement and facilitate convenient self-evaluation. Students can assess their understanding, reinforce learning, and identify areas for improvement, facilitate a dynamic and effective learning experience.
- *Free* ***Workbook:*** The main textbook is supported with a workbook, which has the following:
  1. **Clinicoanatomical problems** emphasize early clinical exposure and vertical integration in medical education. By integrating anatomical knowledge with clinical practice from the outset, students gain a holistic understanding of medical concepts. This approach fosters practical skills, enhances diagnostic abilities, and promotes a deeper comprehension of the human body's complexities within clinical contexts.
  2. **Practice figures** aid in preparing students for academic examinations by providing hands-on experience with exam-style preparation. It will help to build confidence in tackling the challenges commonly encountered in academic assessments.
  3. **Multiple choice questions (MCQs)** will serve as potent tools for reinforcing learning, assessing comprehension, and enhancing attention and critical thinking skills. Through MCQs, students engage actively with the curriculum, consolidate understanding, and develop the ability to analyse information critically, ultimately fostering deeper comprehension and retention of knowledge.

4. **Spotters** and **question bank** introduce students to the examination system by familiarising them with the format and types of questions commonly encountered in assessments. These wide ranges of questions will aid the students in preparing for examinations and gaining confidence in tackling examination challenges effectively.

- ***Free MindMaps in Anatomy*:** A separate booklet of MindMaps in Anatomy is included with each volume. These MindMaps will help the students revise and memorise anatomy through visual impact in a precise manner.
- ***Free access to BDC's Anatomy eBook (digital content through CBSiCentral app)*:** It includes the following:
  a. Additional topics and clinical aspects
  b. *Viva voce* questions, and
  c. Topics for further reference and reading.

  This digital resource will enhance the book's utility, providing students with expanded knowledge and resources for comprehensive learning. Accessible supplementary materials will enhance understanding and facilitate deeper exploration, empowering students to excel in their studies and clinical practice.
- **Free Access to CBSiCentral App:** It includes videos of osteology and soft parts and chapter-wise self-assessment MCQ tests. The videos of the dissection will give three-dimensional image descriptions of tissues and organs, which get effectively registered in the brain for a longer time.
- **Wall charts:** Each volume is provided with meticulously crafted wall charts, elegantly designed and tailored to enhance students' comprehension of anatomy. These visually engaging aids can be easily affixed to walls to grasp the visual impressions of anatomy.

Always remember that success is achieved only through diligent effort and hard work.

Chief Editor
Krishna Garg

Executive Editor
Yogesh Ashok Sontakke

Editors
Pragati Sheel Mittal
Mrudula Chandrupatla

Preface to the First Edition (excerpts)

The necessity of having a simple, systematized and complete book on anatomy has long been felt. The urgency for such a book has become all the more acute due to the shorter time now available for teaching anatomy, and also to the falling standards of English language in the majority of our students in India. The national symposium on 'Anatomy in Medical Education' held at Delhi in 1978 was a call to change the existing system of teaching the unnecessary minute details to the undergraduate students.

This attempt has been made with an object to meet the requirements of a common medical student. The text has been arranged in small classified parts to make it easier for the students to remember and recall it at will. It is adequately illustrated with simple line diagrams which can be reproduced without any difficulty, and which also help in understanding and memorizing the anatomical facts that appear to defy memory of a common student. The monotony of describing the individual muscles separately, one after the other, has been minimised by writing them out in tabular form, which makes the subject interesting for a lasting memory. The relevant radiological and surface anatomy have been treated in separate chapters. A sincere attempt has been made to deal, wherever required, the clinical applications of the subject. The entire approach is such as to attract and inspire the students for a deeper dive in the subject of anatomy.

The book has been intentionally split in three parts for convenience of handling. This also makes a provision for those who cannot afford to have the whole book at a time.

It is quite possible that there are errors of omission and commission in this mostly single-handed attempt. I would be grateful to the readers for their suggestions to improve the book from all angles.

I am very grateful to my teachers and the authors of numerous publications, whose knowledge has been freely utilised in the preparation of this book. I am equally grateful to my professor and colleagues for their encouragement and valuable help. My special thanks are due to my students who made me feel their difficulties, which was a great incentive for writing this book. I have derived maximum inspiration from Prof. Inderbir Singh (Rohtak), and learned the decency of work from Shri SC Gupta (Jiwaji University, Gwalior).

I am deeply indebted to Shri KM Singhal (National Book House, Gwalior) and Mr SK Jain (CBS Publishers & Distributors, Delhi), who have taken unusual pains to get the book printed in its present form. For giving it the desired get-up, Mr VK Jain and Raj Kamal Electric Press are gratefully acknowledged. The cover page was designed by Mr Vasant Paranjpe, the artist and photographer of our college; my sincere thanks are due to him. I acknowledge with affection the domestic assistance of Munne Miyan and the untiring company of my Rani, particularly during the odd hours of this work.

BD Chaurasia

Acknowledgements

We have the blessings and good wishes of Prof NA Faruqi (Aligarh); Dr DC Naik (Rewa); Dr SD Joshi and Dr SS Joshi (Indore); Dr (Brig) Rakesh Gupta (Greater Noida); Dr DR Singh (Lucknow); Dr M Kaul; Dr C Anand and Dr I Bahl (Delhi); Dr Mohsin Azmi (Kanpur); Dr Medha Joshi (Ghaziabad); Dr Surbhi Gupta (Delhi); Dr Nitin Nagarkar (Raipur); Dr CK Shukla (Raipur); Dr Shakuntala Pai (Manipal); Dr Manik Chatterjee (Raipur) and Dr SN Kazi (Pune).

We are thankful to Dr Sangeeta Chouhan, Dr Seema Gupta (Jaipur); Dr Surjit Ghatak (Jodhpur); Dr Vinay Sharma (Muzzafarnagar); Dr Deepu Singh Kataria (UP); Dr Anup Singh Gurjar (Pali); Dr Jagmohan Sharma, Dr Deepak Sharma, Dr Rajesh Arora and Dr Sumit Gupta (Kota); Dr Gopal Sharma and Dr Manoj Sharma (Jhalawar); Dr Rekha Parashar (Dausa); Dr Santosh Kumar (Dholpur); Dr Isha Srivastav, Dr Aprajita Raizada, Dr Sajan Skaria, Dr Hitant Vohra, Dr Anjali Jain, Dr Kalpana Sharma, Dr Praveen Ojha, Dr Prakash KG, Dr Seema Prakash (Udaipur); for giving feedback for various sections of the volumes. We are greatful to Dr K Aravindhan, Dr V Gladwin, Dr Raveendranath V, Dr Suman Verma, Dr Sulochana Sakthivel, Dr Rajasekhar SSSN and Dr Vidhya G (Puducherry) for their support.

We are grateful to Dr Anupma Mahajan (Amritsar); Dr Vanita Gupta (Jammu); Dr Vikas Verma (Lucknow) and Dr Tripta Bhagat (Ghaziabad) for editing chapters to enhance the value of the volumes. We are grateful to Dr Sangeeta and Dr Nusrat Jabeen (Jammu); Dr Gurdeep Singh Kalyan (Gajrola); Dr Rajan Singla (Patiala); Dr Aprajita Sikka (Ludhiana); Dr Bashir (Srinagar) and Dr Ritu (Rajouri); Dr Mubeen (Kathua); Dr RK Srivastava (Kanpur); Dr Punita Manik (Lucknow); Dr Binod Kumar; Dr Sunita Nayak and Dr Shambhu Prasad (Patna); Dr AK Dubey (Ranchi); Dr Satyam Khare, Dr Shilpi Jain and Dr Alok Tripathi (Meerut), for promoting the volumes.

We have been getting constant encouragement and support from Dr Ranjana Verma, Dr Muthukrishnan P, Dr Yogesh Yadav, Dr Pullimi Vineel and Dr Nirupma Gupta (Greater Noida); Dr Nisha Kaul (Ghaziabad); Dr Vinay Singhal (Saharanpur); Dr RK Ashoka (Mathura); Dr Vineet Guhia (Khandwa); Dr Manisha Sinha (Raipur); Dr Jahan Shirin (Kanpur); Dr Damyanti (Manipur) and Dr MK Anand (Bhuj).

Our regards and affection to Dr Rewa Choudhry, Dr Shilpa Paul, Dr Smita Kakar, Dr Anita Tuli, Dr Gayatri Rath, Dr Shashi Raheja, Dr A Shariff, Dr SB Ray, Dr Vandana Mehta, Dr Sabita Mishra, Dr Renu Chauhan, Dr Jyoti Arora, Dr Sneh Agarwal, Dr TS Roy, Dr Ruchi Dhuria, Dr Shaifaly Madan Rustagi (Delhi) and Dr Anjoo Yadav for going through the volumes.

We would like to thank Dr Pritha Bhuiyan (Mumbai); Dr Brijendra Singh (Rishikesh); Retd (Brig) Dr Sushil Kumar (Faridabad); Dr AK Srivastava (Lucknow); Dr MK Pant (Dehradun); Dr Simmi Mehra (Rajkot); Dr Fatima M De Souza (Goa); Dr Mukesh Mittal (Shivpuri); Dr Priti Sinha (Saharanpur); Dr Rashmi Malhotra (Rishikesh); Dr Simmi Soni (Aziznagar); Dr Sunita Gupta (Ahmedabad); Dr Raghunandan Ramanathan (Chennai), Dr BK Aghera (Ahmedabad) and many-many other teachers all over the globe, for giving us good wishes.

We also acknowledge Drs Neetu Sivadasan, Rituraj Majumdar, Nandhini R, Nithya D, Kalaivani K, Jakkula Akhil, Ambiga R, S Nikilesh, Udit Narayan, Jayasree S, Bharathy Mohan P, Nandhini S, Aakriti Mehrotra, Sancy Charly, Madhusingh Thakur, Tarakeshwari RB, Dhivyaa Shree R, Thaiyal Nayagi and Prasanna Raj AV (Puducherry) for their support.

Videos of bones and soft parts of human body, prepared at Kathmandu University School of Medical Sciences, have now been added with the respective chapters and are available at our mobile App CBSiCentral. We are grateful to Dr R Koju, CEO of Kathmandu University School of Medical Sciences (KUSMS) and Dhulikhel Hospital, for his generosity.

The moral support of my (chief editor) family members, Late Dr DP Garg, Dr Suvira Gupta, Dr JP Gupta, Mr Manoj, Ms Rekha, Mr Sanjay, Ms Meenakshi, Dr Manish, Dr Shilpa Garg, Dr Naveen Garg, Dr Manoj, Dr Nalini Shukla, Dr Vikas Verma and Dr Swati Gupta, is appreciated.

The magnanimity shown by Mr SK Jain (Chairman) and Mr Varun Jain (Director), CBS Publishers & Distributors, has been always forthcoming. The unquestionable support of Mr YN Arjuna (Senior Vice President—Publishing, Editorial and Publicity) and his entire team comprising Ms Ritu Chawla (GM—Production), Mr Neeraj Prasad (Graphic Artist), Mr Binay Kumar (Editor) and Mr Vikrant Sharma (DTP operator) has made an excellent contribution to bring out this edition. We are really obliged to them and pray for their prosperity.

Editors

Contents

Preface to the Tenth Edition *vii*
Preface to the First Edition *ix*
Index of Competencies *xiii*

1. Organisation of Nervous System 1
2. Peripheral Nerves and Ganglia 12
3. Receptors 18
4. Meninges of the Brain and Cerebrospinal Fluid 22
5. Spinal Cord 30
6. Cranial Nerves 49
7. Brainstem 84
8. Cerebellum 99
9. Fourth Ventricle 109
10. Diencephalon and Third Ventricle 114
11. Cerebrum, Basal Nuclei and White Matter 126
12. Lateral Ventricle and Limbic System 148
13. Some Neural Pathways and Reticular Formation 157
14. Blood Supply of Brain 162
15. Surface Marking and Radiological Anatomy of Nervous System 173
16. Autonomic Nervous System 178
17. Development of Nervous System 185

Appendix: Ventricles, Cranial Nerves and Arteries 193

Index *197*

eSmartQuiz – Online MCQ Test

After attending the class, students should go through the "*eSmartQuiz* – Online MCQ test" for the following reasons:

- *Reinforcement of Learning*: The "*eSmartQuiz* – Online MCQ test" provide an opportunity to reinforce learning after attending a class or reading a book. It helps to assess understanding and retention of concepts, to solidify knowledge and identify areas that need further revision or clarification.
- *Assessment of Comprehension*: The "*eSmartQuiz* – Online MCQ test" is an effective tool to assess comprehension of the subject matter and to demonstrate the ability to apply the concepts learned in the class.
- *Enhancement of Attention and Critical Thinking*: The "*eSmartQuiz* – Online MCQ test" will help to make students attentive for the class and to enhance critical thinking skills by selecting the most appropriate answer among the given options.

Each *eSmartQuiz* test consists of 10 MCQs, mostly image-based, and the students can see their scores at the end of each test. These questions will be modified after a certain interval. Use the given links or scan the QR code (given in each chapter) for the test. One student can solve each test only one time.

Chapter	*Link for* ***eSmartQuiz***
Brain–Neuroanatomy	
1. Organisation of Nervous System	https://forms.gle/q3QXQaymKrN8LpvB8
2. Peripheral Nerves and Ganglia	https://forms.gle/ZdAcAbiBLx22dcP19
3. Receptors	https://forms.gle/1By6ddQt6Y1Vf7saA
4. Meninges of the Brain and Cerebrospinal Fluid	https://forms.gle/KsXnZzsHqy6ghy5XA
5. Spinal Cord	https://forms.gle/M5b5xRmq52m64H24A
6. Cranial Nerves	https://forms.gle/H1ws2DKLCctwm8Gx7
7. Brainstem	https://forms.gle/J5E9oiZZ4sZpZzJV6
8. Cerebellum	https://forms.gle/X1b5HvoSK3TqDHSm6
9. Fourth Ventricle	https://forms.gle/FWf7GEgYhPxzUNSS6
10. Diencephalon and Third Ventricle	https://forms.gle/pAsf7NtBmtYSE51r6
11. Cerebrum, Basal Nuclei and White Matter	https://forms.gle/tYvNGezPahWx5dV56
12. Lateral Ventricle and Limbic System	https://forms.gle/JdLkLaob4K1eMdzy8
13. Some Neural Pathways and Reticular Formation	https://forms.gle/E4fzgQp2NKfNkb3W9
14. Blood Supply of Brain	https://forms.gle/8pbcViRGCJ1N67kK6
15. Surface Marking and Radiological Anatomy of Nervous System	https://forms.gle/K5rzTmY6hD8pM6nn9
16. Autonomic Nervous System	https://forms.gle/3q9bCZtNHiA27UDU6
17. Development of Nervous System	https://forms.gle/UMXxbzcC1hA1Rpg88

Index of Competencies

As per the latest NMC Guidelines | Competency Based Medical Education (CBME)
Curriculum under Graduate Medical Education Regulation

Code	Competency	Chapter	Page no.
AN31.5	Explain the anatomical basis of oculomotor, trochlear and abducent nerve palsies along with strabismus	6	59
AN56.1	Describe and identify various layers of meninges with its extent and modifications	4	22
AN56.2	Describe formation, circulation and absorption of CSF with its applied anatomy	4	28
AN57.1	Identify external features of spinal cord	5	32
AN57.2	Describe extent of spinal cord in child and adult with its clinical implication	5	30
AN57.3	Draw and label transverse section of spinal cord at midcervical and midthoracic level	5	38
AN57.4	Enumerate ascending and descending tracts at mid thoracic level of spinal cord	5	38
AN57.5	Describe the anatomical basis of clinical conditions affecting the grey and white matter of spinal cord (Brown-Séquard syndrome, poliomyelitis, amyotrophic lateral sclerosis or motor neuron disease, syringomyelia, hereditary sensory neuropathy, subacute combined degeneration, transverse myelitis, paraplegia)	5	46
AN58.1	Identify external features of medulla oblongata	7	84
AN58.2	Describe transverse section of medulla oblongata at the level of: (1) pyramidal decussation, (2) sensory decussation, (3) inferior olivary nucleus	7	87
AN58.3	Enumerate cranial nerve nuclei in medulla oblongata with their functional group	7	87
AN58.4	Describe the anatomical basis of clinical conditions affecting the medulla oblongata (medial and lateral medullary syndromes, crossed diplegia)	7	89
AN59.1	Identify external features of pons	7	91
AN59.2	Draw and label transverse section of pons at the upper and lower level	7	91
AN59.3	Enumerate cranial nerve nuclei in pons with their functional group	7	91
AN60.1	Describe and demonstrate external and internal features of cerebellum	8	99
AN60.2	Describe connections of cerebellar cortex and intracerebellar nuclei	8	103
AN60.3	Describe anatomical basis of cerebellar dysfunction	8	107
AN61.1	Identify external and internal features of midbrain	7	95
AN61.2	Describe internal features of midbrain at the level of superior and inferior colliculus	7	95
AN61.3	Describe the anatomical basis of clinical conditions affecting the midbrain (Weber's syndrome, Benedikt syndrome, Parinaud syndrome)	7	98
AN62.1	Enumerate cranial nerve nuclei with its functional component. Also describe the effects of damage to various functional areas of cerebral cortex	6	49
AN62.2	Describe and demonstrate surfaces, sulci, gyri, poles, and functional areas of cerebral hemisphere	11	128
AN62.3	Describe the white matter of cerebrum. Also describe the effects of damage to corpus callosum and different parts of internal capsule	11	140
AN62.4	Enumerate parts and major connections of basal ganglia/ nuclei and limbic lobe. Also explain the anatomical basis of Parkinson's disease, chorea, athetosis and ballismus	11, 12	137, 151
AN62.5	Describe boundaries, parts, gross relations, major nuclei and connections of dorsal thalamus, hypothalamus, epithalamus, metathalamus and subthalamus	10	114
AN62.6	Describe and identify formation, branches and major areas of distribution of circle of Willis	14	165
AN63.1	Describe and demonstrate parts, boundaries and features of IIIrd, IVth and lateral ventricle	9, 10, 12	109, 123, 148
AN63.2	Describe anatomical basis of congenital hydrocephalus	4	29

(Contd.)

(Contd.)

Code	Competency	Chapter	Page no.
AN63.3	Describe the olfactory, visual, auditory and gustatory pathways	6	52
AN64.1	Describe and identify the microanatomical features of spinal cord, cerebellum and cerebrum	8, 11	106, 136
AN64.2	Describe the development of neural tube, spinal cord, medulla oblongata, pons, midbrain, cerebral hemisphere and cerebellum	17	185
AN64.3	Describe various types of open neural tube defects with its embryological basis	17	190
AN68.1	Describe and identify multipolar and unipolar neurons, ganglia, peripheral nerve	2	12
AN68.3	Describe the ultrastructure of nervous tissue	2	12

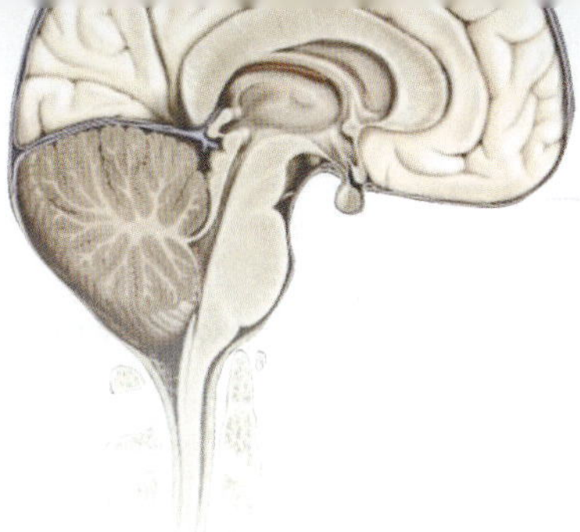

Chapter 1

Organisation of Nervous System

Understanding neuroanatomy is crucial for comprehending the nervous system, the primary controlling and coordinating system of the body. It is responsible for judgement, intelligence and memory. It adjusts the body to the surroundings and regulates all bodily activities both voluntary and involuntary. The sensory part of the nervous system collects information from the surroundings and helps in gaining knowledge and experience, whereas the motor part is responsible for responses of the body.

Average weight of adult brain in air is 1500–2000 grams. Since brain floats in cerebrospinal fluid, it only weighs 50 grams which is comfortable. There are about 180–200 billion neurons in an adult brain.

DIVISIONS OF NERVOUS SYSTEM

Anatomical Divisions

It is divided into CNS and PNS (Flowchart 1.1).

Central nervous system (CNS): It which comprises brain and spinal cord. It is responsible for integrating, coordinating the sensory information and ordering appropriate motor actions. CNS is the seat of learning, memory, intelligence and emotions.

Peripheral nervous system (PNS): It includes 12 pairs of cranial nerves and 31 pairs of spinal nerves. These provide afferent impulses to CNS and carries efferent impulses to muscles, glands and blood vessels.

Functional Divisions

Peripheral nervous system functionally has two components:

1. ***Afferent component*** provides sensory information to CNS.
2. ***Efferent component*** carries motor information to muscles, glands, blood vessels and heart via:
   a. ***Somatic nervous system*** for the control of skeletal muscles.
   b. ***Autonomic nervous system*** for control of heart, smooth muscle of the organs, glands and blood vessels. It is subdivided into sympathetic and parasympathetic parts.

CELLULAR ARCHITECTURE

The nervous tissue is made up of:

1. Nerve cells or neurons (Fig. 1.1).
2. Neuroglial cells (neuroglia), forming the supporting (connective) tissue of the CNS. In peripheral nervous system, these are replaced by Schwann's cells.

Both types of cells are supplied by abundant blood vessels.

NEURON

Each neuron is made up of the following (Fig. 1.1):

1. ***Cell body***: Collectively forms grey matter, the nuclei in the CNS, and ganglia in the peripheral nervous system.

Flowchart 1.1: Divisions of nervous system

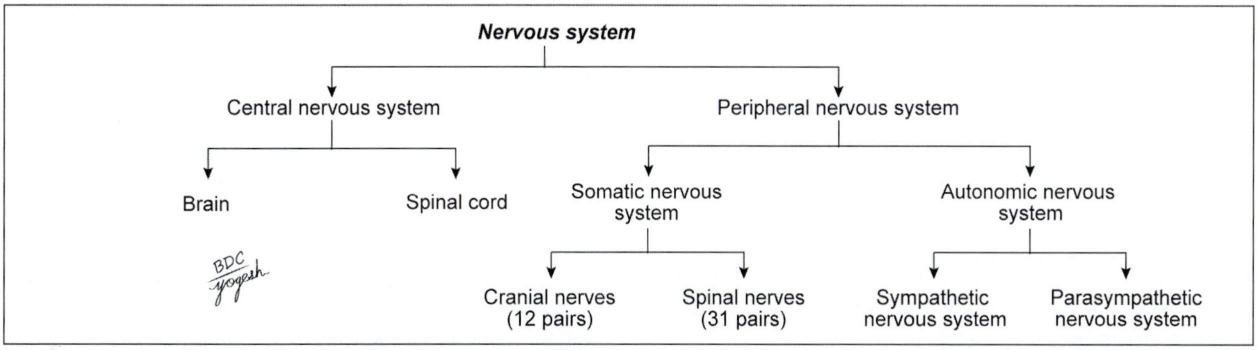

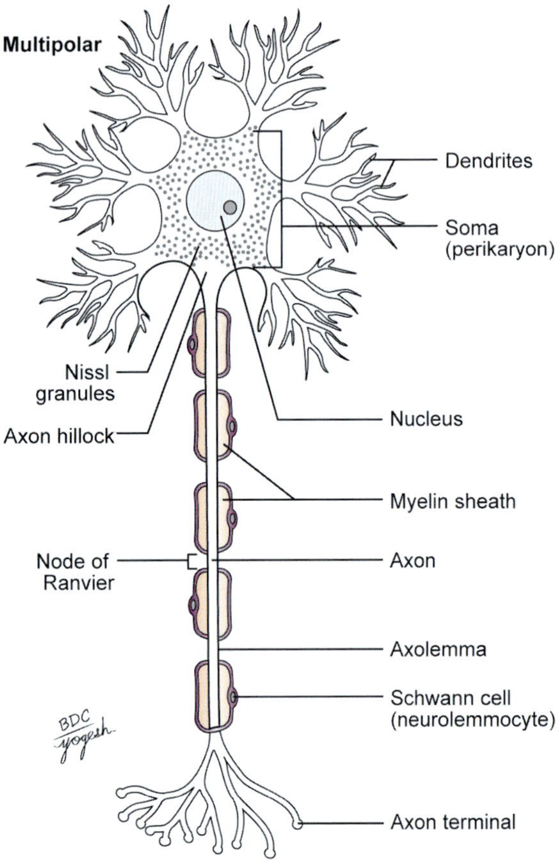

Fig. 1.1: Multipolar neuron

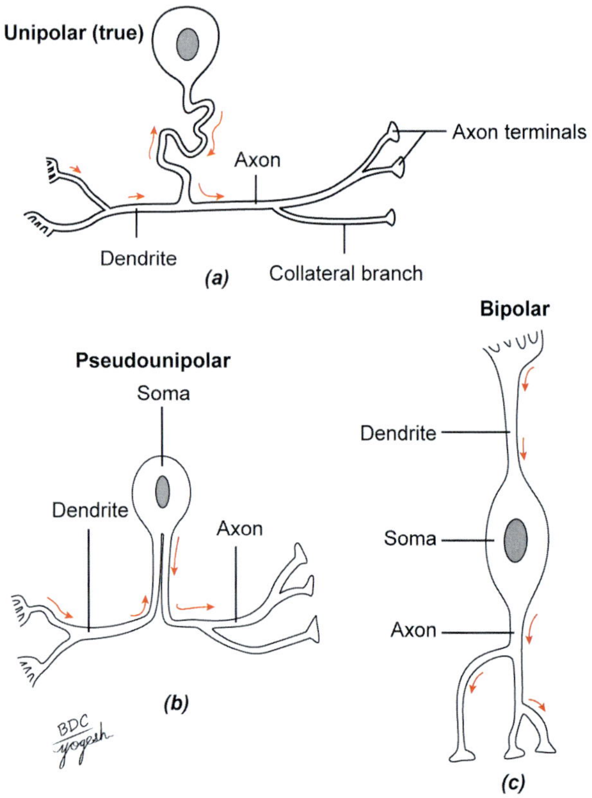

Figs 1.2a to c: Types of neurons (schematic)

Flowchart 1.2: Classification of neurons

Neurons

Based on number of processes

Unipolar: Mesencephalic nucleus of nerve V
Pseudounipolar: Dorsal root ganglia, sensory ganglia of cranial nerves
Bipolar: Retina, VIII nerve ganglia
Multipolar: Purkinje cells, pyramidal cells, anterior horn cells

Based on axon length

Golgi type I: Long axons
Golgi type II: Short axons

Note: Physiologically, neurons are classified as sensory and motor neurons.

2. ***Cell processes*** of two varieties:
   a. ***Dendrites*** (Greek *branch of a tree*) are many, short, richly branched and often varicose (Fig. 1.1).
   b. ***Axon*** is a single elongated process. Collectively the axons form tracts (white matter) in the CNS, and nerves in the peripheral nervous system. The branches of axons often arise at right angles and are called the collaterals.

Note: Functionally, each neuron is specialized for sensitivity and conductivity. The impulses can flow in them with great rapidity, in some cases about 125 meters per second. A neuron shows *dynamic polarity* in its processes. The impulse flows towards the cell body in the dendrites, and away from the cell body in the axon.

Classification of Neurons (Flowchart 1.2)

According to the Number of their Processes

1. ***Unipolar neurons:*** They are present in the mesencephalic nucleus of trigeminal nerve and also occur during foetal life. These cells are more common in lower vertebrates (Fig. 1.2a).
2. ***Pseudounipolar neurons:*** They are actually unipolar to begin with but become bipolar functionally and are found in dorsal nerve root ganglia and sensory ganglia of the cranial nerves (Fig. 1.2b).

   Note: New concept: Unipolar and pseudounipolar neurons are under the same category [Pawlina, Histology, 7th edition].
3. ***Bipolar neurons:*** They are confined to the first neuron of the retina, ganglia of 8th cranial nerve, and the olfactory mucosa (Fig. 1.2c).
4. ***Multipolar neurons:*** Most of the neurons in human are multipolar, e.g. all motor and internuncial neurons (Fig. 1.1).

According to Length of Axon

Golgi type I: These neurons have long axons and numerous short dendrites. These are seen in pyramidal cells of cerebral cortex, Purkinje cells of cerebellum (Fig. 1.3) and anterior horn cells of spinal cord.

Golgi type II: These are neurons with short axons, and establish synapses with neighbouring neurons. These are also seen in cerebral and cerebellar cortices.

Note: ***Amacrine neurons*** are without axon, only with dendrite. They are seen in retina of eyeball.

Mature neuron is incapable of dividing. Recently some neurons in olfactory region and hippocampus have been seen to divide. Brain tumours arise chiefly from the neuroglial cells.

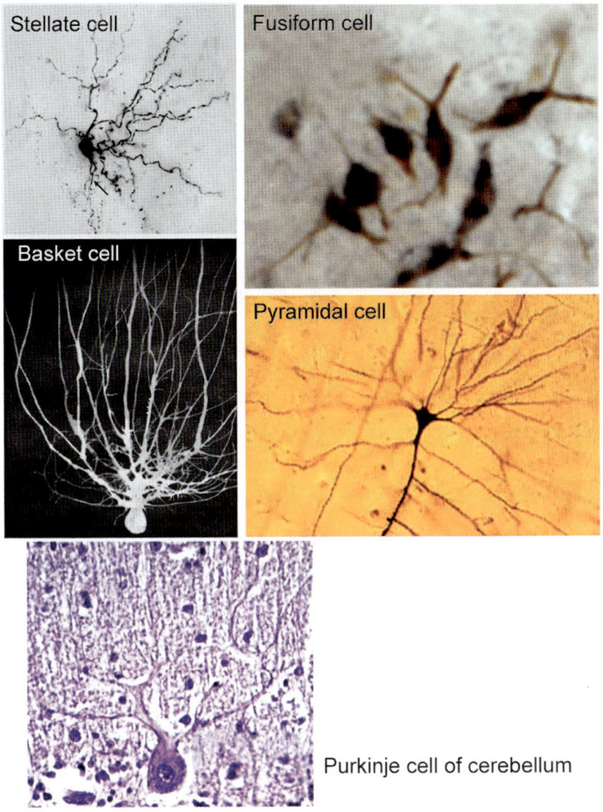

Fig. 1.3: Types of neurons (photomicrograph)

Functional Classification

Neurons are classified into sensory neurons, motor neurons and autonomic neurons, i.e. parasympathetic and sympathetic neurons.

Sensory neurons: They receive impulses and carry signals to the nervous system. These are of three types:

1. *Primary or 1st order sensory neurons* are present as spinal or sensory neurons in the dorsal root ganglion of spinal nerves.
2. *Secondary or 2nd order sensory neurons* are present in the grey matter of spinal cord and in brainstem.
3. *Tertiary or 3rd order sensory neurons* are seen in thalamus.

Motor neurons: These carry impulses from CNS to distal part of the body. These somatic motor neurons are of two types:

1. *Upper motor neurons* are situated in motor area of brain. These synapse with cranial nerve nuclei and anterior horn of spinal cord.
2. *Lower motor neurons* are located in cranial nerve nuclei and anterior horn of spinal cord. Nerves emerging from these nuclei supply the various skeletal muscles.

Parasympathetic neurons (autonomic)

1. Preganglionic neurons are located in cranial nerves III, VII, IX and X, also in sacral 2–4 segments of the spinal cord.
2. Postganglionic neurons are located close to the wall or within the wall of the viscera.
3. Parasympathetic outflow is called 'craniosacral outflow'.

Sympathetic neurons (autonomic)

1. Preganglionic neurons are located in the lateral horn of thoracic, and first and second lumbar segments of the spinal cord.
2. Postganglionic neurons are situated in the ganglia of the sympathetic trunk away from the viscera.
3. Sympathetic outflow is called 'thoracolumbar outflow'.

Note: The neurons can be classified according to shape as stellate, basket, fusiform, and pyramidal.

These can be also classified according to size as *macroneuron* (>7 μm size), e.g. Betz cells and *microneuron* (< 7 μm size), e.g. granular cells.

Structure of Neuron

A neuron has a body, axon, dendrites, and synaptic junctions (Fig. 1.1).

Body/Perikaryon

1. The cell body of a neuron is also called perikaryon or soma. It consists of the nucleus, perinuclear cytoplasm, and cell membrane.
2. ***Cytoplasm*** contains a large central vesicular nucleus, numerous mitochondria, rough endoplasmic reticulum, and Golgi complex. The nucleus is euchromatic (lightly stained) with 1–2 nucleoli.

   Note: New concept: Neurons have centrioles, but they cannot divide (*Previous concept*: Neurons do not have centrioles).
3. *Nissl bodies/substance/granules:* The cytoplasm of neurons shows the presence of granular *basophilic* cytoplasmic material (blue coloured on *H&E staining*) called Nissl bodies. On electron microscopy, Nissl bodies are stacks of the rough endoplasmic reticulum.
4. The neuron contains many *neurofibrils* (microtubules and microfilaments). Centrioles may help in the production of neurofibrils. Some of the neurons also contain melanin pigment (substantia nigra) and lipofuscin pigments.

Neurites

The processes arising from the cell body of a neuron are called *neurites*. They are axons and dendrites.

Dendrites

These are multiple, short, thick, tapering processes. Nissl granules extend into the dendrites. The branching pattern of dendrites (*arborization*) is called *dendritic tree*. Dendrites receive information and carry it toward the body of the cell.

Axons

1. Axon is a single, long, and thin process of neuron. Axons carry information away from the neuron body and have a uniform diameter. Axon is devoid of Nissl granules.
2. *Axoplasm* is cytoplasm in axon and *axolemma* is its cell membrane.
3. *Axoplasmic transport* (axonal transport system): As axons do not contain rough endoplasmic reticulum,

the protein synthesized in the cell body needs to be transported across axon.

Note: New concept: Periaxoplasmic plaques – these are axon terminals that have protein synthesis machinery (rER). These are involved in the process of neuronal cell memory.

4. *Axon hillock*: It is a part of cell body that is devoid of Nissl granules and gives rise to axon.

Note: New concept: Some cells of the olfactory bulb and dentate gyrus of the hippocampus are neural stem cells and they can generate new neurons [*Pawlina, Histology, 7th edition*].

5. *Initial segment*: It is the initial *nonmyelinated* part of axon between axon hillock and myelinated part of axon. An action potential is generated at initial segment.

The differences between axons and dendrites are listed in Table 1.1.

SYNAPSE

The neurons are connected to one another by their processes, forming long chains along which the impulses are conducted. The site of contact (contiguity without continuity) between the nerve cells is known as *synapse* (Greek *together*) (Fig. 1.4).

One cell may establish such contacts through its dendrites with as many as 1000 axonal terminals. However, it must be remembered that each neuron is an independent unit and the contact between neurons is by contiguity and not by continuity ('neuron theory' of Waldeyer, 1891). The impulse is transmitted across a synapse through biochemical neurotransmitters (acetylcholine).

Morphological Classification

Depending on components of the synapse, they are classified as follows (Fig. 1.4):

1. *Axodendritic synapse*: It is the most common type of synapse. In the axodendritic synapse, the axon of one neuron synapses with the dendrite of another neuron.
2. *Axosomatic synapse*: Axon conveys impulses to soma (body) of another neuron.
3. *Axoaxonic synapse*: It is the synapse between two axons.
4. *Dendroaxonic synapse*: It is the synapse between dendrite of presynaptic neuron and axon of postsynaptic neuron. It is seen in some parts of thalamus.

TABLE 1.1: Differences between axon and dendrites

Axon	*Dendrites*
It is a single, long, thin process of neuron	These are multiple, short, thick processes of neuron
It carries signal away from nerve cell body	It carries signal toward nerve cell body
Axon rarely branches Branches of axon form axon terminals	Branches of dendrite form dendritic tree
Diameter: Uniform	Diameter: Taper toward distal end (away from neuron)
Does not contain Nissl granules	Contain Nissl granules

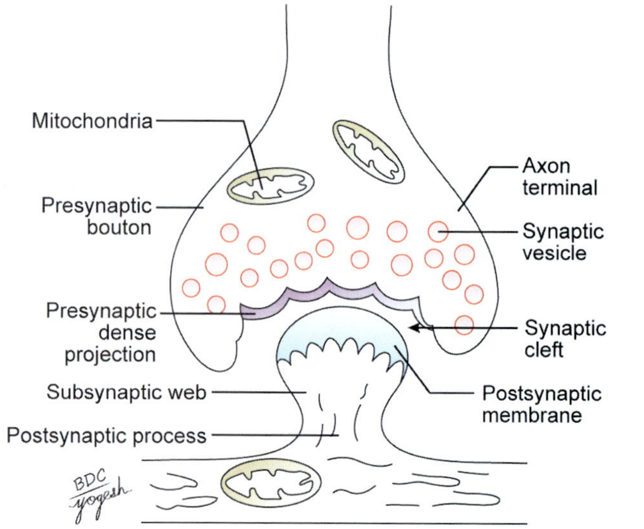

Fig. 1.4: Structure of a synapse neurotransmitters (acetylcholine)

5. *Dendrodendritic synapse*: It is the synapse between two dendrites.
6. *Somatosomatic synapse*: It is the synapse between bodies of neurons.
7. *Somatodendritic synapse*: It is the synapse between soma and dendrite of postsynaptic neurons.

Note: Synapse is not distinguishable on *H&E staining*.

Boutons en passant: Presynaptic neuron makes several contacts with postsynaptic neuron. These contacts are called boutons en passant (means *buttons in passing* in French).

Silver staining (Golgi method): Synapse is visible as oval bodies.

Bouton terminal: Enlarged terminal end of axon is called bouton terminal (means *terminal button* in French).

Chemical and Electric Synapses

Based on mechanism of conduction of nerve impulses, synapses are classified as chemical or electrical.

Chemical synapses

The chemical synapse involves release of chemical (neurotransmitter) from preganglionic neurons for conduction of impulse.

Structure of chemical synapse (Fig. 1.4): The components of chemical synapse are as follows:

1. *Presynaptic element* (*presynaptic knob*) is the part of presynaptic neuron that releases neurotransmitter. Presynaptic element stores neurotransmitter in synaptic vesicles.
2. *Synaptic cleft* is a narrow gap (20–30 nm) between presynaptic and postsynaptic neurons. Neurotransmitter needs to cross synaptic cleft.
3. *Postsynaptic membrane/process* is a membrane of postsynaptic neuron that has receptors for neurotransmitters.

Note: *New concept*: *Porocytosis* is a process of secretion of neurotransmitters through pores created by calcium ions between secretory vesicles and presynaptic membrane (*Previous concept*: Secretory vesicle fuses with presynaptic membrane for the release of neurotransmitter).

Electrical synapses

The electric synapse involves the passage of electric signal from one cell to another cell by gap junctions. Electrical synapses do not involve neurotransmitter release.

Examples: Gap junctions of cardiac and smooth muscles.

NEUROGLIAL CELLS

The supporting cells of the nervous system are called *neuroglia* or *glia*. They are grouped as follows (Flowchart 1.3, Plate 1.1, and Table 1.2):

1. Central neuroglia (neuroglia of the central nervous system).
2. Peripheral neuroglia (neuroglia of the peripheral nervous system).

Flowchart 1.3: Types of neuroglia

Neuroglia

Central neuroglia (in brain and spinal cord)	***Peripheral neuroglia*** (in peripheral nervous system)
Astrocytes Protoplasmic (in grey matter) Fibrous (in white matter) Oligodendrocytes (myelination in CNS) Microglia Ependymal cells	Schwann cells (myelination in PNS) Satellite cells

Central Neuroglia

These are supporting cells of the central nervous system. There are four types of central neuroglia:

Astrocytes, oligodendrocytes, microglia, and ependymal cells. These cells support embryonic (developing) neurons as well as provide physical support after development.

Astrocytes

These are star-shaped cells (largest neuroglia) and they have numerous processes. There are two types of astrocytes: Fibrous and protoplasmic.

1. *Fibrous astrocytes* have fewer and thin processes and are mostly found in the white matter of the CNS.
2. *Protoplasmic astrocytes* have numerous, short, thick, branching cytoplasmic processes. They are mostly found in grey matter.

Functions of astrocytes

- They provide physical support to neurons.
- They maintain a favourable metabolic environment for neurons by removing neurotransmitters from synapses. They store glycogen.
- They help in the maintenance of the blood-brain barrier.
- Astrocytes maintain K^+ ion concentration in extracellular spaces of the brain and spinal cord by potassium spatial buffering.

Note: Glia limitans is the membrane-like barrier on external surfaces of brain and spinal cord. It is produced by protoplasmic astrocytes. *Gliosis* is the proliferation of astrocytes to heal the damaged zones of nervous tissue. *Fibrous astrocytoma* (tumour) accounts for about 80% of brain tumours in adults.

Oligodendrocytes

The oligodendrocytes are small, round cells and have a few cytoplasmic processes (*oligo* = scanty, in Greek). They produce myelin in CNS. One oligodendrocyte myelinates many adjacent axons or sometimes the same axons at different places. The gap between adjacent processes of oligodendrocytes that myelinate an axon is called node of Ranvier. The myelin sheath in CNS differs from that of PNS in protein expression.

Function: Oligodendrocytes produce myelin sheaths in CNS.

Note: The myelin in CNS has fewer *Schmidt–Lanterman clefts* because astrocytes provide favourable metabolic environment to neurons. Oligodendrocytes do not have external lamina (as it is present in Schwann cells). Nonmyelinated neurons are not enclosed by processes of oligodendrocytes in CNS.

Microglia

These are the smallest neuroglial cells. These are involved in phagocytosis when they become active (reactive microglial cells). These are derived from mesoderm (bone marrow). They are small cells with few cytoplasmic processes and elongated nuclei.

Function: Microglia are phagocytic cells. They proliferate specifically in nervous tissue injuries and diseases. Microglia form a part of mononuclear phagocytic system in CNS.

Note: *Current update*: Microglia remove bacteria, cancer (neoplastic) cells, and dead nerve cells. *Gitter* or *Hortega cell* is a lipid-laden microglial cell observed at the edge of healing brain infarcts. It is also called compound granule cell, gitterzelle, mesoglea, or perivascular glial cell.

Ependymal Cells

The cavities of the nervous system are lined by epithelium-like *ependymal cells*. Ependymal cells are cuboidal to columnar in shape and arranged in a single layer. These cells are derived from neural tube.

There are three types of ependymal cells: Ependymocytes, choroid epithelial cells, and tanycytes.

Functions

1. Exchange of substances between the brain and cerebrospinal fluid at the brain–CSF barrier.
2. Choroid plexus secretes CSF.
3. Tanycytes: Respond to glucose concentration changes.

Note: Most of the brain cavities are lined by ependymocytes except at:

1. Choroid plexuses are lined by *choroid epithelial cells* that secrete cerebrospinal fluid.
2. Floor of third (not fourth) ventricle is lined by *tanycytes* (specialized ependymal cells). These cells are *sensitive to changes in glucose concentration* and monitor levels of metabolites.

Plate 1.1: Types of neuroglial cells

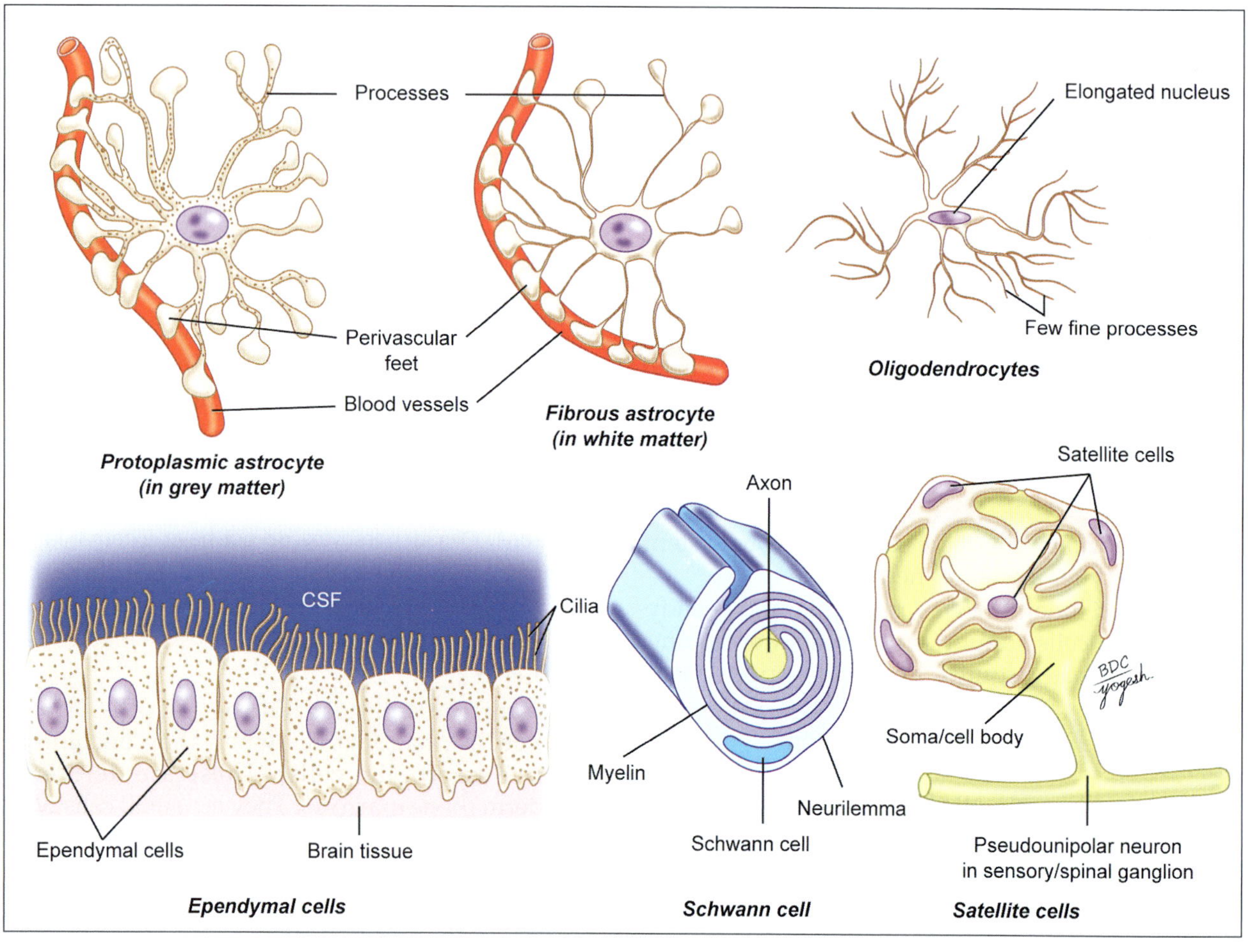

TABLE 1.2: Types of neuroglial cells

	Protoplasmic astrocyte	*Fibrous astrocyte*	*Oligodendrocyte*	*Microglia*
Cell size	Large	Large	Medium	Small, elongated
Shape of nucleus	Oval, light stained	Oval, light stained	Small, spherical, dark stained	Small, elongated, dark stained
Cytoplasmic processes	Many, short and thick	Many long slender	Few, short, beaded	Short, thin, spinous
Cytoplasm	Granular	Fibrillar	—	—
Situation	Grey matter	White matter	White matter	Grey and white matters
Function	Blood–brain barrier (BBB)	BBB	Myelination	Phagocytosis
Embryological origin	Neural crest	Neural crest	Neural crest	Mesoderm

Peripheral Neuroglia

Schwann Cells

These are also called *neurolemmocytes*. These are present only in peripheral nervous system. These cells are flattened cells with a flattened nucleus that is surrounded by abundant cytoplasm. They are derived from neural crest cells.

Functions: Schwann cells produce myelin in peripheral nervous system.

Satellite Cells

In the ganglia (collection of neuronal cell bodies outside the CNS), neuronal bodies are surrounded by a layer of flat cuboidal cells called satellite cells. These cells work similar to Schwann cells but do not produce myelin.

Satellite cell capsule gives passage to nerve cell processes. In sensory ganglia, the satellite cell capsule is nearly complete as sensory neurons do not synapse in ganglia. In autonomic ganglia, the satellite cell capsule is not complete as autonomic neurons have synapses in the ganglia.

Functions: Protection and support ganglionic neurons.

CLINICAL NEUROANATOMY

- ***Gliosis***: Proliferation of glial cells is called the 'gliosis'. A CNS lesion heals by gliosis. A spontaneous gliosis is an indication of a degenerative change in the nervous tissue.
- ***Brain tumours***: Since the glial cells are capable of dividing, they can form CNS tumours.

GREY MATTER AND WHITE MATTER

Unit of nervous tissue is the neuron, comprising of cell body, dendrites and axon. Neurons are supported by neuroglia and blood vessels.

Grey matter is the part of nervous tissue containing the cell body (soma), neuroglial cells and abundance of blood vessels. It covers the outer aspect of brain and is known as the cortex. Grey matter present within the depth of white matter is called ganglia/nuclei.

White matter comprises only the fibres, i.e. axons, dendrites, neuroglial cells and fewer blood vessels. In the brain, the white matter lies deep to the cortex of brain. In the spinal cord, the white matter lies superficial to the deeply placed 'H-shaped' grey matter.

REFLEX ARC

A reflex arc is the functional unit of the nervous system. In its simplest form (monosynaptic reflex arc), it consists of:

1. Receptor, e.g. the skin/muscle
2. Sensory neuron
3. Motor neuron
4. Effector, e.g. the muscle.

An involuntary motor response to a sensory stimulus is known as the *reflex action*. These are of two types:

1. Cortical responses which are voluntary in nature.
2. Subcortical responses which are involuntary.

Reflex action is chief function of spinal cord. Knee jerk and ankle jerk are monosynaptic reflex arcs (Figs 1.5 and 1.6). Some common reflex arcs are shown in Table 1.3.

PARTS OF THE NERVOUS SYSTEM

CENTRAL NERVOUS SYSTEM (CNS)

Components of Central Nervous System

Spinal cord: It receives sensory information from the skin, joints, and muscles of the trunk and limbs and contains

TABLE 1.3: Some common reflexes

Name of reflex	*Way of eliciting*	*Result*	*Comment*
Biceps jerk	Striking biceps brachii tendon	Flexion of the elbow joint	C5, C6 segments intact Tendon jerks may be exaggerated in upper motor neuron lesion or lost in lower motor neuron lesion
Triceps jerk	Striking triceps brachii tendon	Extension of the elbow joint	C7, C8 segments intact
Knee jerk (Fig. 1.5)	Striking the ligamentum patellae	Extension of the knee joint	L3, L4 segments of spinal cord intact
Ankle jerk	Striking tendo calcaneus	Plantar flexion of the ankle joint	S1, S2 segments intact
Abdominal reflex	Striking a quadrant of abdomen	Contraction of abdominal muscles	Positive reflex indicates normal pyramidal tract with T7–T12 nerves intact
Plantar reflex	Scratching the sole of foot from lateral side towards big toe	Plantar flexion of the great toe and other toes	A normal plantar response indicates intact pyramidal tract
Babinski's sign (Fig. 1.6)	Same as in plantar reflex	Dorsiflexion of the great toe and fanning of other toes	Babinski's sign indicates pyramidal tract injury, except in infants

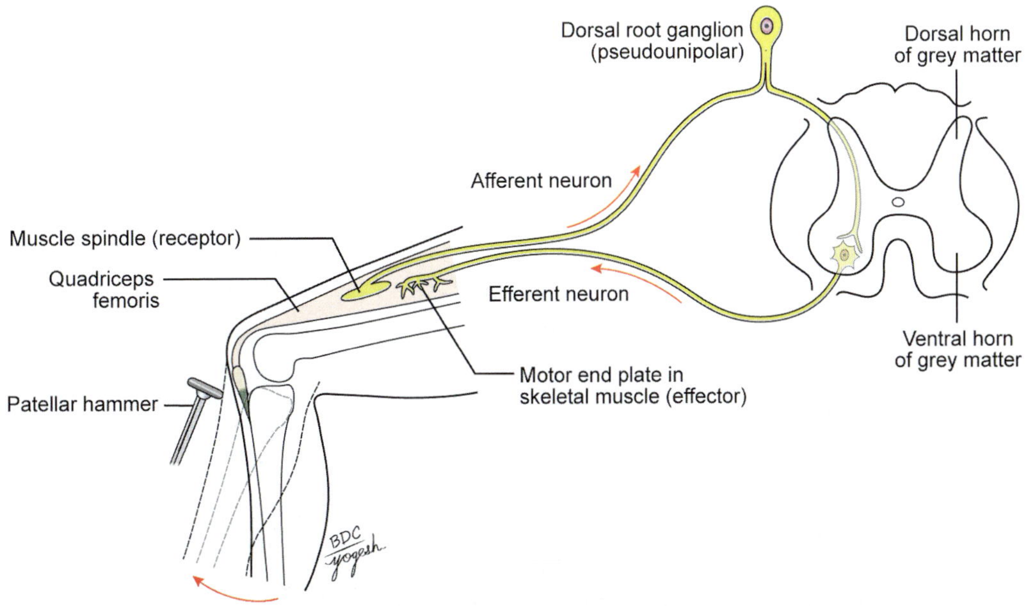

Fig. 1.5: Components of the knee jerk

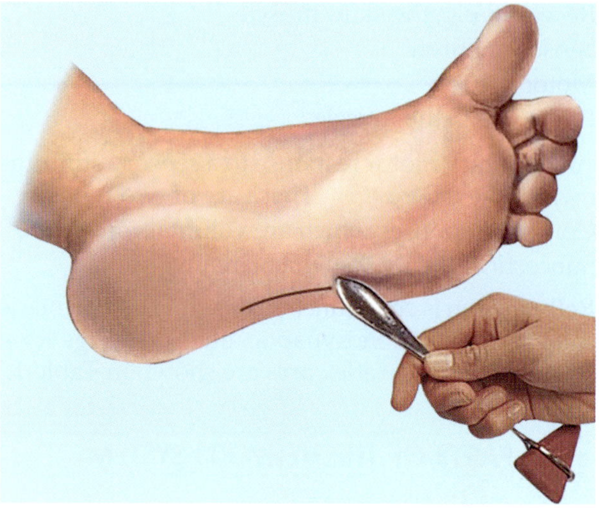

Fig. 1.6: Babinski's sign

the motor neurons responsible for both voluntary and reflex movements. It has central grey matter and peripheral white matter.

Brainstem: It includes:

a. *Medulla*: This is the direct rostral extension of the spinal cord.
b. *Pons*: It lies rostral to the medulla.
c. *Midbrain*: This is the smallest brainstem component which lies rostral to the pons.

Cerebellum: The cerebellum lies dorsal to the pons and medulla. The cerebellum plays a major role in the control of tone, equilibrium and posture, including head and eye movements.

Diencephalon: It includes the thalamus, hypothalamus epithalamus and metathalamus. It is present between the cerebral hemispheres and the midbrain. The hypothalamus lies ventral to the thalamus.

Cerebral hemispheres: This is the largest region of the brain. It consists of the cerebral cortex/grey matter and the fibres which form white matter with deeply located nuclei: The basal ganglia, the hippocampal formation and the amygdala. Each hemisphere comprises 4 lobes, e.g. frontal, parietal, temporal and occipital lobes. Each hemisphere has a flat medial surface which lie adjacent to each other separated by a longitudinal fissure. In the lower part of the fissure is present a thick band of fibres—the corpus callosum. The hemisphere shows infoldings in the form of sulci and gyri, giving more space for the neurons.

Ventricles of brain: Ventricles are continuous cavities in various parts of brain as follows:

1. *Lateral ventricle* is cavity of each cerebral hemisphere.
2. *Third ventricle* is present between the two thalami. It continues as *aqueduct* of midbrain.
3. *Fourth ventricle* is cavity of hindbrain, i.e. pons, medulla and cerebellum and continues downwards as *central canal of spinal cord*.

CSF circulation in the ventricles and subarachnoid space provides nourishment to the components of brain.

Protective coverings: Brain and spinal cord are covered by 3 meninges with intervening spaces. The outermost is the dura mater, middle layer is delicate cobweb-like arachnoid mater and the inner one is the pia mater. The subdural space is very narrow while the subarachnoid space is big containing very important cerebrospinal fluid.

PERIPHERAL NERVOUS SYSTEM

Somatic (cerebrospinal) nervous system: It is made up of 12 pairs of cranial nerves and 31 pairs of spinal nerves. Its efferent fibres reach the effectors without interruption (Fig. 1.7a).

Autonomic (splanchnic) nervous system: It consists of sympathetic and parasympathetic systems. Its efferent fibres first relay in a ganglion, and then the postganglionic fibres pass to the effectors (Figs 1.7b and c).

GROSS STUDY OF BRAIN

Learning neuroanatomy is beginning of a journey in gaining knowledge of our own brain. The knowledge of the nervous system will be helpful in the field of medicine for understanding neurophysiology, neuropathology, neuropharmacology, and many diseases that will encounter during clinical practice.

The brain can be studied by viewing it from different views such as superior, inferior, anterior, posterior, lateral, and medial (Plate 1.2).

For the study purposes, the brain can be cut in the following planes (Plate 1.3):

1. *Coronal plane* – When brain is cut through dorsal and ventral surfaces in the coronal plane.
2. *Horizontal plane* – When it is cut from side-to-side.
3. *Sagittal plane* – When brain is cut in relation to longitudinal axis, i.e. from anterior to posterior aspect.
4. *Oblique plane* – When brain is cut at an angle from cerebral cortex down through the brainstem.

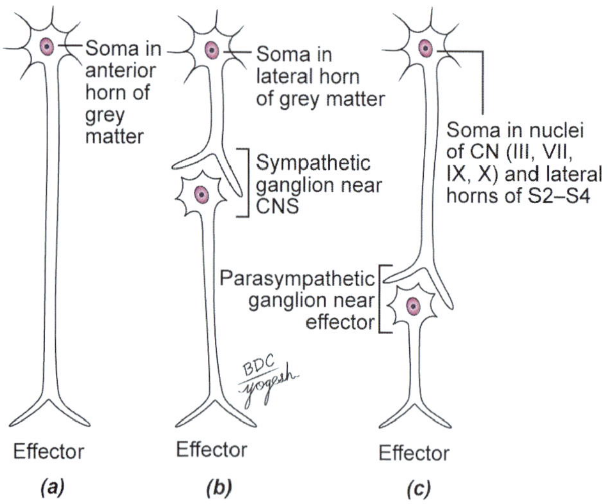

Figs 1.7a to c: Types of peripheral nervous system: (a) Somatic, (b) sympathetic and (c) parasympathetic

Plate 1.2: Various views of the brain

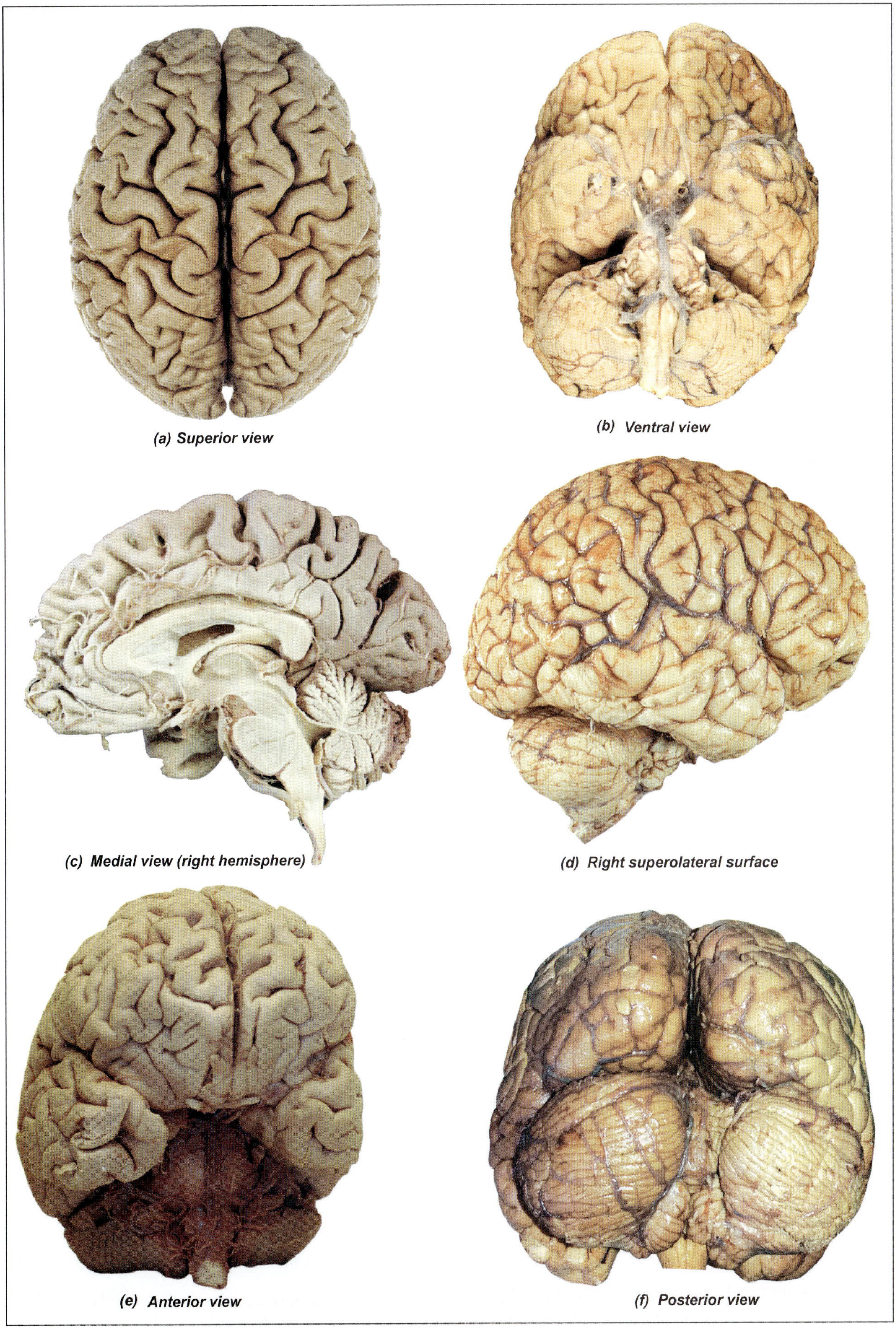

(a) Superior view

(b) Ventral view

(c) Medial view (right hemisphere)

(d) Right superolateral surface

(e) Anterior view

(f) Posterior view

Plate 1.3: Sections of brain in different planes: A to C—coronal sections; D—horizontal section; E and F—sagittal sections; G—oblique section

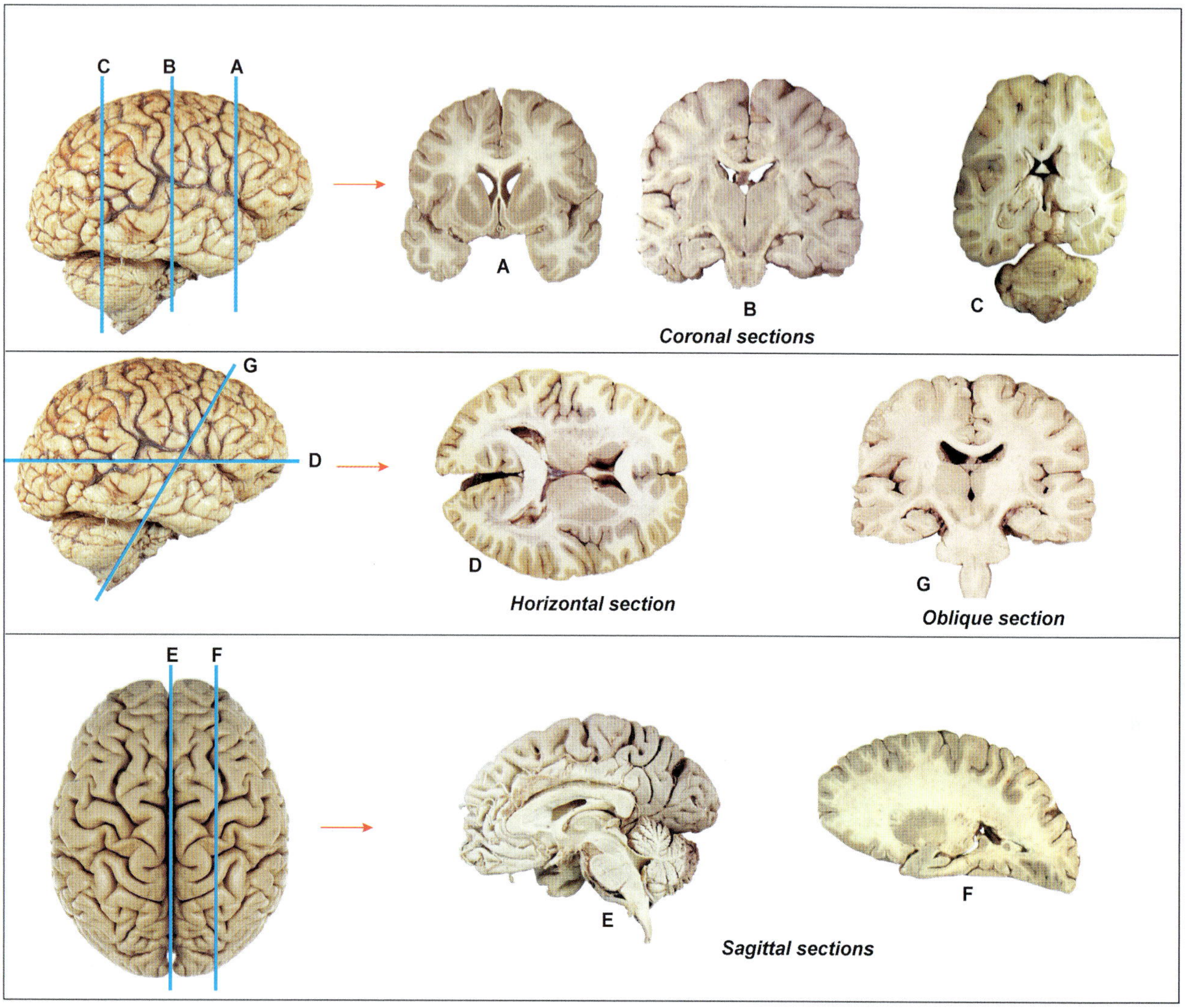

PARTS OF BRAIN

The brain has forebrain, midbrain and hindbrain. The main parts and their subdivisions of the forebrain are shown in Table 1.4, and Figs 1.8 and 1.9. The brainstem includes the midbrain, pons and medulla. Hindbrain includes pons, medulla and cerebellum.

The dilated part of the central canal of spinal cord within the conus medullaris is known as the terminal ventricle. Similarly, the cavity of septum pellucidum is sometimes called the fifth ventricle.

TABLE 1.4: Parts of brain and their subdivisions

Parts	*Subdivisions*	*Cavity*
1. Forebrain (prosencephalon)	A. Telencephalon (cerebrum), made up of two cerebral hemispheres and the median part in front of the interventricular foramen	Lateral ventricle
	B. Diencephalon (thalamencephalon), hidden by the cerebrum, consists of: a. Thalamus b. Hypothalamus c. Metathalamus, including the medial and lateral geniculate bodies, and d. Epithalamus, including the pineal body, habenular trigone and posterior commissure e. Subthalamus	Third ventricle
2. Midbrain (mesencephalon)	Crus cerebri, substantia nigra, tegmentum, and tectum, from before backwards	Cerebral aqueduct
3. Hindbrain (rhombencephalon)	A. Metencephalon, made up of pons and cerebellum B. Myelencephalon or medulla oblongata	Fourth ventricle

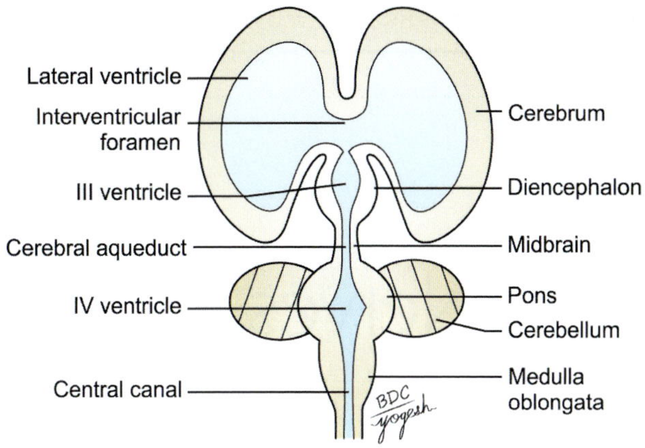

Fig. 1.8: Parts of the brain

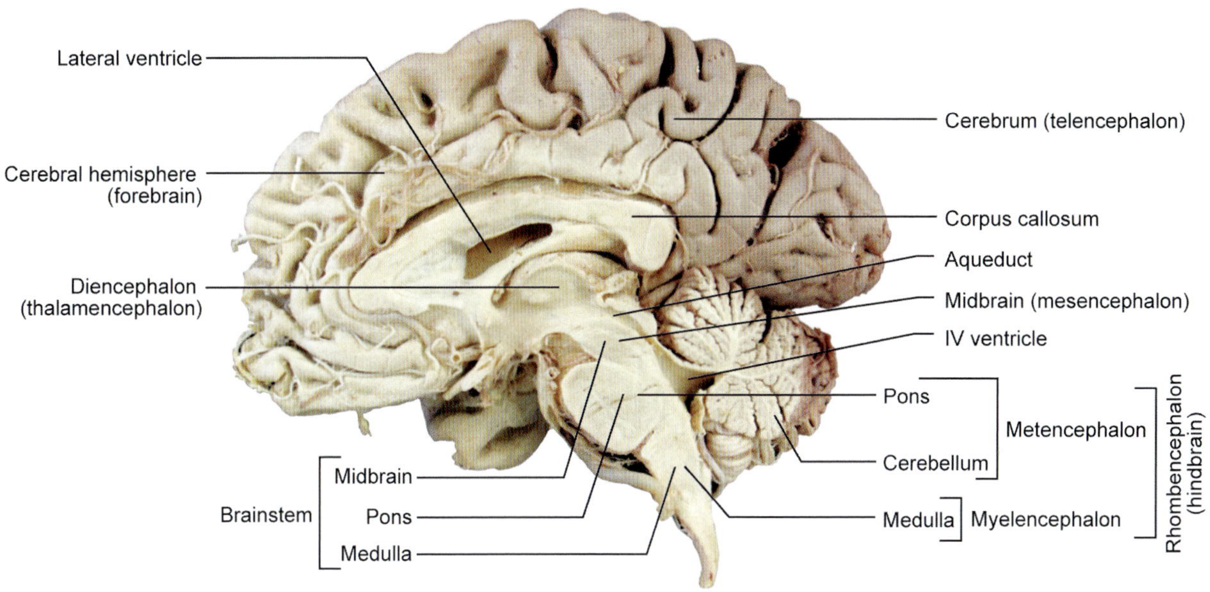

Fig. 1.9: Parts of the brain (dissection)

Facts to Remember

- Neurons in human brain are about 180–200 billion.
- Unipolar neurons are present only in the mesencephalic nucleus of 5th cranial nerve.
- Nissl granules are the rough endoplasmic reticulum. They are absent in the axon hillock and axon.
- Mature neurons do not divide after birth except in olfactory region and in hippocampus.
- Impulse travels from dendrite to cell body and then into axon.
- Contact between neurons is by contiguity (like hand shake) and not by continuity.
- Ependymal cells are responsible for the formation of cerebrospinal fluid. Astrocytes form the blood–brain barrier.

BDC's Anatomy *e*-book

1. Further reading
2. Viva voce questions

Chapter

2

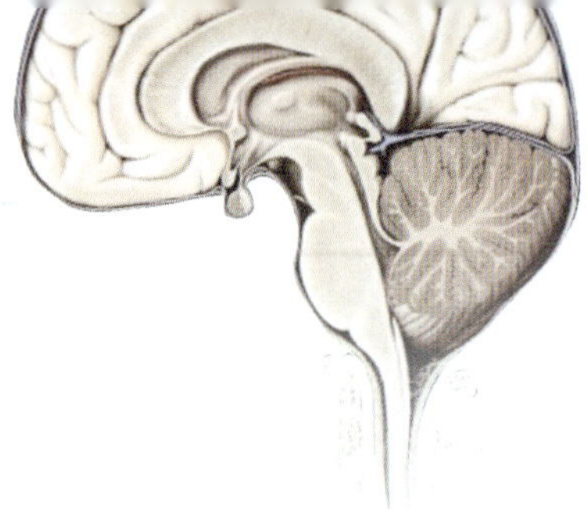

Peripheral Nerves and Ganglia

The peripheral nerves form a communication between the organs and the central nervous system. It consists of two components:

1. Somatic nerves
2. Autonomic (splanchnic or visceral) nerves.

The peripheral nerves include:

- 12 pairs of cranial nerves
- 31 pairs of spinal nerves
- Autonomic (splanchnic) nerves: Sympathetic and parasympathetic nerves.

The peripheral nerve contains the following nerve fibres:

1. *Somatic afferent (sensory) fibres* to carry sensory inputs from skin, bones, muscles, and joints to the CNS.
2. *Somatic efferent (motor) fibres* to carry motor impulses to the skeletal muscles.
3. *Visceral afferent (sensory) fibres* to carry input from the organ and blood vessels to the CNS.
4. *Visceral efferent (motor) fibres* to carry impulses from CNS to glands, smooth muscle of organs and blood vessels, and cardiac muscles.

Note: The bundle of nerve fibres in CNS is called *tract*.

Competencies:

AN68.1: Describe and identify multipolar and unipolar neurons, ganglia, peripheral nerve under the microscope.

AN68.3: Describe the ultrastructure of nervous tissue.

STRUCTURES OF PERIPHERAL NERVE

The peripheral nerve is a collection of many nerve fibres held together by connective tissue. The concept of nerve fibre is confusing as it does not mean a connective tissue fibre.

Nerve fibre indicates:

1. *Motor or efferent nerve fibres* are axons that carry impulses from CNS to muscle or glands. Cell bodies of motor neurons lie in CNS, especially in the grey matter of the spinal cord and brainstem.
2. *Afferent or sensory nerve fibres* are nerve processes that carry impulses or information toward CNS.
3. Nerve cell bodies of afferent fibres lie in the sensory ganglia.

Ganglion is a collection of nerve cell bodies outside the CNS.

Examples: Dorsal root ganglion, autonomic ganglion.

Basic Structure of Peripheral Nerve

(Flowchart 2.1, Fig. 2.1)

The *nerve fibre* with Schwann cells and basal lamina is the basic structural unit of the peripheral nerve. Each single *nerve fibre* is surrounded by a thin connective tissue called the *endoneurium*. The *endoneurium* consists of the loose connective tissue with collagen fibril, few fibroblasts, occasional mast cells, and macrophages.

Note: In peripheral nerve section, 90% of nuclei are of Schwann cells and only 10% belongs to connective tissue cells.

A group of nerve fibres forms a *nerve fascicle* or bundle. Each *nerve fascicle* is surrounded by a layer of specialized connective tissue called perineurium.

The *perineurium* is made-up of flattened (squamous) perineurial cells. They may be arranged in two or more perineurial cell layers and externally covered by a *basal lamina*. The perineurial cells are connected with each

Flowchart 2.1: Peripheral nerve

Peripheral nerve

- ***Each nerve fibre***
  - Axon
  - Schwann cells
  - Basal lamina
- ***Endoneurium***
  - Surrounds individual nerve fibre
  - Loose connective tissue
- ***Perineurium***
  - Surrounds nerve fascicle
  - Squamous perineurial cells
  - Forms blood–nerve barrier
- ***Epineurium***
  - Surrounds nerve bundles and entire nerve
  - Dense connective tissue

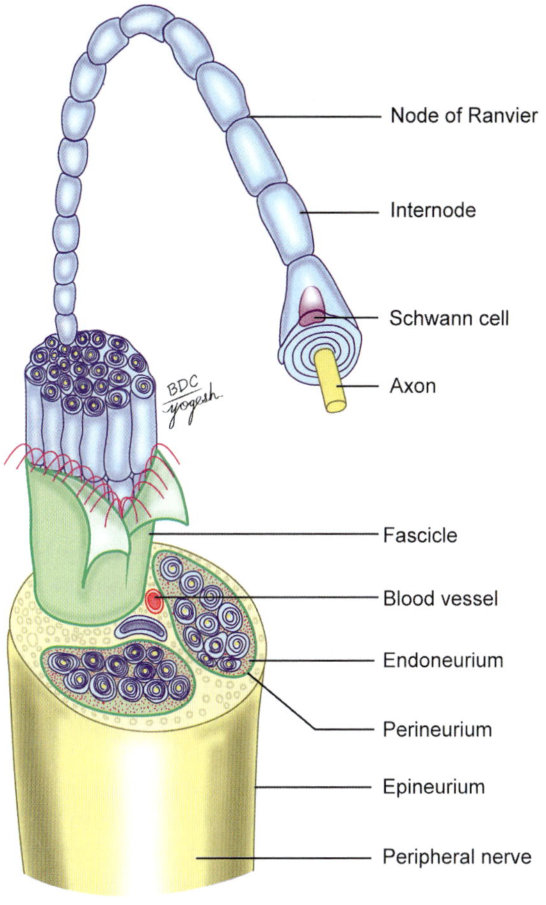

Fig. 2.1: Structure of peripheral nerve

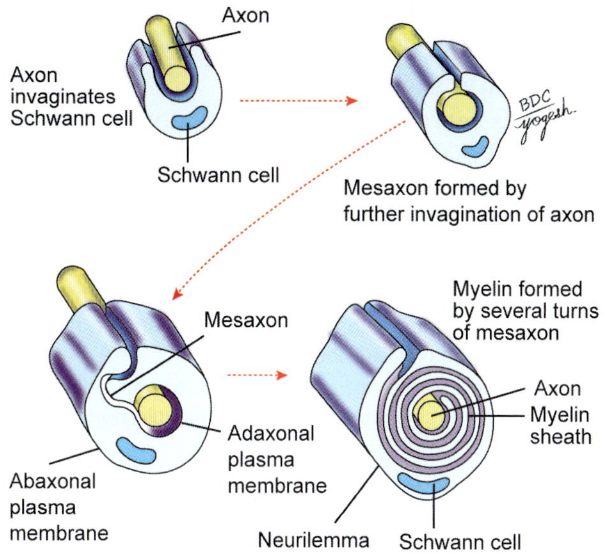

Fig. 2.2: Process of myelination

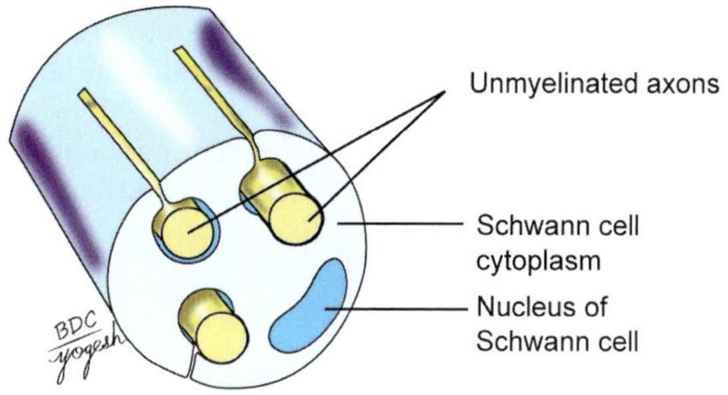

Fig. 2.3: Role of Schwann cell in the protection of nonmyelinated axon

Note: One Schwann cell surrounds multiple nonmyelinated nerve fibres.

other by tight junctions and hence, form a *blood–nerve barrier*.

Many fasciculi are held together by dense irregular connective tissue called epineurium. It surrounds entire peripheral nerve. It contains blood vessels that supply the nerve.

Note: Blood vessels (*vasa nervorum*) are present only in epineurium and perineurium. Endoneurium does not have blood vessels. Nerve fibres receive nutrition by diffusion through endoneurium.

H&E staining – axons, endoneurium, perineurium, and epineurium is stained. Myelin gives an empty appearance (Fig. 2.2). The osmium tetroxide is a special stain used for myelin. Myelin is washed away during preparation for *H&E stain*. Hence, osmium tetroxide staining method is used. In osmium tetroxide staining method, myelin sheath stains black (Fig. 2.3).

MYELIN SHEATH

The myelin is an insulating sheath surrounding the axons of myelinated nerve cells. Myelin is produced by oligodendrocytes in CNS and Schwann cells in PNS.

Formation of Myelin Sheath (Fig. 2.2)

In process of myelination, the axon initially lies in a groove of a Schwann cell. The cell membrane of Schwann cell is converted into three zones:

1. *Abaxonal plasma membrane* – exposed to an external environment
2. *Adaxonal/periaxonal plasma membrane* – lies in contact with axon
3. ***Mesaxon*** is a double membrane fold that connects abaxonal and adaxonal membranes.

The sheet-like extension of mesaxon surrounds axon spirally and cytoplasm of mesaxon gets squeezed.

Thus, it results in the formation of myelin sheath (lipid layer) around axon. Outside the myelin sheath, thin layer of cytoplasm of Schwann cell is present along with surrounding cell membrane of Schwann cells, now called ***neurilemma*** or *neurilemmal sheath*. The myelin consists of lipids (80%), proteins, and water.

Around a single axon, many Schwann cells form the myelin sheath. The gap between the segment of myelin and between adjacent Schwann cells is called ***nodes of Ranvier*** or ***incisura myelini***. These nodes increases the rate of nerve conduction by saltatory conduction.

The ***internode*** is a segment of myelin sheath between adjacent nodes of Ranvier. The thickness of myelin sheath depends on axon diameter of axon and not on Schwann cell. Myelin sheath thickness is regulated by neuregulin (NRG1) growth factor that is expressed on axolemma of the axon.

Functions of Myelin Sheath

1. Protection and physical support to axons
2. Insulation of axons
3. Increases nerve conduction by saltatory conduction
4. Neurilemmal sheath plays a major role in nerve regeneration.

Note:
- *Schmidt-Lanterman clefts*: These are the small pockets of cytoplasm in the inner layers of the myelin sheath. Usually, cytoplasm gets squeezed out of the myelin sheath during the wrapping of mesaxon around the axon.
- Nonmyelinated axons are covered by Schwann cells in PNS. Single Schwann cell is invaginated by multiple nonmyelinated axons.
- One Schwann cell can produce a myelin sheath around a small segment of one axon. One oligodendrocyte can produce a myelin sheath around many axons. Hence, the neurilemmal sheath is present only in the peripheral nervous system (cell membrane of Schwann cell) and not in CNS as a single oligodendrocyte does not cover one axon. Because of the absence of neurilemmal sheath in CNS, regeneration of neuron is not possible in CNS.
- A single Schwann cell protects many nonmyelinated axons (Fig. 2.3). The nerve fibres in the peripheral nerve may be myelinated or nonmyelinated, most of the fibres in the peripheral nerve are myelinated.
- Nonmyelinated fibres include fine sensory nerve fibres and postganglionic autonomic fibres. These are called *type C fibres*.

CLINICAL NEUROANATOMY

Enuresis (bed-wetting). It is observed in the first 3–6 years of life. It occurs up to the completion of myelination of corticospinal tract fibres that control the emptying of the urinary bladder. *Embryological basis*: The myelination begins before birth and continues for a few years after birth. Enuresis is normal in infants.

CONDUCTION OF ACTION POTENTIAL

The ionic concentration within the neuron and extracellular fluid creates *resting membrane potential* across the neuronal plasma membrane (RMP). At resting membrane potential, the neuronal plasma membrane is polarized. Resting membrane potential is always negative (–70 mV).

The resting membrane potential is negative because of the high concentration of cations (for example, Na^+ ions) outside the nerve fibres in the extracellular fluid.

Action potential is a sequential change in membrane potential that develops on activation or stimulation of the nerve cell. The rise in membrane potential soon comes back to resting membrane potential. It involves two phases:

1. ***Depolarization*** – increase in membrane potential up to +40 mV
2. ***Repolarization*** – decrease in or restoration of membrane potential.

The action potential is generated at one point of the neuronal plasma membrane, and it propagates across this

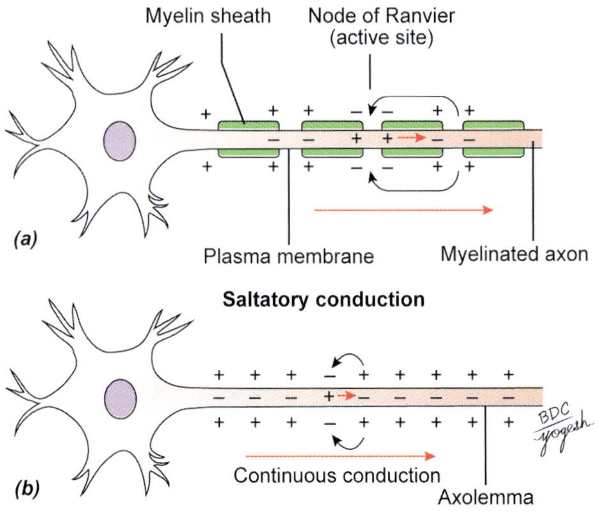

Figs 2.4a and b: Conduction of action potential along an axon: (a) In myelinated axon and (b) in nonmyelinated axon

membrane (Figs 2.4a and b). The speed of conduction of action potential depends on the myelination of the nerve fibres. The thickness of myelin is directly proportional to the conduction of action potential.

Saltatory conduction (*saltare* = to leap in Latin) is jumping conduction of action potential from one node of Ranvier to other nodes of Ranvier. In thick myelinated motor fibres (alpha fibres), the speed of conduction is very high (70–120 meters per second).

CLASSIFICATION OF NERVE FIBRES

Based on the diameter of the nerve fibres, they are grouped as follows (Table 2.1):

Group A: Highly myelinated fibres
Group B: Thinly myelinated fibres (up to 3 μm thick)
Group C: Nonmyelinated fibres (about 0.2–1.5 μm thick).

CLINICAL NEUROANATOMY

Nerve injuries: Based on the severity of the damage, nerve injuries are classified as:

1. *Neurotmesis* – both axon and myelin sheath damaged
2. *Axonotmesis* – only axon is damaged, myelin sheath is intact
3. *Neuropraxia* – both axon and myelin sheath are preserved.

- Nerve regeneration occurs in the peripheral nerve in case of ***neuropraxia*** and ***axonotmesis***, but in case of *neurotmesis*, nerve regeneration does not occur.

Nerve degeneration and regeneration: The injury to the axon with myelin sheath follows two events:

1. Degeneration of nerve fibre
2. Regeneration of nerve fibre.

Rate of nerve regeneration/growth is 3.5 to 4.5 mm per day. A proper nutrition is essential for faster nerve regeneration.

TABLE 2.1: Classification of peripheral nerve fibres

Type of fibre	*Example*	*Maximum diameter*	*Myelin*	*Conduction velocity (m/s)*
Group A fibres				
Afferent (sensory) fibres				
Type Ia	Annulospiral endings of muscle spindle	20 μm	Present	18–120
Type Ib	Golgi tendon	20 μm	Present	80–120
Type II	Flower-spray ending in muscle spindle Cutaneous mechanoreceptors (touch, pressure)	12 μm	Present	33–75
Type III	Free nerve endings for pain and temperature	5 μm	Thin	30
Efferent (motor) fibres				
Alpha (α) motor neurons	Supply extrafusal muscle fibres	20 μm	Present	120
Beta (β) motor neurons	Supply extrafusal fibres and muscle spindle	12 μm	Present	70
Gamma (γ) motor neurons	Supply intrafusal muscle fibres	8 μm	Present	24
Group B fibres	Preganglionic fibres	5 μm	Present	15
Group C fibres	Postganglionic autonomic fibres	1.5 μm	Absent	2

Degeneration of nerve fibre: These are the changes that occur in the nerve cell following the injury. These include changes in the nerve cell body and changes in the nerve fibre (Fig. 2.5).

- *Changes in nerve fibre*: These include:
  1. *Wallerian degeneration*: These are changes in the distal segment. It includes disintegration of myelin and degeneration of nerve fibres.
  2. Degeneration of proximal segment up to the nearest node of Ranvier.
- *Changes in the nerve cell body*: Due to loss of neural activity after injury, the cell body undergoes the following changes:
  1. Chromatolysis – disintegration of Nissl bodies
  2. Cell swelling
  3. Nucleus shifts to an eccentric position.

Regeneration of nerve fibre: The regeneration of nerve fibres is a very slow process. It begins after two weeks after injury. It involves (Fig. 2.5):

1. In the process of regeneration, macrophages remove the degenerated debris by phagocytosis.
2. Schwann cell proliferation: The Schwann cells proliferate and fill the empty space created by disintegration of axon and the myelin. Schwann cells also fill the gap between proximal and distal segments of axon.
3. Axonal growth: The ends of the axon give rise to multiple sprouts that enter the *endoneurial tube* of proliferated Schwann cells.
4. Elongation of axon: One of the axonal sprouts continues elongation under the guidance of Schwann cells to reach the end organ.
5. Regeneration of myelin: Surrounding Schwann cells reform the myelin sheath to restore the function completely.

Neuroma is a benign tumour. Sometimes, if the distance between the cut ends of nerve fibres is more, then the gap is filled with fibrous tissue which contains growing axonal sprouts. This mass forms neuroma. It is painful.

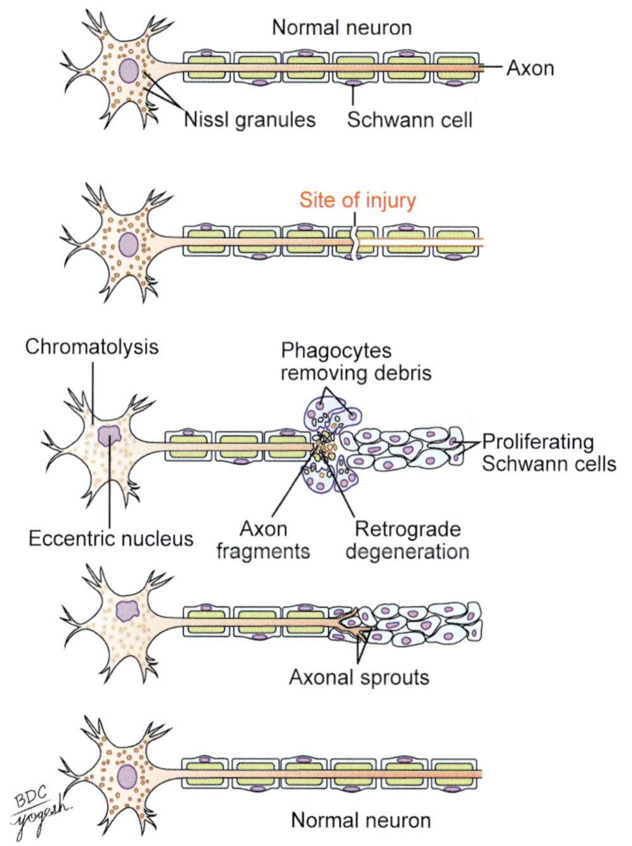

Fig. 2.5: Degeneration and regeneration of a nerve fibre (Wallerian degeneration)

GANGLIA

The ganglion is the aggregation of the cell bodies of neurons outside the central nervous system.

Ganglia are of two types: Sensory and autonomic.

Sensory Ganglia

The sensory ganglia are present just outside the CNS. The neurons of sensory ganglia carry impulses toward CNS (Plate 2.1, Flowchart 2.2).

Plate 2.1: Histology of dorsal root/sensory ganglion

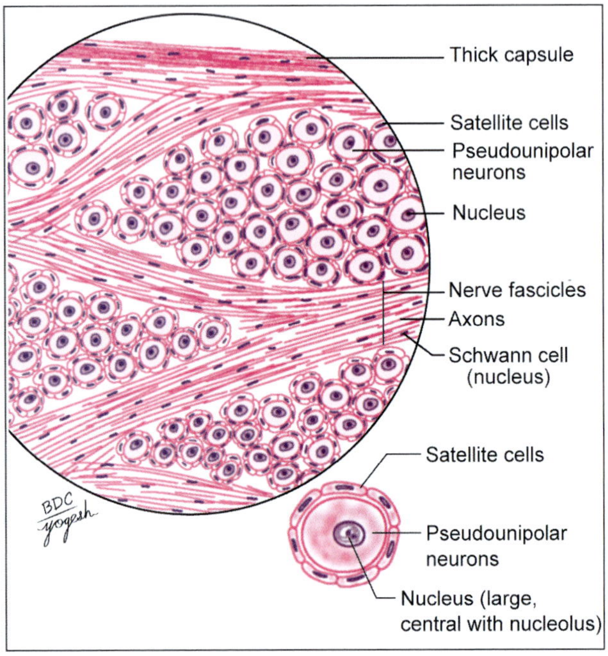

Examples:

1. Dorsal root ganglia of spinal nerves
2. Sensory ganglia of cranial nerves: Trigeminal, facial, vestibulocochlear, glossopharyngeal, and vagus nerves.

Structure of Sensory Ganglia

The sensory ganglia have *pseudounipolar neurons* (except vestibulocochlear ganglia that has bipolar neurons). These neurons have a peripheral process that carries information from the sensory receptor and a central process that passes received information to CNS.

A section of sensory ganglia shows *large neurons that are present in groups*, mostly at the periphery of ganglia. The nuclei of neurons are large, vesicular, and *centrally placed*. The group of neurons are separated by bundles of myelinated nerve fibres. Each neuronal body is surrounded by a *complete capsule* of satellite or capsular cells which are flattened cells (low cuboidal). The ganglion is covered by a fine connective tissue capsule.

Plate 2.2: Histology of autonomic/sympathetic ganglion

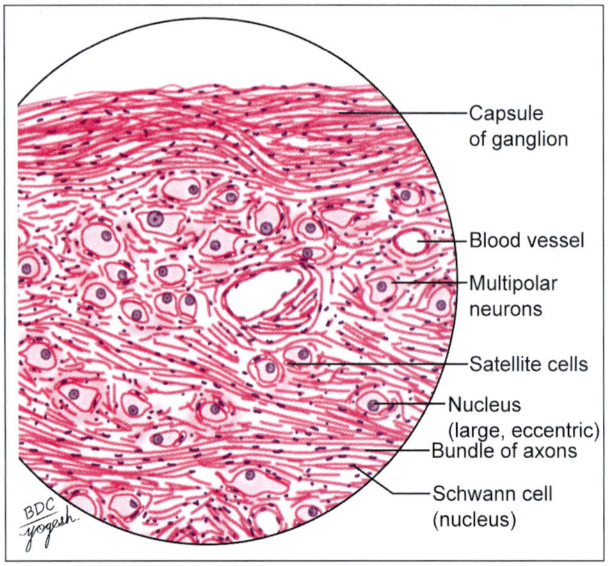

Autonomic Ganglia

The autonomic ganglia supply smooth muscles and glands. The autonomic nervous system shows two neurons (Plate 2.2, Flowchart 2.2):

1. *Preganglionic neuron*: It lies in CNS and its axons extend from CNS up to autonomic ganglia.
2. *Postganglionic neuron*: It lies in autonomic ganglia and its axon supplies smooth muscle cells and glands.

Examples:

1. *Sympathetic ganglia*: Sympathetic trunk, paravertebral ganglia (celiac, superior mesenteric, inferior mesenteric, and aorticorenal ganglia), and adrenal medulla.
2. *Parasympathetic ganglia*: Ciliary ganglion, submandibular ganglion, otic ganglion, pterygopalatine ganglion, and terminal ganglia that lie near the organs.

Structure of Autonomic Ganglia

Usually, the sympathetic ganglion is easy to obtain and sufficiently large for teaching purposes; hence, its slide (section) is given for practical demonstration as a prototype of autonomic ganglia. The autonomic ganglia are smaller than the sensory ganglia.

Flowchart 2.2: Ganglia

Ganglia

Dorsal root ganglion
Dorsal root ganglia of spinal nerves
Sensory ganglia of cranial nerves

- ***Neuron***
  - Pseudounipolar
  - Large, spherical
  - Nucleus – central
  - Present in groups
- ***Satellite cells***
  - Flat cells
  - Forms complete ring
- ***Nerve fibres***
  - Myelinated
  - Run in bundles among group of neurons

Note: Usually, clusters of neurons are seen in peripheral part of ganglion.

Sympathetic (autonomic) ganglion
Sympathetic ganglia
Parasympathetic ganglia

- ***Neuron***
  - Multipolar
  - Large, irregular
  - Eccentric nucleus
  - Scattered
- ***Satellite cells***
  - Flat cells
  - Do not form complete ring
- ***Nerve fibres***
  - Preganglionic – myelinated
  - Postganglionic – nonmyelinated
  - Runs in bundles among groups of neurons

BDC yogesh

TABLE 2.2: Differences between sensory and autonomic ganglia

Criteria	*Sensory (dorsal root) ganglion*	*Autonomic (sympathetic) ganglion*
Neuron	Pseudounipolar	Multipolar
Neuron-body shape	Large spherical	Small irregular
Types of neurons	Sensory	Postganglionic autonomic/sympathetic neuron
Nucleus	Large, vesicular, centrally placed	Large, vesicular, eccentrically placed
Satellite cells	Complete ring around the neuronal body	Few satellite cells, do not form a complete ring around the neuronal body
Neuronal groups	Neurons are present in groups (clusters)	Neurons are scattered
Nerve fibres	Nerve fibres are present in bundles that separate clusters of neurons	Nerve fibres are present between scattered neurons

The *multipolar postganglionic neurons* of autonomic ganglia are scattered throughout the ganglion. These neurons are separated from each other by discrete bundles of nerve fibres (nonmyelinated and thin). The *nuclei* of neurons are large, pale-staining with the prominent nucleolus, and *eccentrically placed* in the cytoplasm. Few satellite cells are seen to surround each nerve cell body, but these cells *do not form a complete capsule*. The ganglion is surrounded by a connective tissue capsule.

As postganglionic autonomic neurons synthesize catecholamines, Nissl granules are prominently seen in their cytoplasm. Silver staining is useful for better visualization of processes of neurons.

The difference between sensory and autonomic ganglia are listed in Table 2.2.

CLINICAL NEUROANATOMY

- *Peripheral neuropathy:* It is a disease or injury that affects the functions of the peripheral nerve. It may have acute (rapid) onset or chronic (slower onset) progressive course. The signs and symptoms depend on the nerves involved. It may be:
  1. Mononeuropathy – involves a single nerve
  2. Polyneuropathy – involves many nerves

  It may result in the numbness, paralysis, imbalance, gait, impairment, and muscle atrophy and burning, itching, tingling, or pricking sensation due to nerve irritation.
- ***Radiculopathy*** involves compression of the nerve root (typical spinal nerve) in case of spondylitis or disc prolapse.
- **Entrapment syndrome** results due to compression of peripheral nerve in a narrow passage. For example, compression of the median nerve in the carpal tunnel.
- ***Multiple sclerosis*** (*encephalomyelitis disseminate*) is an autoimmune disease that results in degeneration of the myelin sheath. It causes numbness, impairment of muscular coordination, blurred vision, and severe fatigue due to impaired nerve conduction.

Facts to Remember

- Myelin is produced by oligodendrocytes in CNS and Schwann cells in PNS.
- Schmidt-Lanterman clefts are the small pockets of cytoplasm in the inner layers of the myelin sheath.
- One Schwann cell can produce a myelin sheath around a small segment of one axon. One oligodendrocyte can produce a myelin sheath around many axons.
- Because of the absence of neurilemmal sheath in CNS, regeneration of neuron is not possible in CNS.
- Thickness of myelin is directly proportional to the conduction of action potential.
- Sensory ganglia have pseudounipolar neurons (except vestibulocochlear ganglia that has bipolar neurons)

BDC's Anatomy *e*-book

1. Further reading
2. Viva voce questions

Chapter

3

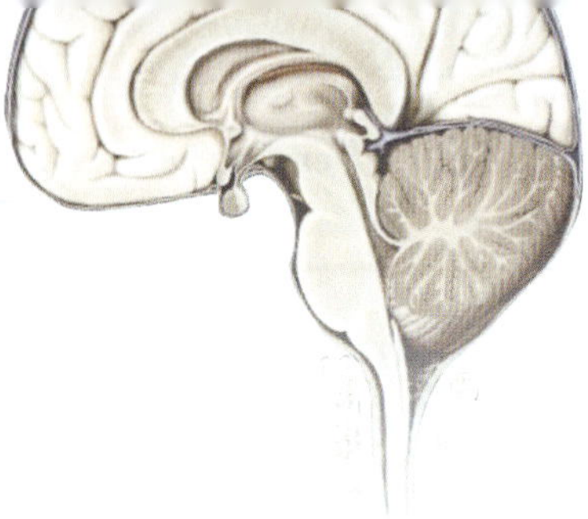

Receptors

The peripheral endings of sensory (afferent/ascending) and motor (efferent/descending) nerves are called receptors.

Classification of Receptors

The receptors are classified into various groups based on:
1. ***Functional basis:*** Exteroceptors, proprioceptors, and interoceptors.
2. ***Stimulus that activates them:*** For example, mechanoreceptors, chemoreceptors, and so on (Table 3.1).
3. ***Anatomical basis:*** Encapsulated and nonencapsulated.
4. ***Location:*** Cutaneous receptors, muscle receptors, tendon receptors, joint receptors.

Functional Classification of Receptors

1. ***Exteroceptors*** are receptors that get stimulated by the stimuli from outside the body. They are located in the skin and called cutaneous receptors.
2. ***Proprioceptors*** are receptors that receive stimuli of the position of body parts such as joints, muscles, and tendons.
3. ***Interoceptors*** are receptors that receive information from blood vessels (increase or decrease in blood pressure) and from viscera (expansion, collapse, and so on).

Anatomical Classification of Receptors

Anatomically, the sensory receptors are classified as (Table 3.2, Fig. 3.1):

A. Encapsulated receptors:
   1. Meissner's corpuscles
   2. Pacinian corpuscles
   3. End bulb of Krause
   4. Ruffini's corpuscles.

B. Nonencapsulated receptors:
   1. Free nerve endings
   2. Peritrichial or root hair plexus
   3. Merkel disc.

SENSORY AFFERENT RECEPTORS

The peripheral endings of afferent fibres which receive impulses are known as receptors.

TABLE 3.1: Type of receptors based on the stimuli

Receptor type	*Stimulus*
Mechanoreceptors	Mechanical deformation
Chemoreceptors	Chemical change (such as pH)
Thermoreceptors	Change in temperature
Nociceptors	Damaged tissue (induces pain and discomfort)
Osmoreceptors	Change in osmotic pressure

TABLE 3.2: Receptors and their activating stimulus

Receptor	*Stimulus*
Free nerve endings	Fine touch, heat, cold, pain sensation, hair-movement senses
Merkel disc	Mechanoreceptors
Meissner's corpuscles	Light touch
Pacinian corpuscles	Deep pressure, vibration
End bulb of Krause	Cold, temperature
Ruffini's corpuscles	Stretch, torque sensation
Peritrichial or root hair plexus	Fine touch

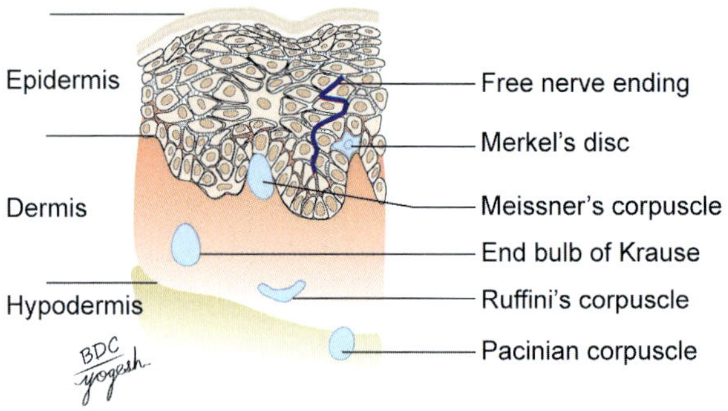

Fig. 3.1: Location of receptors in the skin

Nonencapsulated Receptors

Here the sensory nerve endings do not show any particular specialisation of structure and are directly applied to the tissue cells or may lie freely in the extracellular spaces.

1. ***Free nerve endings:*** Sensory nerve endings which repeatedly form plexuses or terminate with fewer branches constitute free nerve endings. Such types of endings are found in connective tissue, dermis of skin, fasciae, tendons, ligaments, joints, capsules, peritoneum, perichondrium and sheaths of blood vessels. These are particularly numerous in relation to hair follicles.

   These endings respond to temperature, touch and stretch. So these are thermoreceptors and mechanoreceptors. They respond to pain also (Fig. 3.2).

2. ***Merkel (disc-shaped) endings:*** The nerve fibres of these structures expand into a disc applied closely to the base of a specialised non-nervous cell (the Merkel cell) which is inserted into the basal cells of epithelium of the epidermis. These are also found around apical ends of certain hair follicles. These are responsive to pressure sensations.

Encapsulated Nerve Endings

These are special end organs. These have one feature in common that is the termination of nerve is enveloped by a capsule. These may be present in dermis, joints, muscles and tendons (Fig. 3.2).

1. ***Tactile corpuscles of Meissner:*** These are found in the dermal papillae of skin of hand, feet, front of forearm, lips and mucous membrane of tip of tongue. They are cylindrical in shape with long axis perpendicular to deep surface of epidermis and are about 80 µm long and 30 µm broad. Each corpuscle consists of a capsule with central core. The capsule consists of elastic fibres oriented along the long axis of corpuscle and interspersed with fibrocytes. The elastic fibres anchor the corpuscle to the epidermis. The capsule contains number of lamellae of flattened cells with associated basement membrane. The core of corpuscle is supplied by several myelinated nerve fibres and a few unmyelinated nerve fibres. These are responsible for touch.

2. ***Lamellated (Pacinian) corpuscles:*** These are found in subcutaneous tissue on the palmar aspects of hand, plantar aspect of foot and digits, in the genital organs of both sexes, arms, nipple, neck and in mesentery. These are relatively big in comparison to other end organs and are about 2 mm in length and 100 to 200 µm in width.

   The centre of the core generally contains a single nerve fibre, the end of which is expanded into a bulb. Lamellated corpuscles are pressure receptors.

3. ***Ruffini's corpuscles:*** These are also encapsulated nerve endings. They contain collagen bundles which emerge at each end of the thin perineurial capsule. They are slowly adapting and give a sustained response when the skin is stretched in their long axes. These occupy deep dermis and respond when heavy objects are gripped.

Note: Functional application: The encapsulated nerve endings and tactile menisci are all mechanoreceptors. Meissner's and Pacinian corpuscles are rapidly adapting tactile menisci. In medical practice, five modalities are easily tested. These are deep touch, vibration, light touch, temperature (warm or cold) and pain. Ruffini's corpuscles are slowly adapting.

4. ***Krause's end bulb:*** Mainly found in the mucocutaneous regions, e.g. lips and external genitalia. The bulb is spheroidal in shape, about 50 µm in diameter. Its capsule is continuous with the endoneurium. The nerve fibres branch into the bulb. It probably receives thermal impulses.

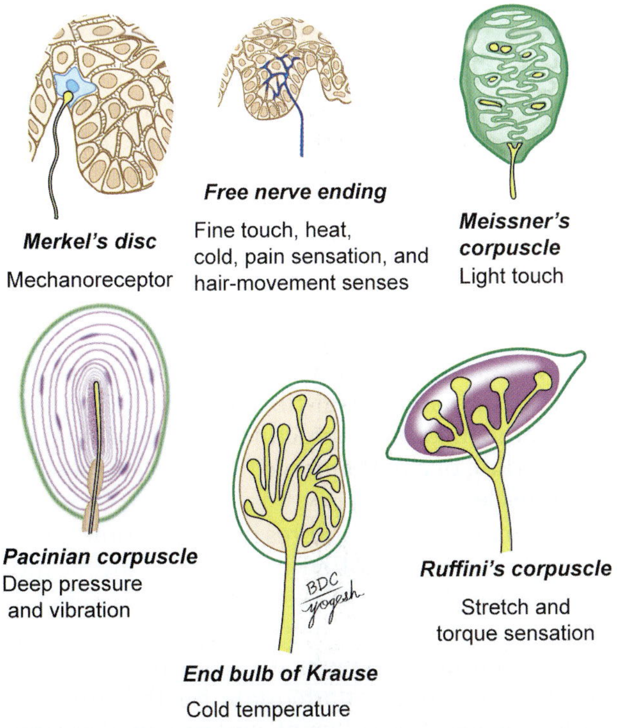

Fig. 3.2: Structure of the receptors located in the skin

Joints, Muscles and Tendons

The afferent endings are proprioceptors and furnish the central nervous system with information required for the performance of properly coordinated movements. In addition, proprioceptive information reaches consciousness so that there is awareness of the position of body parts and of their movements. Pain arising in muscles, tendons and bones is detected by free nerve endings in connective tissue. These are known as nociceptive fibres. The receptors in tendons and muscles are: neurotendinous spindle of Golgi and neuromuscular spindle.

Neurotendinous Spindle of Golgi

The *Golgi tendon organ* (*GTO*) is a fusiform-shaped receptor located at sites where muscle fibres insert into the tendon (Fig. 3.3). It consists of interlacing intrafusal collagen bundles enclosed in connective tissue capsule. It is innervated by type A sensory fibres. Each nerve fibre pierces the capsule and branches into numerous terminals that are interposed among the intrafusal collagen bundles.

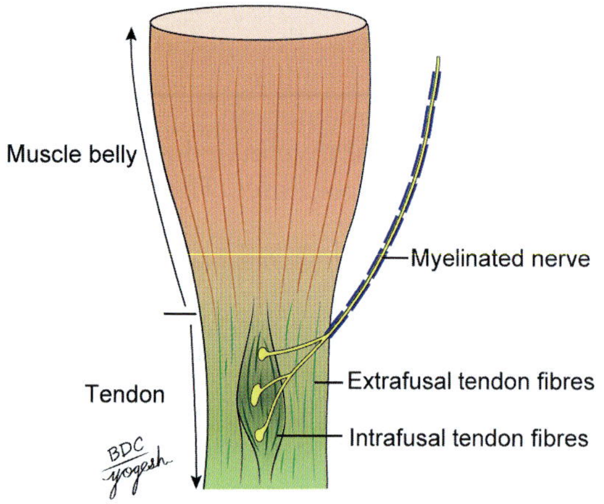

Fig. 3.3: Golgi tendon organ (a neurotendinous spindle)

Function

Golgi tendon organ monitors the tension produced during muscle contraction. It inhibits the activity of α-motor neuron that produces muscle contraction (through interneurons).

Neuromuscular Spindles

The muscle (neuromuscular) spindle is a spindle-shaped sensory end organ of skeletal muscles (Plate 3.1).
Length: 5–10 mm
Diameter: 100 µm.

Structure

It consists of capsules, sensory neuron, gamma motor neurons, and intrafusal muscle fibres. The muscle spindle is enclosed within fusiform connective tissue fibres.

It has ***intrafusal muscle fibres*** that are enclosed within the capsule. The extrafusal fibres form the main bulk of the muscle.

There are two types of intrafusal fibres:

1. *Nuclear bag fibres*: Many nuclei are located in the middle of the fibres.
2. *Nuclear chain fibres*: Nuclei are arranged in a single row.

Nuclear bag fibres are long and extend outside the capsule up to the endomysium of adjacent extrafusal fibres.

Nerve supply of muscle spindle:

- Muscle spindle is supplied by gamma motor neurons and sensation is carried by sensory afferent nerve fibres (type Ia and II). Extrafusal (main muscle) fibres are supplied by alpha motor neurons.
- Type Ia fibres have annulospiral nerve endings that surround the central area of the nuclear chain and bag fibres.
- Type II fibres have floral spray endings that are present in the peripheral part of bag fibres.
- The sensory neurons get stimulated on the stretching of muscle fibres.

Functions

During muscle contraction, stretching of muscle spindle stimulates sensory nerve fibres (type Ia and type II).

Plate 3.1: Muscle spindle

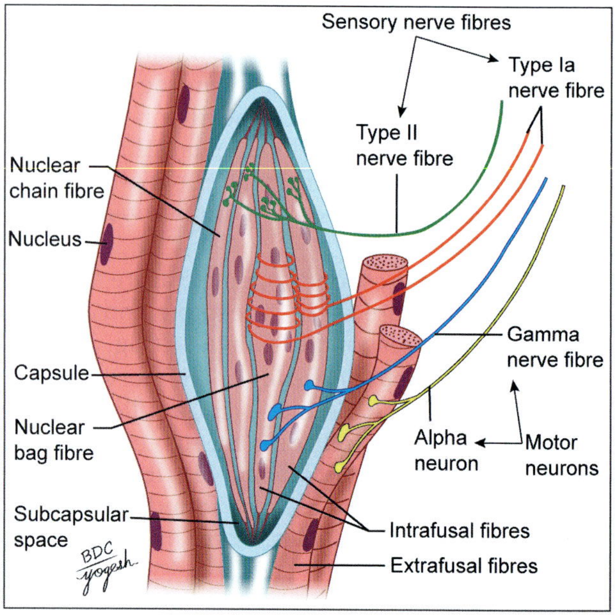

These sensory fibres provide inputs to the CNS about muscle stretch and help to modulate the activity of motor neurons supplying the same muscle.

CLINICAL NEUROANATOMY

***Myotatic* or *stretch reflex*:** Elongation of the spindle on stretching the skeletal muscle produces reflex rapid contraction of the muscle. This is called the *stretch reflex*.
Components: Muscle stretch → stimulation of type I and type II sensory nerve fibres of muscle spindle → synapse with alpha (α) motor neuron → skeletal muscle contraction (Plate 3.1).

EFFECTOR NERVE ENDINGS

The effector nerve endings or motor efferent endings controls the activity of the skeletal or smooth muscles.

Somatic Effectors

The somatic effectors are the terminals of myelinated motor neurons. These are lower motor neurons.

Motor Innervation of Skeletal Muscle

The myoneural junctions or motor end plates on extrafusal and intrafusal fibres of skeletal/striated muscles are synapse-like structure with two components, i.e. the ending of a motor nerve fibre and subjacent part of the muscle.

The number of muscle fibres in a motor unit (number of muscle fibres supplied by a single alpha motor neuron) varies from one to several hundred depending upon the size and function of a muscle.

A large **motor unit** in which a single neuron supplies many muscle fibres, is adequate for the function of muscles such as those of trunk and proximal portion of limbs. However, in extraocular and intrinsic muscles

Plate 3.2: Neuromuscular junction

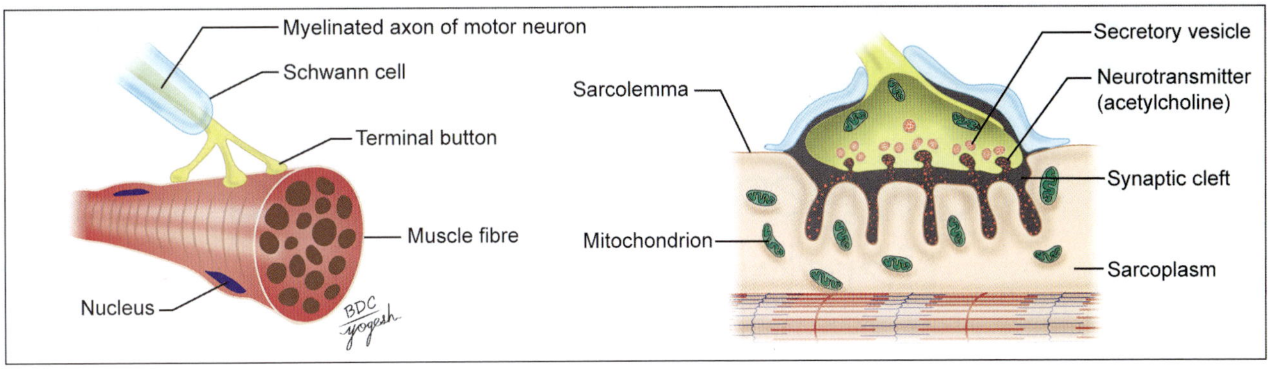

of hand which function with precision, the motor unit includes only a few muscle fibres.

Each branch of nerve fibre gives up its myelin sheath on approaching a muscle fibre and ends as several branchlets that constitute the neural component of **end plate** (Plate 3.2).

In the majority of muscles, the terminals of the nerve end in a small localised area of muscle fibre forming a so-called motor end plate. In this region, the sarcoplasm contains many nuclei rich in mitochondria and has granular appearance. This region of sarcoplasm is known as soleplate. There is an interval of 20–50 µm, constituting a synaptic cleft between surface of nerve terminal and that of muscle fibre. The sarcolemma of muscle fibre has a wavy outline where they oppose the nerve terminal, with irregularities being known as junctional folds. Axon terminal in this region is rich in mitochondria and contains vesicles similar to those seen in the region of synapse. There is no protoplasmic continuity between the axoplasm and sarcoplasm.

The vesicles in axoplasm contain the neurotransmitter acetylcholine that is released when nervous impulse reaches myoneural junction. Acetylcholine creates a wave of depolarisation in the sarcolemma resulting in contraction of muscle fibres. Thereafter, acetylcholine is quickly destroyed by an enzyme called cholinesterase.

Innervation of Smooth Muscles and Glands

The contact between nerve ending and smooth muscle is not as close as in skeletal muscle. Axon terminal contains vesicles. In most cases of sympathetic terminals, these vesicles contain adrenaline or noradrenaline. In case of parasympathetic terminals, they contain acetylcholine. Similarly, the nonmyelinated nerve endings come in contact with the secretory cells.

CLINICAL NEUROANATOMY

- ***Myasthenia gravis***: It is a consequence of autoimmune destruction of nicotinic postsynaptic receptors for acetylcholine. Thymus abnormality occurs in 80% of patients.

  Clinical features: Limb and trunk: Weakness of neck muscles resulting in rolling of head. Proximal limb muscles are preferentially affected. Limb reflexes are hyperactive. Muscle wasting occurs in 15% cases.

  Diagnosis: Acetylcholine receptor antibodies are detected in majority of patients.
- ***Myotatic or stretch reflex***: Elongation of the spindle on stretching the skeletal muscle produces reflex rapid contraction of the muscle. This is called the stretch reflex.

  Components: Muscle stretch → stimulation of type I and type II sensory nerve fibres of muscle spindle → synapse with alpha motor neuron → skeletal muscle contraction (Fig. 3.4).

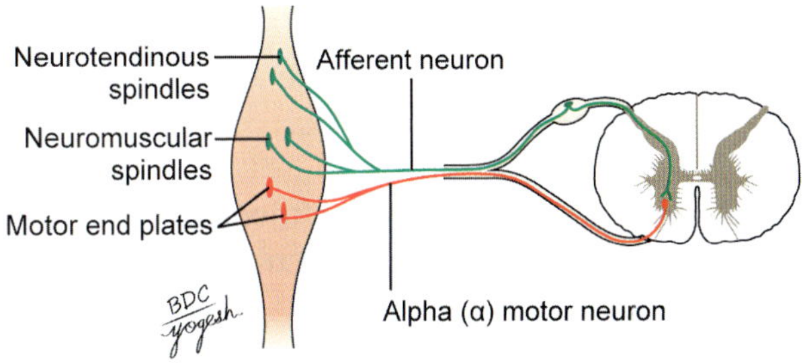

Fig. 3.4: Stretch reflex. A simple reflex arc consisting of an afferent neuron that is arising from neuromuscular spindle or neurotendinous spindle and an efferent alpha motor neuron stimulating extrafusal muscle fibres

Facts to Remember

- Meissner's corpuscles – Light touch
- Pacinian corpuscles – Deep pressure, vibration
- End bulb of Krause – Cold, temperature
- Ruffini's corpuscles – Stretch, torque sensation
- Free nerve endings – Fine touch, heat, cold, pain sensation, hair-movement senses
- Merkel disc – Mechanoreceptors
- Peritrichial or root – Fine touch hair plexus

BDC's Anatomy *e*-book

1. Further reading
2. Viva voce questions

Chapter

4

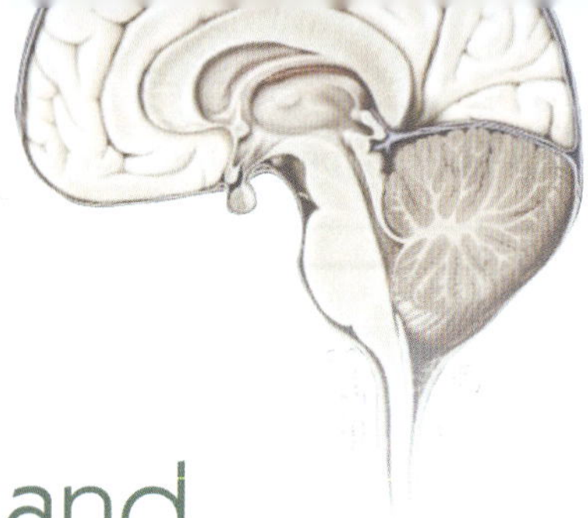

Meninges of the Brain and Cerebrospinal Fluid

The brain is a very important delicate organ. It is protected by the following coverings.

1. Bony covering of the cranium
2. Three membranous coverings (meninges):
   a. Outer dura mater (pachymeninx)
   b. Middle arachnoid mater
   c. Inner pia mater.

   Note: The arachnoid and pia are together known as the leptomeninges.

   [*Mnemonics*: ***PAD:*** **P** – Pia mater; **A** – Arachnoid mater; **D** – Dura mater]
3. The spaces in relation to meninges are:
   a. Extradural/epidural
   b. Subdural
   c. Subarachnoid
4. The cerebrospinal fluid (CSF) fills the space between the arachnoid and the pia maters (subarachnoid space) and acts as a water cushion.

Competency:

AN56.1 Describe and identify various layers of meninges with its extent and modifications.

MENINGES

DURA MATER

The cerebral or cranial dura mater is the thickest, toughest, and outermost fibrous covering of brain (*dura* = hard, *mater* = mother).

The cerebral dura mater is made up of two layers: Outer endosteal and inner meningeal layers, and enclosing the cranial venous sinuses between these two.

The ***endosteal layer*** is attached to the inner surfaces of the cranial bones and is continuous through the sutural ligaments, and around the margins of the foramina with the periosteum on the external surface of the cranium. It provides *sheaths* for the cranial nerves, the sheaths fuse with the epineurium outside the skull.

The ***meningeal layer*** forms four folds:

1. Falx cerebri
2. Tentorium cerebelli
3. Falx cerebelli
4. Diaphragma sellae.

These folds divide the cranial cavity into intercommunicating compartments for different parts of the brain (Table 4.1, Figs 4.1 and 4.2). The meningeal layer is continuous with the ***spinal dura*** mater.

The details of cerebral dura mater are described in Chapter 12, Volume 3.

Folds of Dura Mater

Falx Cerebri

The falx cerebri is a large sickle-shaped fold of dura mater occupying the median longitudinal fissure between the two cerebral hemispheres (Plate 4.1).

Tentorium Cerebelli

The tentorium cerebelli is a tent-shaped fold of dura mater, forming the roof of the posterior cranial fossa. It separates the cerebellum from the occipital lobes of the cerebrum, and broadly divides the cranial cavity into supratentorial and infratentorial compartments. The infratentorial compartment is the posterior cranial fossa containing the hindbrain and the lower part of the midbrain.

Its anterior free margin *forms the* U-shaped ***tentorial notch*** which is occupied by the midbrain and the anterior part of the superior vermis.

Falx Cerebelli

The falx cerebelli is a small sickle-shaped fold of dura mater projecting forwards into the posterior cerebellar notch.

Diaphragma Sellae

The diaphragma sellae is a small circular, horizontal fold of dura mater forming the roof of the hypophyseal fossa. The diaphragma has a ***central aperture*** through which the stalk of the hypophysis cerebri passes.

Blood Supply

The outer layer is richly vascular. It is supplied by the middle meningeal, anterior ethmoidal, posterior ethmoidal, ophthalmic, accessory meningeal, internal carotid, ascending pharyngeal artery, vertebral, and occipital arteries.

TABLE 4.1: The meningeal layer sends inward following folds of dura mater

Folds	*Shape*	*Attachments*	*Venous sinuses enclosed*
Falx cerebri	Sickle-shaped, separates the right from left cerebral hemisphere	Superior, convex margins are attached to sides of the groove lodging the superior sagittal sinus Inferior concave margin is free Anterior attachment is to crista galli and frontal crest Posterior attachment is to upper surface of cerebelli tentorium	Superior sagittal sinus Inferior sagittal sinus Straight sinus
Tentorium cerebelli	Tent-shaped, separates the cerebral hemispheres from hindbrain and lower part of midbrain Lifts off the weight of occipital lobes from the cerebellum	Has a free anterior margin. Its ends are attached to anterior clinoid processes Rest is free and concave Posterior margin is attached to the lips of groove containing transverse sinuses, superior petrosal sinuses and to posterior clinoid processes	Transverse sinuses, Superior petrosal sinuses
Falx cerebelli	Small sickle-shaped fold partly separating two cerebellar hemispheres	Base is attached to posterior part of inferior surface of tentorium cerebelli Apex reaches till foramen magnum	Occipital sinus
Diaphragma sellae	Small horizontal fold	Anterior attachment is to tuberculum sellae Posterior attachment is to dorsum sellae; laterally continuous with dura mater of middle cranial fossa	Anterior and posterior intercavernous sinuses

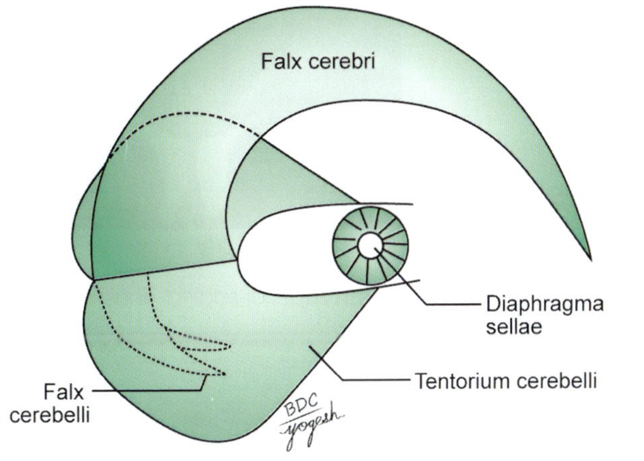

Fig. 4.1: Various folds of meningeal layer of dura mater

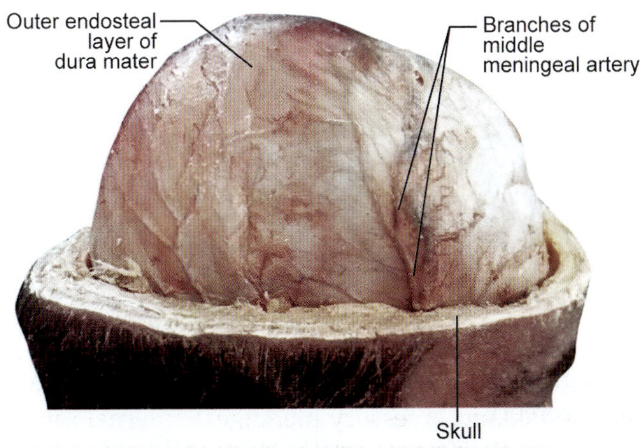

Fig. 4.2: Endosteal layer of dura mater

DISSECTION

Cut through the fused endosteum and dura mater on the ventral aspect of brain from the inferolateral borders extending along the superolateral margin. Pull upwards the endosteum along with the fold of dura mater present between the adjacent medial surfaces of cerebral hemispheres, extending from the frontal lobe till the occipital lobe. This is falx cerebri. Pull backwards a similar but much smaller fold between two adjacent lobes of cerebellum—the falx cerebelli.

Separating the cerebrum and the cerebellum is another fold of dura mater called the tentorium cerebelli. Pull it on a horizontal plane. Thus, the fused endosteum and dura mater get separated from the underlying subarachnoid mater, pia mater and the brain.

Identify various venous sinuses between the endosteum and folds of dura mater. Underneath the dura mater and separated by a flimsy subdural space is the cobweb-like arachnoid mater. It is separated from the underlying pia mater by the subarachnoid space, containing cerebrospinal fluid and blood vessels of the brain. Cranial nerves also pass through this space. Near the superior sagittal sinus, arachnoid mater forms arachnoid villi. The subarachnoid space is dilated around the brainstem and at the base of the brain forming the subarachnoid cisterns.

ARACHNOID MATER

The arachnoid (Latin *cobweb-like*) mater is a thin transparent membrane that loosely surrounds the brain *without* dipping into many of its sulci (Figs 4.3a and b

Plate 4.1: Dural folds and dural venous sinuses enclosed within them, viewed from superolateral aspect

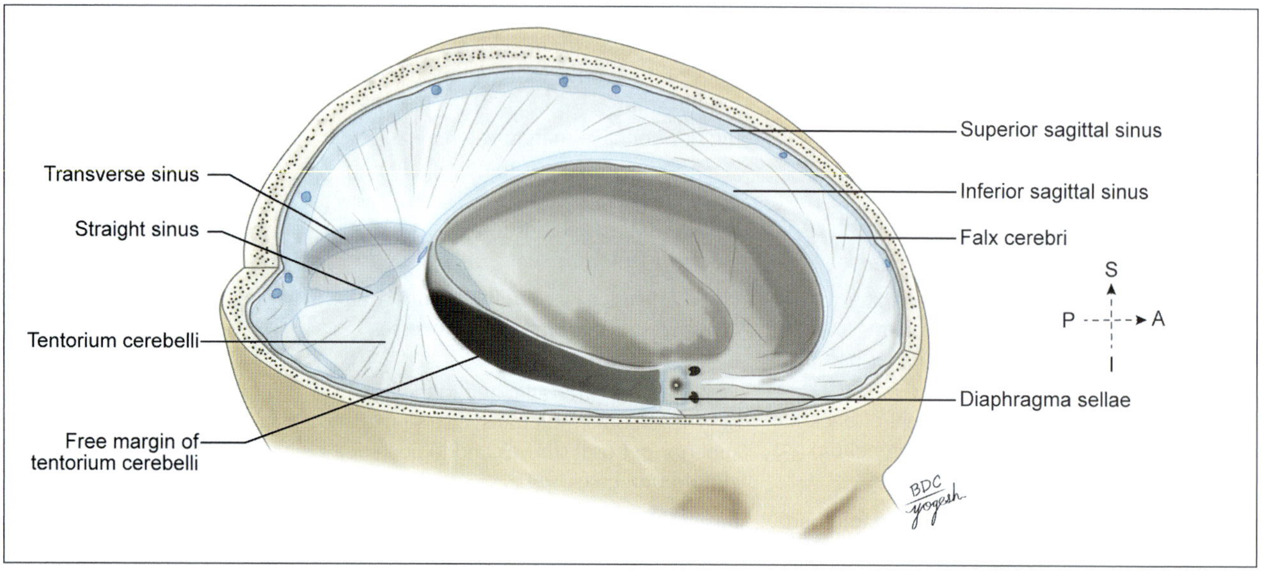

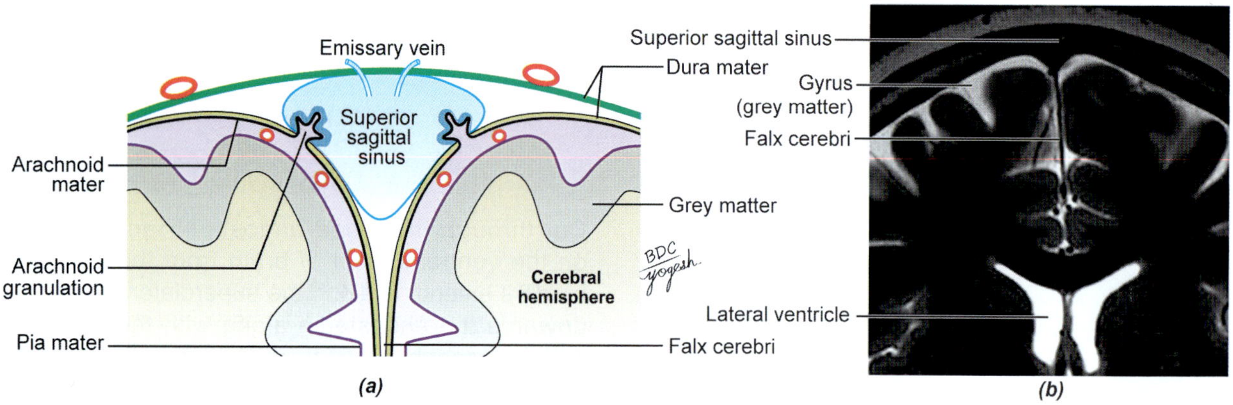

Figs 4.3a and b: (a) Arachnoid granulation and (b) MRI of coronal section through superior sagittal sinus

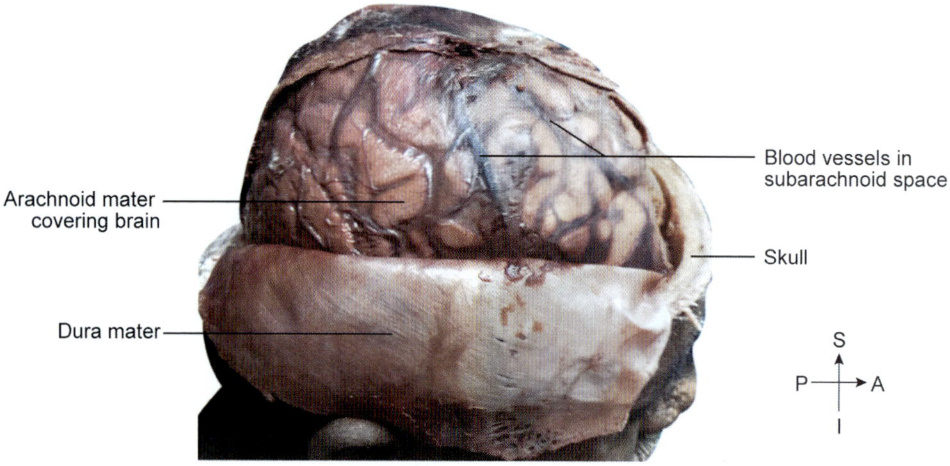

Fig. 4.4: Arachnoid mater

and 4.4). Thus, it bridges all irregularities of the brain. It enters the following sulcus/fissure:

1. Stem of lateral sulcus where it is pushed by lesser wing of sphenoid.
2. Longitudinal cerebral fissure where it is carried in by falx cerebri.

Note: The arachnoid mater cannot be identified in the hypophyseal fossa.

Relations

It is separated from the dura by the ***subdural space***, and from the pia by the ***subarachnoid space*** containing cerebrospinal fluid (CSF) and blood vessels.

Prolongations

1. It provides sheaths for the cranial nerves as far as their exit from the skull.
2. ***Arachnoid villi*** are small, finger-like processes of arachnoid tissue, projecting into the cranial venous sinuses. They absorb CSF.
3. With advancing age, the arachnoid villi enlarge in size to form pedunculated tufts, called ***arachnoid granulations***. These granulations may produce depressions in bone.

Note: Cerebrospinal fluid formed by choroid plexuses flows through the ventricles of the brain into the subarachnoid space to be absorbed via subarachnoid villi into the superior sagittal sinus.

PIA MATER

The pia (Latin *loving mother*) mater is a thin vascular membrane that closely invests the brain, dipping into various sulci and other irregularities of its surface. It comprises epi-pia and pia-glia (Fig. 4.5).

On the cerebellum, pia mater dips and forms folds in relation to larger fissures of cerebellum. It is pierced by blood vessels to nourish the brain and spinal cord.

Prolongations

1. ***Perivascular sheaths***: The pia mater provides sheaths around the vessels entering or leaving the brain substance.

   Note: ***Perivascular space*** (*Virchow-Robin's space*): The blood vessels in the substance of brain are surrounded by a sheath of external pia mater and inner arachnoid mater. The space between these two layers is called perivascular space.
2. ***Tela choroidea of ventricles***: These are folds of pia mater surrounded by ependymal lining.
3. ***Choroid plexus***: The tuft of capillaries and tela choroidea together forms choroid plexus. It produces CSF.
4. Sheaths around cranial nerves.

EXTRADURAL (EPIDURAL) AND SUBDURAL SPACES

The extradural or epidural space is a potential space between the inner aspect of skull bone and the endosteal layer of dura mater. Vertebral epidural space is present between vertebral column and spinal dura mater. The subdural space is also a potential space between the dura and arachnoid maters. These become actual spaces in pathological conditions.

The subdural space is traversed by cerebral veins on their path for draining into dural venous sinuses.

SUBARACHNOID SPACE

This is the space between the arachnoid and the pia maters. It is traversed by a network of arachnoid trabeculae which give it a ***sponge-like appearance*** (Fig. 4.5).

It surrounds the brain and spinal cord, and ends below at the lower border of the 2nd sacral vertebra.

The subarachnoid space contains CSF, and large vessels of the brain. Cranial nerves pass through the space.

Larger arteries lie in subarachnoid space. Smaller ones carry sheaths of pia. Subarachnoid space and perivascular spaces are separated by layer of pia mater.

Space between the nervous tissue and fold of pia mater with arterioles is known as ***Virchow-Robin perivascular space***.

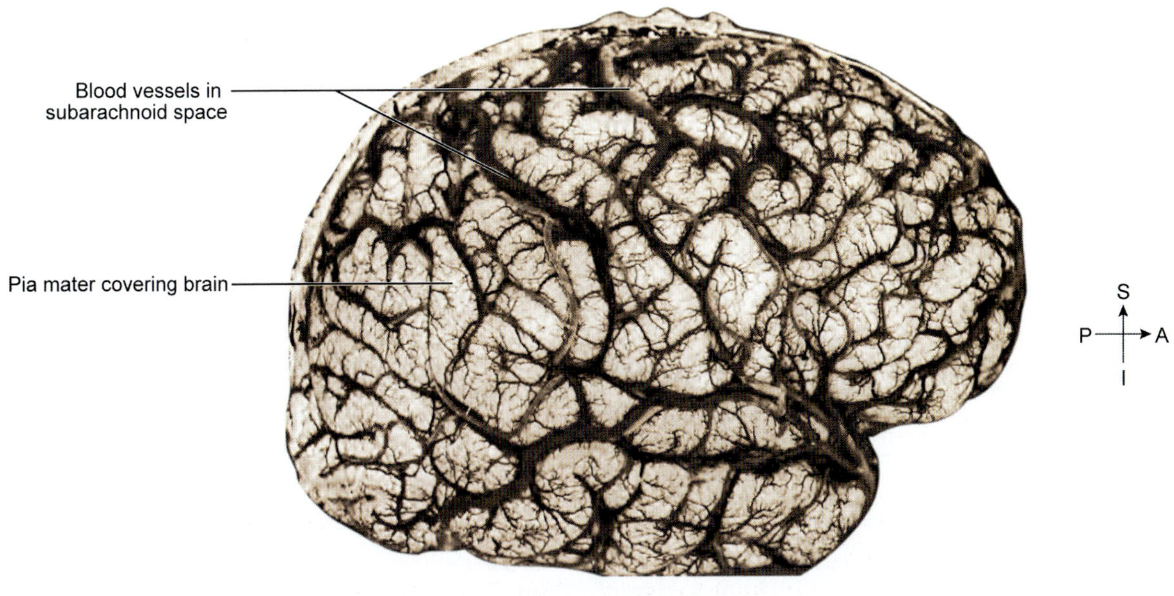

Fig. 4.5: Pia mater

Subarachnoid Cisterns

At the base of the brain and around the brainstem, the subarachnoid space forms intercommunicating pools, called *cisterns* (Latin *reservoir*). These reinforce the protective effect of CSF on the vital centres situated in the medulla. The subarachnoid cisterns are as follows (Flowchart 4.1 and Plate 4.2):

1. ***Cerebellomedullary cistern or cisterna magna:*** It is the largest cistern lying in the angle between medulla oblongata, cerebellum and occipital bone. It is triangular in section. It bridges the interval between inferior surface of cerebellum and medulla oblongata (Figs 4.6a and b). It receives CSF from the 4th ventricle via the median foramen of Magendie and the paired lateral foramina of Luschka.
   Contents:
   a. Vertebral artery and the origin of the posteroinferior cerebellar artery (PICA)
   b. Ninth (IX), tenth (X), eleventh (XI) and twelfth (XII) cranial nerves
   c. Choroid plexus.
2. ***Cisterna pontis:*** It is present on the ventral aspect of the pons. It is continuous with interpeduncular cistern cranially, with cerebellomedullary cistern behind and with spinal subarachnoid space caudally.
   Contents:
   a. Basilar artery and the origin of the anteroinferior cerebellar artery (AICA)
   b. Origin of the superior cerebellar arteries
   c. Sixth (VI) cranial nerve.
3. ***Interpeduncular cistern:*** This is a large cistern as the arachnoid mater passes across the two temporal lobes. The cistern is continuous with the subarachnoid spaces around anterior, middle and posterior cerebral arteries.
   Contents:
   a. Optic chiasma
   b. Bifurcation of the basilar artery
   c. Peduncular segments of the PCA
   d. Peduncular segments of the superior cerebellar arteries
   e. Perforating branches of the PCA
   f. Posterior communicating arteries (PCoA)
   g. Basal vein of Rosenthal
   h. Third (III) cranial nerve, which passes between the posterior cerebral and superior cerebellar arteries.
4. ***Cistern of lateral sulcus:*** It lies in front of each temporal pole and is formed due to bridging of arachnoid mater over the lateral sulcus. This cistern contains middle cerebral vessels.
5. ***Cistern of great cerebral vein (cisterna ambiens):*** This cistern lies in the space between splenium of corpus callosum and superior surface of cerebellum. It contains pineal gland and great cerebral vein of Galen.
6. ***Lumbar cistern:*** This is a large subarachnoid space in the lumbar region of the vertebral column distal to the termination of the spinal cord. In the space between L3 and L4 (which is part of the lumbar cistern), lumbar puncture is done to obtain a sample of CSF.

Note: The arterial pulsations within the cisterns help to force the CSF from the cisterns onto the superolateral surface of the hemispheres. The cisterns themselves form cushions around the medulla.

Communications

The subarachnoid space communicates with ventricular system of brain at:

1. A median foramen of Magendie
2. Two lateral foramina of Luschka, situated in the roof of the fourth ventricle. The CSF passes through these foramina from the fourth ventricle to subarachnoid space.

Prolongations

1. The space is prolonged into the arachnoid sheaths around nerves where it communicates with the neural lymphatics, particularly around the 1st, 2nd and 8th cranial nerves.
2. The space also extends into the pial sheaths around the vessels entering the brain substance (perivascular space). Thus, CSF comes into direct contact with nerve cells.

Flowchart 4.1: Subarachnoid space and cisterns

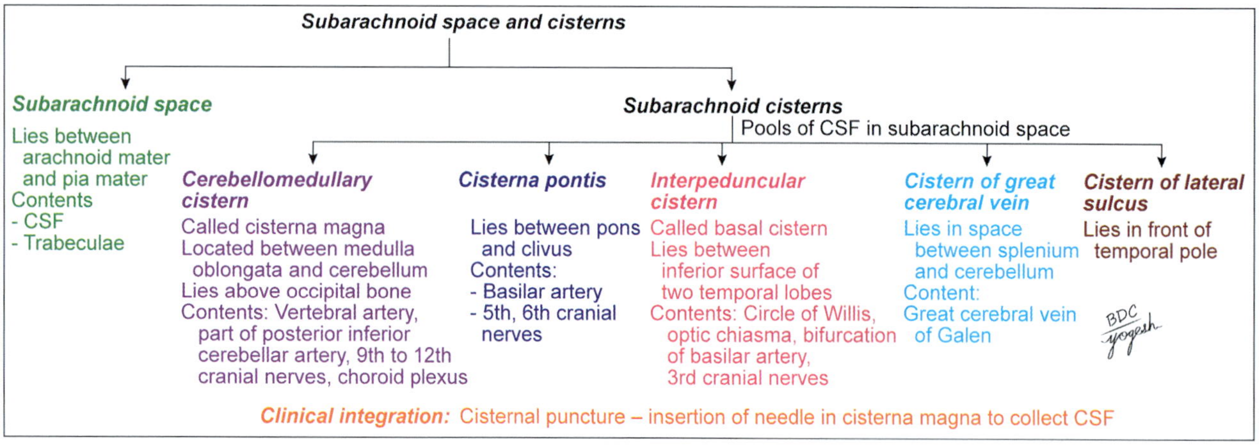

Plate 4.2: Location of principal subarachnoid cisterns (midsagittal section, right medial view)

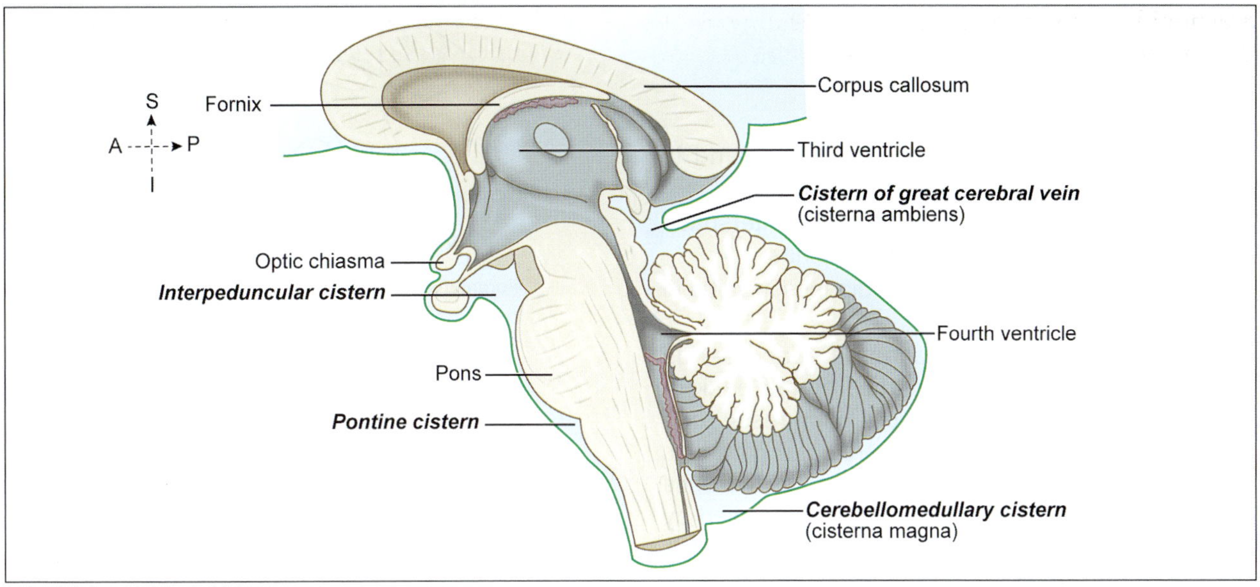

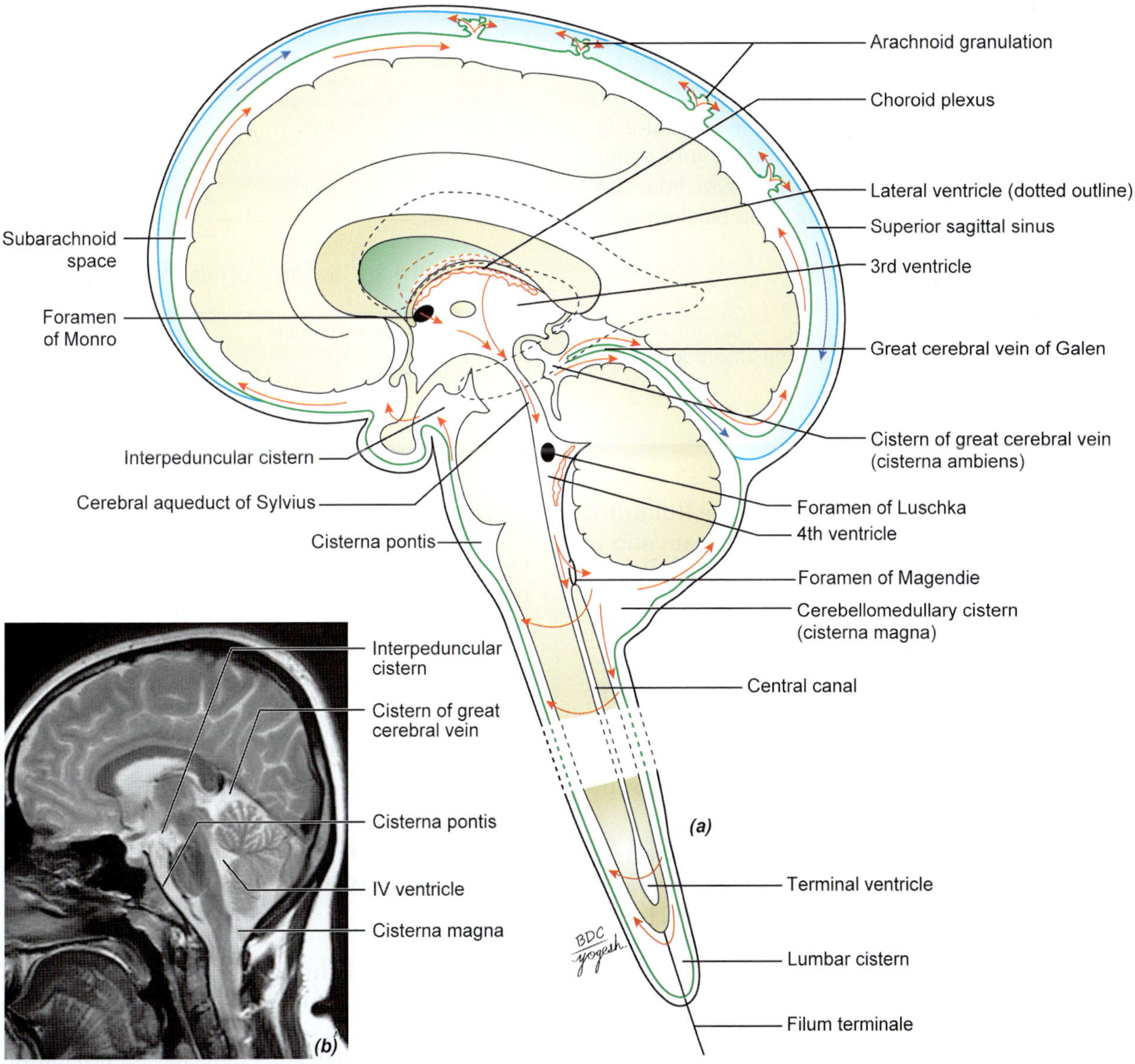

Figs 4.6a and b: CSF circulation: (a) Various cisterns of the brain including formation, circulation and absorption of cerebrospinal fluid. Arrows show the direction of flow of CSF and (b) MRI depicting the cisterns

CLINICAL NEUROANATOMY

- CSF can be obtained by:
  a. Lumbar puncture
  b. Cisternal puncture
  c. Ventricular puncture.

  Lumbar puncture is the easiest method and is commonly used.

  It is done by passing a needle in the interspace between the third and fourth lumbar spines.
- Biochemical analysis of CSF is of diagnostic value in various diseases.
- ***Papilloedema:*** The subarachnoid space sends extensions along the optic nerves till the back of eyeball. Increased CSF pressure compresses the wall of retinal vein leading to forward bulging of optic disc with oedema of the disc. Oedema of the optic disc is known as *papilloedema*. It can be viewed by an ophthalmoscope.
- ***Lumbar epidural space:*** The epidural space is the space between vertebral canal and dura mater. The procedure is same as lumbar puncture, the needle should reach only in the epidural space and not deep to it in the dura mater. Epidural space is utilized for giving anaesthesia or analgesia.
- Inflammation of pia mater and arachnoid mater is known as ***meningitis***. This is commonly tubercular or pyogenic. It is characterised by fever, marked headache, neck rigidity, and a changed biochemistry of CSF.

Competency:

AN56.2 Describe formation, circulation and absorption of CSF with its applied anatomy.

CEREBROSPINAL FLUID (CSF)

The cerebrospinal fluid is a modified tissue fluid. It is contained in the ventricular system of the brain and in the subarachnoid space around the brain and spinal cord. CSF replaces lymph in the CNS (Fig. 4.7, Flowchart 4.2).

Formation

1. Bulk of the CSF is formed by the *choroid plexuses* of the lateral ventricles and lesser amounts by the choroid plexuses of the 3rd and 4th ventricles (Fig. 4.7).
2. Possibly, it is also formed by the capillaries on the surface of the brain and spinal cord.

The total quantity of CSF is about 150 ml. It is formed at the rate of about 20 ml per hour or 500 ml per day.

The normal pressure of CSF is 60 to 100 mm H_2O.

Circulation

CSF passes from each lateral ventricle to the 3rd ventricle through the interventricular foramen of Monro. From the 3rd ventricle, it passes to the 4th ventricle through the cerebral aqueduct. From the 4th ventricle, the CSF passes to the subarachnoid spaces of the cerebrum and the vertebral canal through the median and lateral apertures of the 4th ventricle (Flowchart 4.3). Some of it passes down the central canal of spinal cord.

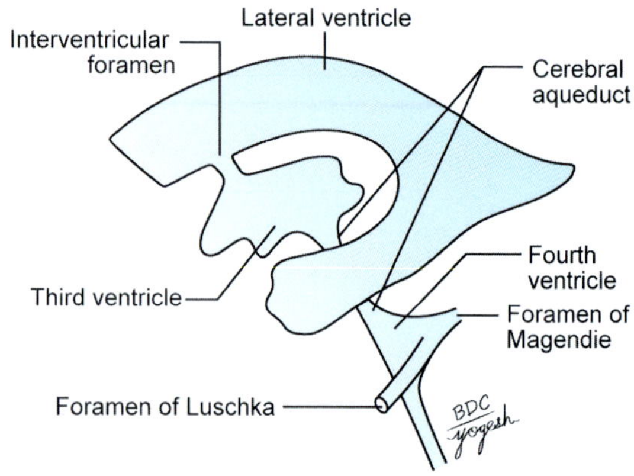

Fig. 4.7: Ventricular system of brain

Flowchart 4.2: Cerebrospinal fluid

Cerebrospinal fluid (CSF)
Total volume: 150 ml
Clear, colourless, slightly alkaline fluid

Definition	*Composition*	*Formation*	*Functions*
Modified tissue fluid that lies in ventricles of brain, central canal of spinal cord, subarachnoid space	Specific gravity: 1005–1008 Proteins: 25 mg/dl Glucose: 50 mg/dl Chloride: 120 mEq/L Lymphocytes: 0–5/mm^3	By choroid plexuses of ventricles 500 ml/day Normal CSF pressure 6–10 cm of water	Protection shock-absorption Nutrition Waste product removal

Flowchart 4.3: Circulation of cerebrospinal fluid (CSF)

Lateral ventricle
↓
Interventricular foramen of Monro
↓
3rd ventricle
↓
Cerebral aqueduct of Sylvius
↓
4th ventricle
↓ Central canal of spinal cord
↓ Through foramen of Magendie, two foramina of Luschka
Subarachnoid space
↓ Flows upward around cerebellum and cerebrum through tentorial notch
Subarachnoid granulation
↓ Absorption
Venous blood of superior sagittal sinus

Absorption

1. CSF is absorbed chiefly through the arachnoid villi and granulations, and is thus drained into the cranial venous sinuses.
2. It is also absorbed partly by the perineural lymphatics around the first, second and eighth cranial nerves.
3. It is also absorbed by veins related to spinal nerves.

Composition

CSF is a clear, colourless, slightly alkaline fluid.

Specific gravity: 1005–1008

Proteins: 25 mg/dl

Glucose: 50 mg/dl

Chloride: 120 mEq/L

Lymphocytes: 0–5/mm^3.

Functions of CSF

1. CSF decreases the sudden pressure or forces on delicate nervous tissue.
2. CSF ***nourishes*** nervous tissue. Only CSF comes in contact with neurons. Even blood cannot directly come in contact with neurons. It provides nourishment and returns products of metabolism to the venous sinuses.
3. Neurons cannot live without glucose and oxygen for more than 3–5 minutes. These are constantly provided by CSF.
4. Pineal gland secretions reach pituitary gland via CSF.
5. A major function of CSF is to ***cushion*** the brain within its solid vault. The brain and CSF have approximately the same specific gravity, so that the brain simply floats in the fluid.
6. There is no CSF–brain barrier, so drugs can reach the neurons through CSF.
7. There is blood–CSF barrier. There are no antibodies in CNS, making infections of brain very serious entity.

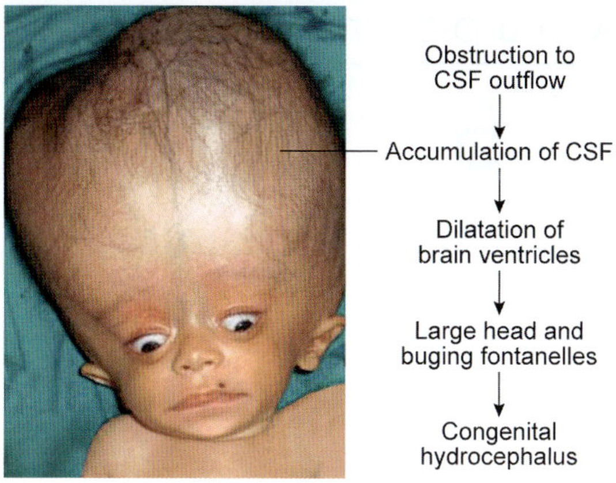

Fig. 4.8: Hydrocephalic child

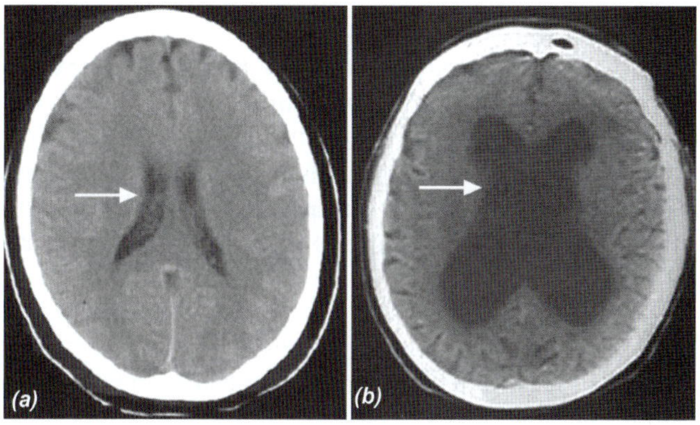

Figs 4.9a and b: (a) Normal ventricles and (b) dilated ventricles in hydrocephalic child (Ventricles are dark in colour and marked by arrow)

Competency:

AN63.2 Describe anatomical basis of congenital hydrocephalus.

CLINICAL NEUROANATOMY

- Drainage of CSF at regular intervals is of therapeutic value in ***meningitis***. Certain intractable headaches of unknown aetiology are also known to have been cured by a mere lumbar puncture with drainage of CSF.
- Obstruction in the vertebral canal produces ***Froin's syndrome*** or *loculation syndrome*. This is characterised by yellowish discolouration of CSF (xanthochromia) below the level of obstruction, and its spontaneous coagulation after withdrawal due to a high protein content. Biochemical examination of such fluid reveals that the protein content is raised, but the cell content is normal. This is known as *albuminocytologic dissociation*.
- ***Hydrocephalus***: It is the dilatation of the ventricular system and occurs due to obstruction of CSF circulation. It may be of the following types (Figs 4.8 and 4.9):
  a. ***Communicating hydrocephalus:*** If the obstruction is outside the ventricular system, usually in the subarachnoid space or arachnoid granulations, it is termed *communicating hydrocephalus*. This occurs due to fibrosis following meningitis.
     It is also called external hydrocephalus.
     Clinical features are:
     - Head size is rather large.
     - Tense anterior fontanelle
     - Dilated veins over thin scalp.
  b. ***Non-communicating hydrocephalus:*** If the obstruction is within the ventricular system, it is called *non-communicating* or *internal hydrocephalus*. This is usually caused by a tumour or inflammation. A shunt procedure is employed to divert the CSF from the ventricular system into the peritoneal cavity.

Facts to Remember

- Leptomeninges = arachnoid mater + pia mater
- Dura mater is toughest and pia mater is most delicate among the meninges.
- CSF is present in the subarachnoid space, ventricles of brain, and central canal of spinal cord.
- CSF is produced by choroid plexuses and absorbed by subarachnoid granulations.
- Increased formation or decreased absorption or any obstruction in its flow leads to hydrocephalus.

BDC's Anatomy *e*-book

1. Anatomical basis of hydrocephalus
2. Further reading
3. Viva voce questions

Chapter

5

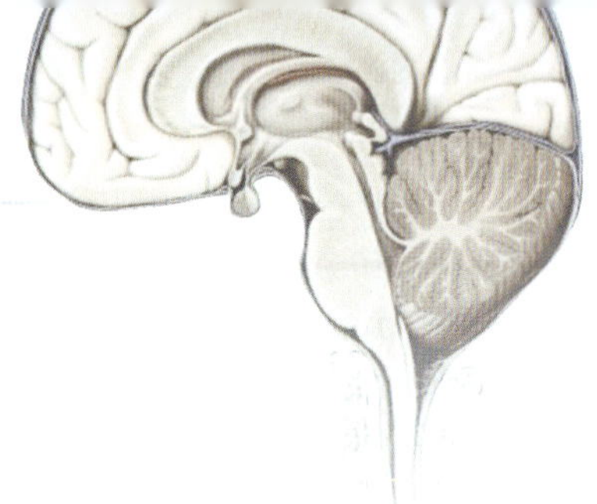

Spinal Cord

The spinal cord is the long cylindrical lower part of central nervous system. It is the main pathway for information connecting the brain and peripheral nervous system.

It occupies upper two-thirds of vertebral canal and is enclosed in the three meninges. It gives rise to 31 pairs of spinal nerves and retains the basic structural pattern.

> *Competency:*
> **AN57.2** Describe extent of spinal cord in child and adult with its clinical implication.

Features

It is cylindrical and slightly flattened anteroposteriorly.

Measurements

Length: 18 inches or 45 cm in an adult male
42 cm in adult female.

Weight: 30 g.

It is surrounded by the three meninges (Fig. 5.1).

Extent

It extends from upper border of atlas vertebra to the lower border of first lumbar vertebra in an adult. In newborn, it extends up to L3 vertebra. Superiorly, it is continuous with the medulla oblongata; inferiorly, it terminates as conus medullaris. The spinal cord extends in the lower part of 1st lumbar vertebra as *conus medullaris.*

SPINAL MENINGES

The spinal cord is surrounded by three meninges (Fig. 5.2):

1. *Dura mater*: It is the outermost covering and extends from the foramen magnum to the lower border of second sacral vertebra.
2. *Arachnoid mater* (cobweb-like in Latin) is the middle layer and a thin transparent membrane that loosely surrounds the spinal cord. It also extends up to the lower border of S2 vertebra.
3. *Pia mater* (loving mother in Latin): It is the innermost layer and a thin vascular membrane that closely invests the spinal cord.

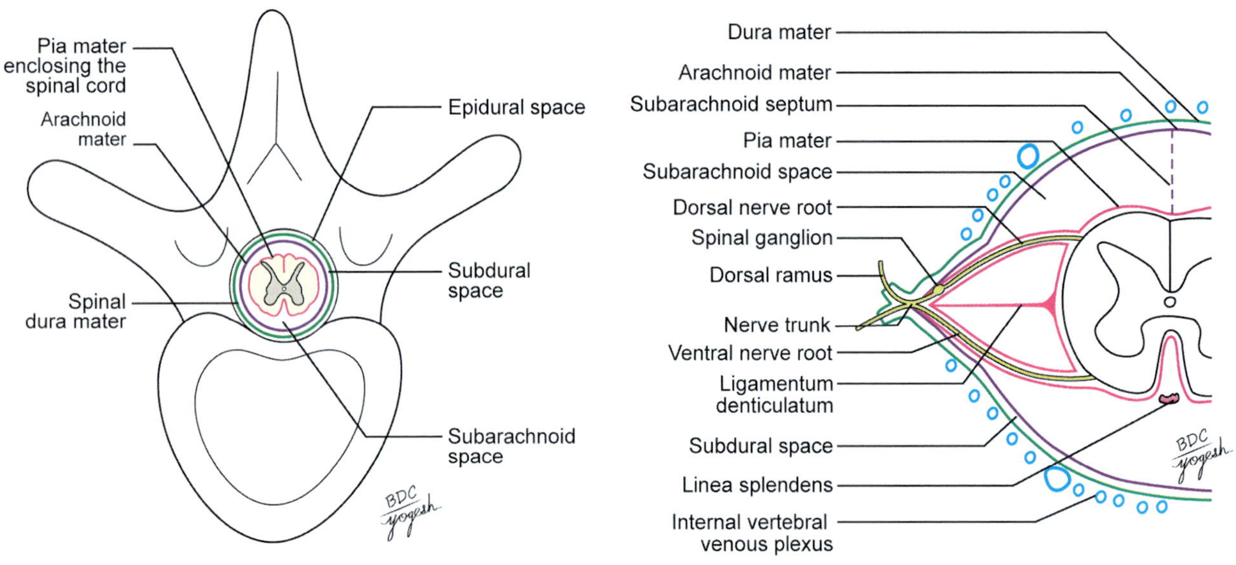

Fig. 5.1: Spinal cord with its meninges

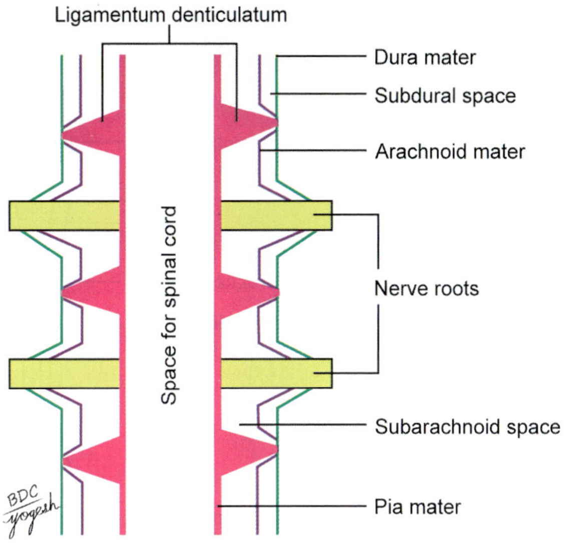

Fig. 5.2: Ligamentum denticulatum and its relationship to the dura mater and to the arachnoid mater

Modifications of Pia Mater

The spinal pia mater undergoes **modification** as follows to keep the spinal cord in position during the movements of the vertebral column.

1. ***Ligamenta denticulata:*** They are 21 pairs of teeth-like projections. They fuse laterally with the arachnoid and dura maters midway between the exits of the roots of adjacent spinal nerves. The highest process attaches immediately superior to foramen magnum. The ligamentum denticulatum keeps the spinal cord in position.
2. ***Filum terminale:*** Below the level of conus medullaris, only pia mater is continued as a thin fibrous cord, the ***filum terminale***. It is 20 cm long and after leaving through sacral hiatus ends by getting attached to the periosteum of dorsal surface of first segment of coccyx. It consists of two parts:
   a. *Filum terminale internum*, the upper part which is 15 cm long which extends up to lower border of second sacral vertebra.
   b. *Filum terminale externum*, the lower part which is outside the dura mater and is attached to the first segment of the coccyx.

   Note: Between the lower border of L1 and S2 vertebrae, the subarachnoid space contains spinal nerve roots which constitute the cauda equina. It is due to this feature that lumbar puncture is done below L2 vertebra without any danger to spinal cord.
3. ***Subarachnoid septum:*** It is the midline septum of pia mater which connects the posterior surface of spinal cord with arachnoid mater.
4. ***Linea splendens:*** It is a thickening seen at the anteromedian sulcus in the lower part of the spinal cord.

Spaces Surrounding the Spinal Cord

1. ***Epidural space:*** The spinal cord is enclosed only by the meningeal layer of dura mater. The space between the meningeal layer and endosteum of the vertebral canal is called *epidural space*, where epidural anaesthesia can be given. The epidural space is filled with adipose tissue, and it contains a network of blood vessels.
2. ***Subdural space:*** The space between dura mater and arachnoid mater is called *subdural space*. The arachnoid and pia maters are separated by subarachnoid space which contains cerebrospinal fluid.
3. ***Subarachnoid space:*** It is the space between arachnoid mater and pia mater. It is filled with cerebrospinal fluid (CSF).

   Note: The dura and arachnoid along with subarachnoid space containing CSF extend up to 2nd sacral vertebra.
4. ***Lumbar cistern:*** In the lower part of the vertebral column below the lower end of spinal cord, the subarachnoid space forms a pool of CSF. It is called lumbar cistern.

CLINICAL NEUROANATOMY

- ***Epidural anaesthesia***: In this, anaesthetic agent is injected in the epidural space to block the pain in a particular region of the body, that is, to anesthetise a particular part. It is useful for lower extremity, gynaecological surgeries, caesarean section, and so on (Fig. 5.3).
- In ***lumbar puncture*** or spinal tap a needle is introduced to withdraw cerebrospinal fluid from the subarachnoid space, usually from the lumbar region of the spine (Fig. 5.4).

  The lumbar puncture in a child is done at a lower level—L4 vertebra as spinal cord extends till L3 vertebra at birth. As it ascends till level of L1 vertebra in adult, lumbar puncture is done at level of L3 vertebra to prevent injury to spinal cord.

  Indications: Lumbar puncture is performed to collect CSF for diagnostic purpose in meningitis, subarachnoid haemorrhage, and other neurological disorders or for therapeutic purpose to reduce raised intracranial pressure.

  Contraindications: It should be avoided in the following conditions:
  – Infection at the site of lumbar puncture
  – Cases with signs of increased intracranial pressure
  – Severe thrombocytopenia or other bleeding disorders.

  Position of a patient: Patient lying down on one side (or sitting) with fully flexed spine. It will raise the lower level of spinal cord.
- ***Ligamentum denticulatum – surgical guide***: In cordotomy surgery: A part of spinal cord behind the ligamentum denticulatum is sectioned to relive pain. A part of spinal cord anterior to ligamentum denticulatum is sectioned to paralyze muscles. The 1st lumbar nerve lies just below the last pair of ligamentum denticulatum. It helps for identification of desired spinal nerves.

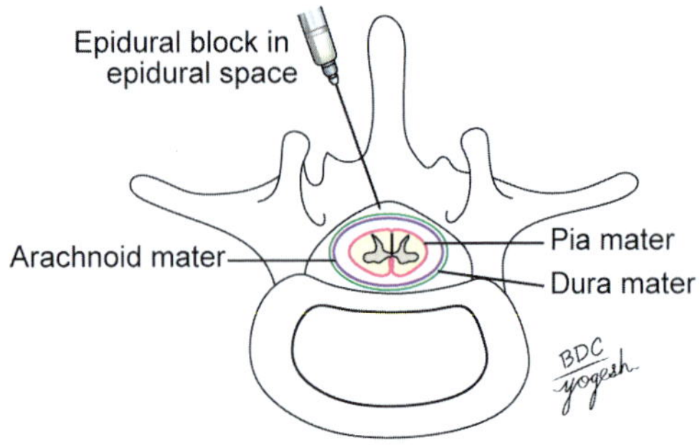

Fig. 5.3: Lumbar epidural anaesthesia

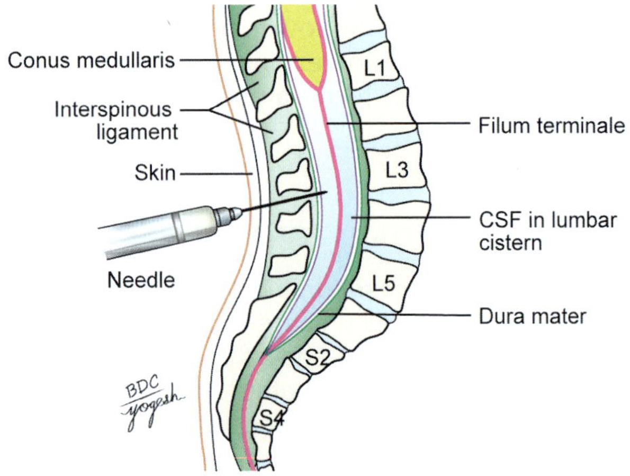

Fig. 5.4: Lumbar puncture in an adult

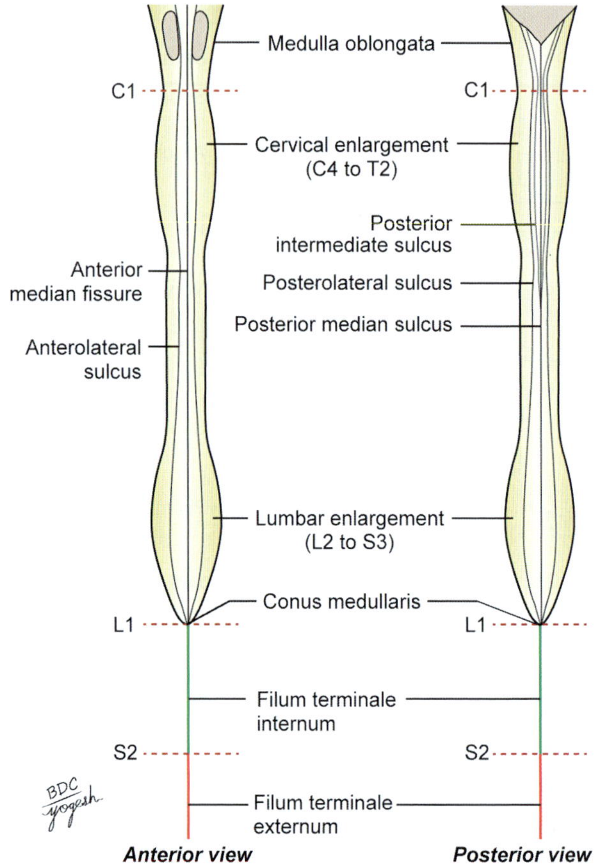

Fig. 5.5: Extent and external features of the spinal cord

Competency:
AN57.1 Identify external features of spinal cord.

EXTERNAL FEATURES OF SPINAL CORD

The external features of spinal cord include (Fig. 5.5):
1. Fissures and sulci
2. Attachments of spinal nerves
3. Enlargements
4. Cauda equina.

Fissures and Sulci

The spinal cord is flat anteroposteriorly. The spinal cord shows the following sulci and fissures:
1. *Anterior median fissure* is a deep groove in the midline anteriorly. It is lined by pia mater. It contains anterior spinal artery.
2. *Posterior median sulcus* is a shallow midline sulcus posteriorly. From it, a septum of neurological tissue (*posterior median septum*) extends into the substance of the spinal cord to a variable extent.
3. *Ventrolateral* (*anterolateral*) *sulcus* is indistinct. The ventral rootlets of the spinal nerve emerge at this sulcus.
4. *Dorsolateral* (*posterolateral*) *sulcus* lies on each side, at about 2 mm from the posterior median sulcus. It corresponds to the attachment of dorsal roots of spinal nerve.
5. *Dorsointermediate* (*posterointermediate*) *sulcus* lies between the posterior median and posterolateral sulcus. It is present only in cervical and upper thoracic levels.

Attachment of Spinal Nerve and Spinal Segments

The 31 pairs of spinal nerves are attached to the spinal cord. These include 8 cervical, 12 thoracic, 5 lumbar, 5 sacral, and 1 coccygeal pairs of nerves (Plate 5.1).

Each spinal nerve is attached to the spinal cord by 2 roots: Ventral and dorsal nerve roots.
- *Ventral* or *anterior motor root* carries motor or efferent fibres from the spinal cord.
- *Dorsal* or *posterior sensory root* carries sensory or afferent fibres. It shows an oval swelling called *dorsal root ganglion*. This ganglion contains pseudounipolar neurons. Their fibres divide in T-shaped manner and give rise to:
  a. Central processes that enter the spinal cord
  b. Peripheral processes that join the ventral root to form a spinal nerve.

Note: As the spinal cord is much shorter than the length of the vertebral column, the spinal segments do not lie opposite the corresponding vertebrae. In estimating the position of a spinal segment in relation to the surface of the body, it is important to remember that a vertebral spine is always lower than the corresponding spinal segment (Table 5.1).

Note: During the third month of embryonic development, the spinal cord extends the entire length of the vertebral canal and both grow

Brain–Neuroanatomy 5

Plate 5.1: Spinal cord with attachment of nerve roots on right side

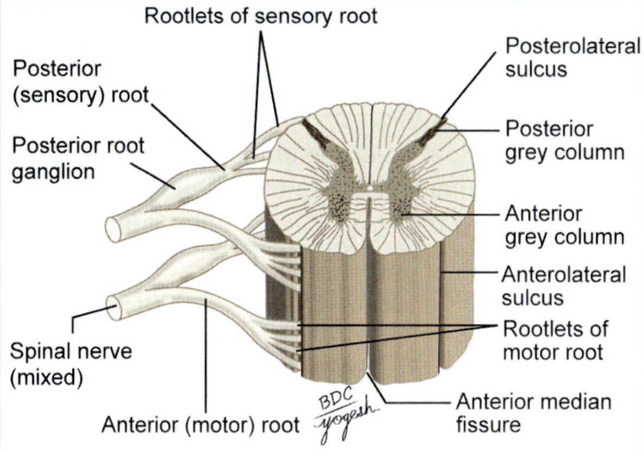

TABLE 5.1: Vertebral level of spinal cord segments

Spinal segment	*Vertebral level*
C1, C2	Same level
C3 to C6	One vertebra above
C7, C8, T1 to T5	Two vertebrae above
T6 to T10	Three vertebrae above
T11, T12	Three to five vertebrae above
L1, L2	At T10 vertebra
L3, L4	At T11 vertebra
L5	At T12 vertebra
Sacral and coccygeal segments	At L1 vertebra

Note: These are approximate levels.

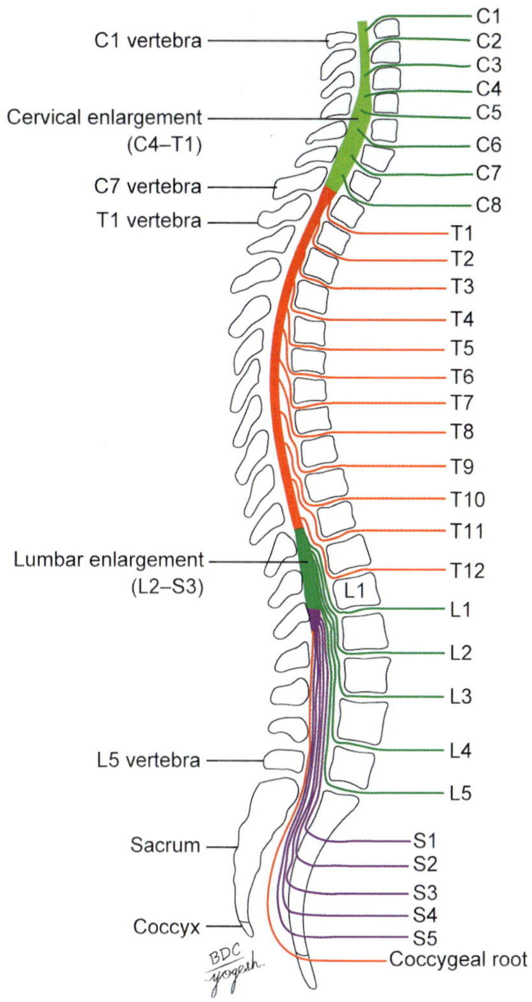

Fig. 5.6: The spinal cord with 31 pairs of spinal nerves

at about the same rate. As development continues, the body and the vertebral column continue to grow at a much greater rate than the spinal cord proper. The outcome of this uneven growth is that the adult spinal cord extends to the level of the first or second lumbar vertebrae, and the nerves grow to exit through the same intervertebral foramina as they did during embryonic development. This growth of the nerve roots occurring within the vertebral canal, results in the lumbar, sacral, and coccygeal roots extending to their appropriate vertebral levels.

Spinal Nerves

Each spinal nerve arises by a series of six to eight dorsal and ventral nerve rootlets. These rootlets unite in or near the intervertebral foramen to form the spinal nerve (Fig. 5.6).

Dorsal root ganglion: As the dorsal rootlets converge, there is a swelling, the dorsal or posterior root ganglion, which houses the cell bodies of all the sensory neurons in that particular nerve. The neurons are pseudounipolar type.

Branches

1. *Dorsal ramus:* It supplies the dorsal one-third of the body wall. Dorsal rami do not supply the limbs.
2. *Ventral ramus:* It supplies the ventral two-thirds of the body wall *including the limbs.*

Enlargements

Limbs form the appendages of the trunk. Their muscles have to be supplied by neurons of spinal cord. Neurons at appropriate levels form enlargements to be able to supply increased musculature. It presents:

a. ***Cervical enlargement*** for supply of upper limb muscles. This extends from C3 to T2 spinal segments with maximum diameter of 38 mm at level of C6 segment (Fig. 5.6, Table 5.2) (*Reference*: Gray's Anatomy, 42nd Edn.).
b. ***Lumbar enlargement*** for supply of muscles of lower limb. It extends from the level of L1 to S3 segments (*Reference*: Gray's Anatomy, 42nd Edn.). Its maximum diameter is 35 mm at the level of S1 segment.

TABLE 5.2: Enlargement of spinal cord

Feature	*Cervical enlargement*	*Lumbar enlargement*
Extent	From C3–T2 spinal segments	From L1 to S3 spinal segments
Maximum diameter and its location	3.8 cm at C6 spinal segment	3.5 cm at T12 vertebral level
Function	Innervation of upper limb	Innervation of lower limb

Cauda Equina

Dorsal and ventral nerve roots of right and left sides of L2 to L5, S1 to S5 and Co1 nerves lie almost vertically around filum terminale. These are called cauda equina as these resemble a horse's tail.

The dorsal and ventral nerve roots of one segment join together at respective intervertebral foramen to exit as the spinal nerve (Fig. 5.7).

Note: There are 40 nerve roots at the beginning of cauda equina. These are dorsal and ventral nerve roots of right and left sides for each segment. So each segment has 4 nerve roots. Thus, there are 4 × 4 = 16 lumbar nerve roots; 4 × 5 = 20 sacral nerve roots; and 4 × 1 = 4 coccygeal nerve roots, making it to 40 nerve roots. One dorsal root and one ventral root joins to form one spinal nerve and leaves through the foramen on one side. So at every intervertebral foramen, 4 nerve roots exit the cauda equina; leaving it thinner. At the end, only filum terminale remains to be attached to the coccyx.

CLINICAL NEUROANATOMY

Conus medullaris syndrome: Due to injury to S2–S4 segments of spinal cord. Features are:

a. Anaesthesia in the perineum. The region is supplied by these three segments.
b. Involvement of bladder and bowel is early as S2–S4 segments carry sacral component of the parasympathetic system which supplies the bladder and lower bowel.
c. Sexual functions are affected as same nerves carry out sexual functions as well.

Cauda equina syndrome: Damage to cauda equina results in:

1. Lower motor neuron paralysis of lower limbs
2. Loss of tendon reflexes of lower limb
3. Severe root pain
4. Saddle-shaped anaesthesia
5. Sexual dysfunction
6. Late involvement of urinary bladder.

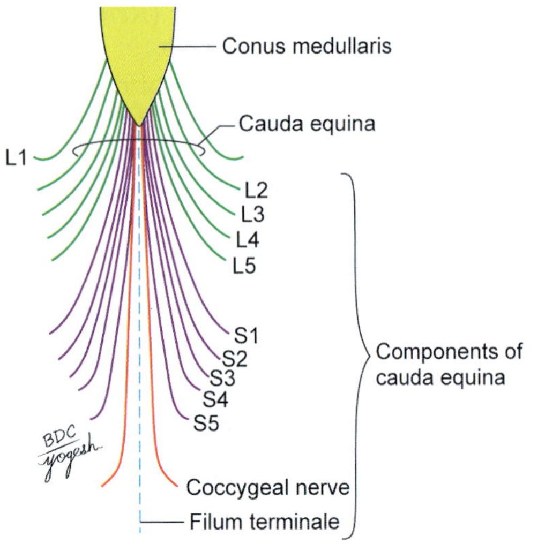

Fig. 5.7: Cauda equina

DISSECTION

Study the spinal cord after it was removed from vertebral canal (*see* Chapter 11, *BD Chaurasia's Human Anatomy, Volume 3*) and separated from the dura mater and arachnoid mater. Identify the dorsal root by the presence of dorsal root ganglion or spinal ganglion. Note the position of cervical enlargement in the upper part and lumbosacral enlargement in the lower part. See the numerous nerve roots surrounding the filum terminale forming the cauda equina.

Cut transverse sections of spinal cord at cervical, thoracic, lumbar, and sacral regions to note the shape and size of the horns in relation to white matter.

INTERNAL STRUCTURE OF SPINAL CORD

Spinal cord consists of (Fig. 5.8):

1. Central grey matter
2. Peripheral white matter
3. Central canal containing CSF. The canal is lined by single layer of ependymal cells.

GREY MATTER OF SPINAL CORD

The grey matter is in the form of 'H' with a grey commissure joining the grey matter of right and left sides.

Grey matter comprises one ***posterior horn*** and one ***anterior horn*** on each side in the entire extent of the cord. Only in T1–L2 and S2–S4 segments, there is an additional ***lateral horn*** for the supply of the viscera. This horn is a part of the autonomic nervous system.

The dorsal horn is found at all spinal cord levels and is comprised of sensory neurons that receive and process incoming somatosensory information. From there, ascending projections emerge to transmit the sensory information to the diencephalon.

The ventral horn comprises *motor neurons* that innervate skeletal muscle. Nerve cells in the grey substance are multipolar, varying much in their morphology.

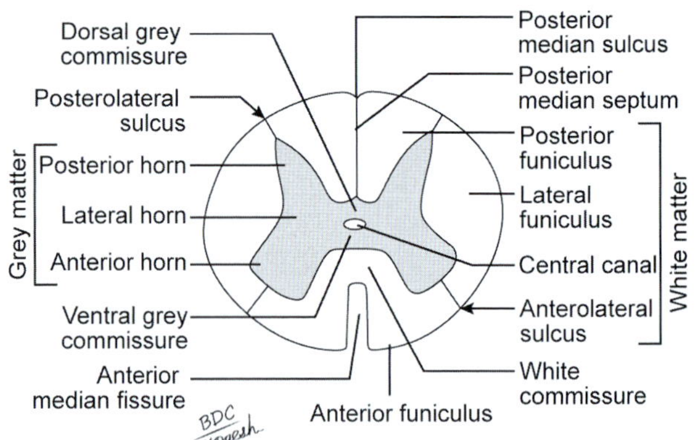

Fig. 5.8: Transverse section of the spinal cord

Structure of Grey Matter

The neurons of grey matter of spinal cord are multipolar and can be grouped functionally as motor neurons, interneurons, and sensory neurons.

Motor Neurons

These are present in anterior and lateral horns. These are of two types: Alpha and gamma neurons.

a. *Alpha neurons*: These are large cells (25 µm or more in diameter). They supply the extrafusal fibres of skeletal muscle.
b. *Gamma neurons*: These are small multipolar neurons (15–25 µm in diameter). They supply the intrafusal fibres of muscle spinal.

Sensory neurons are present in posterior horn. These are small neurons. They receive inputs from the neurons of dorsal root ganglion. Their axons form ascending or intersegmental tracts.

Interneurons (internuncial neurons) are small associated neurons. They connect different type of neurons.

Note: Many of the neurons of the spinal grey matter are Golgi type I and Golgi type II nerve cells. The axons of ***Golgi type I*** are long and pass out of the grey matter into the ventral spinal roots or the fibre tracts of the white matter. The axons and dendrites of the ***Golgi type II*** cells are largely confined to the neighbouring neurons in the grey matter. ***Renshaw cells*** are Golgi type II neurons and located in the anterior horn.

Shape and size of the horns differ in different segments due to functional reasons (Fig. 5.9) and shown in Table 5.3.

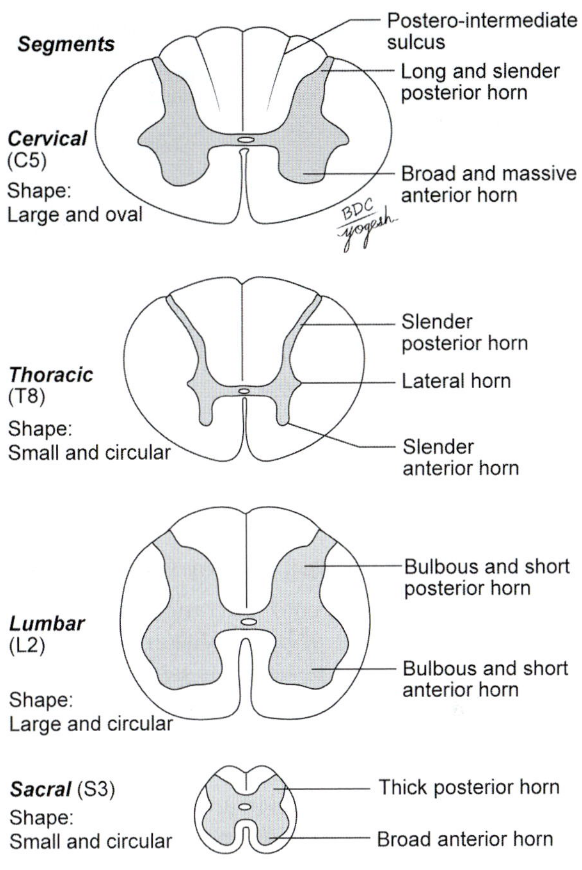

Fig. 5.9: Features of spinal cord at various levels

CLINICAL NEUROANATOMY

- ***Poliomyelitis:*** It is a viral disease which involves anterior horn cells leading to flaccid paralysis of the affected segments. It is a lower motor neuron paralysis (Figs 5.10 and 5.11). Virus passes from the digestive system to neurons via axonal transport. If poliomyelitis affects the upper cervical segments of spinal cord, it may be fatal because of the involvement of C4 segment which supplies the diaphragm through phrenic nerve.
- ***Tabes dorsalis*** (Fig. 5.11): It occurs during tertiary stage of syphilis. There is degenerative lesions of dorsal nerve roots and of posterior white columns. Its feature is severe pain in lower limbs, as the disease occurs in lower thoracic and lumbosacral segments. The lower limbs are mainly affected.

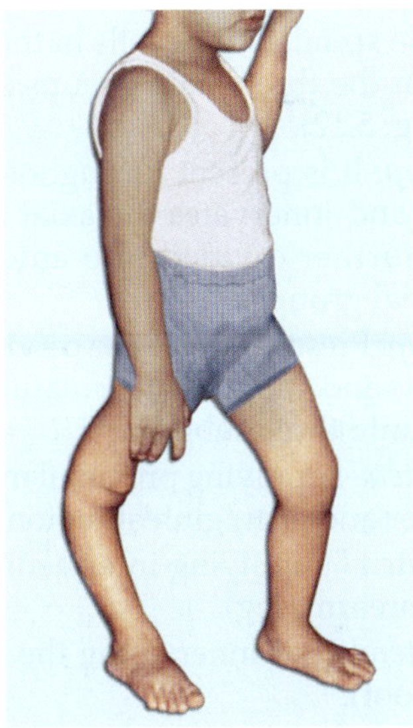

Fig. 5.10: Poliomyelitis of right lower limb

TABLE 5.3: Shape of horns in different segments of spinal cord

Segments of spinal cord	*Posterior horn*	*Lateral horn*	*Anterior horn*
Cervical, oval shape (Fig. 3.4)	Slender	Absent	Narrow in 1–3 segments Broad in C4 to C8 segments for supply of upper limbs
Thoracic, circular shape	Slender	Present for thoracolumbar outflow	Slender in T2–T12 segments, broad in T1 segment
Lumbar, circular shape	Bulbous	Present only in lumbar 1 and 2 segments	Bulbous for supply of lower limbs
Sacral, circular but smaller	Thick	Group of cells in sacral 2–4 segments for sacral outflow	Bulbous for supply of lower limbs

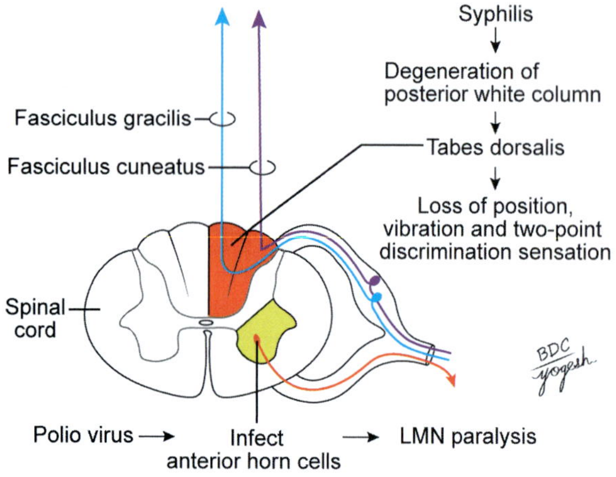

Fig. 5.11: Tabes dorsalis and poliomyelitis

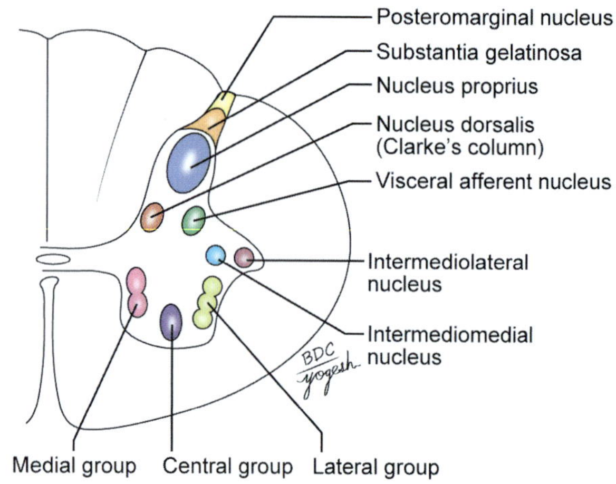

Fig. 5.12: Cell groups in spinal cord

Nerve Cell Groups (Nuclei) of Grey Columns

The grey matter of spinal cord is arranged in three horns. Anterior is motor, lateral being visceral efferent and afferent in function, and posterior is sensory in function.

Nuclei in Anterior Grey Column or Horn

The anterior horn is divided into a ventral part, head and a dorsal part, base. The nuclei in anterior horn innervate the skeletal muscles. Most prominent neurons are alpha neurons. Their axons leave the spinal cord through ventral nerve roots to innervate skeletal muscles. Smaller neurons are gamma neurons. These supply intrafusal fibres of muscle spindles. The cells in the anterior horn are arranged in the three main groups: medial, lateral and central (Fig. 5.12).

1. ***Medial group:*** It is present throughout the extent of spinal cord and innervates the axial muscles of the body. It is further divided into anteromedial and posteromedial groups:
2. ***Lateral group:*** Present only in the cervical and lumbar enlargements and supplies musculature of limbs. It is subdivided into three subgroups.
   a. *Anterolateral* supplying proximal muscles of limbs (shoulder and arm/gluteal region and thigh).
   b. *Posterolateral* supplying intermediate muscles of limbs (forearm/leg).
   c. *Post-posterolateral* innervating the distal segment (hand/foot).
3. ***Central group:*** Only in upper cervical segments as phrenic nerve nucleus and nucleus of spinal root of accessory nerve.

Nuclei in Lateral Grey Column or Horn

Nuclei in lateral horn are as follows (Fig. 5.12):

1. ***Intermediolateral nucleus:*** This acts as both efferent and afferent nuclear columns. This nucleus is seen at two levels.
   a. From T1 to L2 segments—giving rise to preganglionic sympathetic fibres (thoracolumbar outflow).
   b. From S2 to S4 segments—giving rise to preganglionic parasympathetic fibres chiefly for the pelvic viscera.

   At these two levels, the intermediolateral cell column receives visceral afferent fibres.
2. ***Intermediomedial nucleus:*** This is mostly internuncial neuronal column.

Nuclei in Posterior Grey Column or Horn

The four main afferent nuclei are seen in this are (Fig. 5.12):

1. ***Posteromarginal nucleus:*** Thin layer of neurons caps the posterior horn. It receives some of incoming dorsal root fibres.
2. ***Substantia gelatinosa:*** This is found at the tip of posterior horn through the entire extent of spinal cord. Here first order neurons of lateral spinothalamic tract synapse.
3. ***Nucleus proprius:*** It lies subjacent to the substantia gelatinosa throughout the entire extent of cord. 1–3 groups of nuclei are present in laminae I–IV. It is concerned with sensory associative mechanism. The axons originating project to the thalamus via the anterior spinothalamic tract and to the cerebellum via ventral spinocerebellar tract.
4. ***Nucleus dorsalis of Clarke*** also known as thoracic nucleus at the medial part of base of posterior horn extending from C8 to L3 segments. These are situated in laminae V and VI. It contains interneurons.

Laminar Organisation in Spinal Cord

In thick sections, spinal cord neurons appear to have a laminar (layered) arrangement. Ten layers of neurons are recognised, also known as ***laminae of Rexed*** (Table 5.4). These are numbered consecutively by Roman numerals, starting at the tip of the dorsal horn and moving ventrally into ventral horn (Fig. 5.13).

Laminae I to IV, in general, are concerned with exteroceptive sensation and comprise the dorsal horn, whereas laminae V and VI are concerned primarily with proprioceptive sensations. Lamina VII is equivalent to the intermediate zone and acts as a relay between muscle spindle to midbrain and cerebellum, and laminae VIII–IX comprise the ventral horn and contain mainly motor neurons. The axons of these neurons innervate mainly skeletal muscle. Lamina X surrounds the central canal and contains neuroglia.

TABLE 5.4: Rexed laminae

Lamina	*Corresponding grey column*
I	Posteromarginal nucleus
II	Substantia gelatinosa
III	Nucleus proprius
IV	Nucleus proprius
V VI	Base of dorsal horn
VII	Nucleus dorsalis Lateral horn (intermediolateral, intermediomedial nuclei)
VIII	Anterior horn of thoracic region Medial group of anterior horn in cervical and lumbosacral region
IX	Lateral group of nuclei of anterior horn
X	Surrounds the central canal

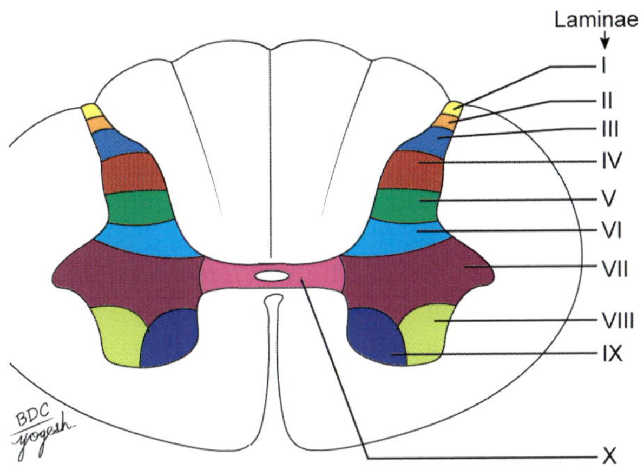

Fig. 5.13: Various laminae in spinal cord

WHITE MATTER OF SPINAL CORD

The white matter of the spinal cord surrounds the grey matter. It appears white due to presence of myelinated nerve fibres.

Divisions of White Matter

The white matter of spinal cord is divided into right and left halves by *anterior median fissure* and *posterior median septum*. Each of the spinal cord shows three column or fasiculi of white matter:

1. *Anterior (ventral) white column (funiculus)* lies between anterior median fissure and the lateralmost fibres of ventral root of spinal nerve.
2. *Lateral white column (funiculus)* lies between the lateralmost fibres of ventral root and posterolateral sulcus.
3. *Posterior or dorsal column (funiculus)* lies between posterior median sulcus and posterolateral sulcus.

Types of Fibres in White Matter

The white matter of spinal contains three types of fibres:

1. *Sensory fibres* include central processes of pseudo-unipolar neurons of dorsal root ganglion and axons of dorsal horn cells that forms ascending tracts.
2. *Motor neurons* include descending fibres from higher centres to the spinal cord and axon of anterior horn cells.
3. *Association fibres* include the fibres that originate and terminate within the spinal cord.

TRACTS OF THE SPINAL CORD

A collection of nerve fibres that connects two masses of grey matter within the central nervous system is called a tract. They are usually named after the masses of grey matter connected by them. Some tracts are called fasciculi or lemnisci.

Classification of Tracts

The tracts of spinal cord are classified into three types (Fig. 5.14):

1. Ascending
2. Descending
3. Intersegmental.

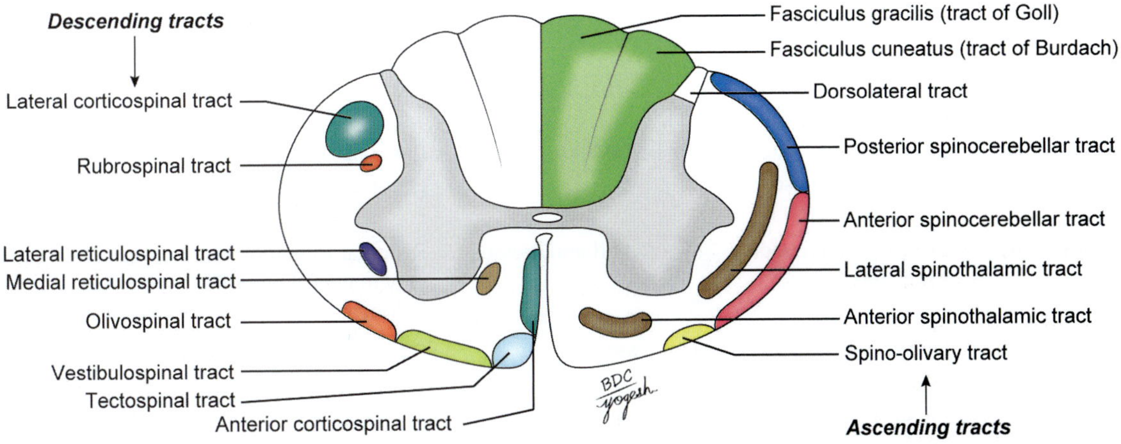

Fig. 5.14: Main descending (motor) tracts in the left half and ascending (sensory) tracts in the right half (transverse section of the spinal cord at mid-cervical region)

Locations of Tracts in Spinal Cord

The tracts are located in the white matter of the spinal cord as follows:

Anterior white column:

- *Ascending tracts*: Anterior spinothalamic
- *Descending tracts*: Anterior corticospinal, vestibulospinal, tectospinal, medial rubrospinal.

Lateral white column:

- *Ascending tracts*: Lateral spinothalamic, anterior spinocerebellar, posterior spinocerebellar, spinotectal.
- *Descending*: Lateral corticospinal, rubrospinal, lateral reticulospinal, hypothalamospinal.

Posterior white column:

Ascending tracts (only): Tract of Goll (fasciculus gracilis), tract of Burdach (fasciculus cuneatus).

Competencies:

AN57.3 Draw and label transverse section of spinal cord at midcervical and midthoracic level.

AN57.4 Enumerate ascending and descending tracts at mid thoracic level of spinal cord.

DESCENDING TRACTS

The descending tracts are of two types: Pyramidal and extrapyramidal (Table 5.5).

Pyramidal or Corticospinal Tracts

Components

It consists of two fibres:

1. *Corticospinal fibres* that terminate at the anterior horn cells of spinal cord.
2. *Corticonuclear fibres* that terminate at the motor nuclei of cranial nerves in the brainstem.

Composition

Pyramidal tract consists of two neurons: Upper and lower (Fig. 5.15). The upper motor neurons are located in motor area (area 4) and premotor area (area 6) of the cerebral cortex. *Motor area* lies in front of central sulcus (precentral gyrus). This area contains giant *pyramidal cells*.

Note: Body is represented upside down in the motor cortex. Leg area is situated uppermost extending on to the medial surface of paracentral lobule. The leg area is followed by thigh, trunk, upper limb, face larynx, lips, jaw, tongue, and pharynx area.

Pathway (Fig. 5.15)

Upper motor neurons

1. The fibres of pyramidal tract originate from the large *pyramidal cells* (UMN) of the motor area.
2. Their axons run in a fan-shaped manner as *corona radiata*. Then these fibres converge and pass through the genu and posterior limb of *internal capsule*.
3. *In midbrain*: Then these fibres pass through the middle three-fifths of the *crus cerebri of midbrain*.

TABLE 5.5: The descending tracts

Name	*Function*	*Crossed and uncrossed*	*Beginning*	*Termination*
Pyramidal tracts				
Lateral corticospinal	Main motor tract for skillful voluntary movements	Crosses in medulla	Motor area of cortex (areas 4, 6)	Anterior grey column cells (alpha motor neurons)
Anterior corticospinal	Facilitates flexors	Crosses in corresponding spinal segment	Motor area of cortex (areas 4, 6)	Anterior grey column cells (alpha motor neurons)
Extrapyramidal tracts				
Tectospinal	Efferent pathway for visual reflexes	Crossed	Superior colliculus	Alpha and gamma motor neurons of anterior grey column cells
Rubrospinal	Efferent pathway for cerebellum and corpus striatum	Crossed	Red nucleus of midbrain	Alpha and gamma motor neurons of anterior grey column cells
Medial reticulospinal	Extrapyramidal tract Facilitates extensors	Uncrossed	Reticular formation of grey matter of pons	Alpha and gamma motor neurons of anterior grey column cells
Lateral reticulospinal	Extrapyramidal tract Facilitates flexors	Uncrossed and crossed	Reticular formation of grey matter of medulla oblongata	Alpha and gamma motor neurons of anterior grey column cells
Lateral vestibulospinal	Efferent pathway for equilibratory control	Uncrossed	Lateral vestibular nucleus	Alpha and gamma motor neurons of anterior grey column cells
Olivospinal	Extrapyramidal tract	Uncrossed	Inferior olivary nucleus	Alpha and gamma motor neurons of anterior grey column cells

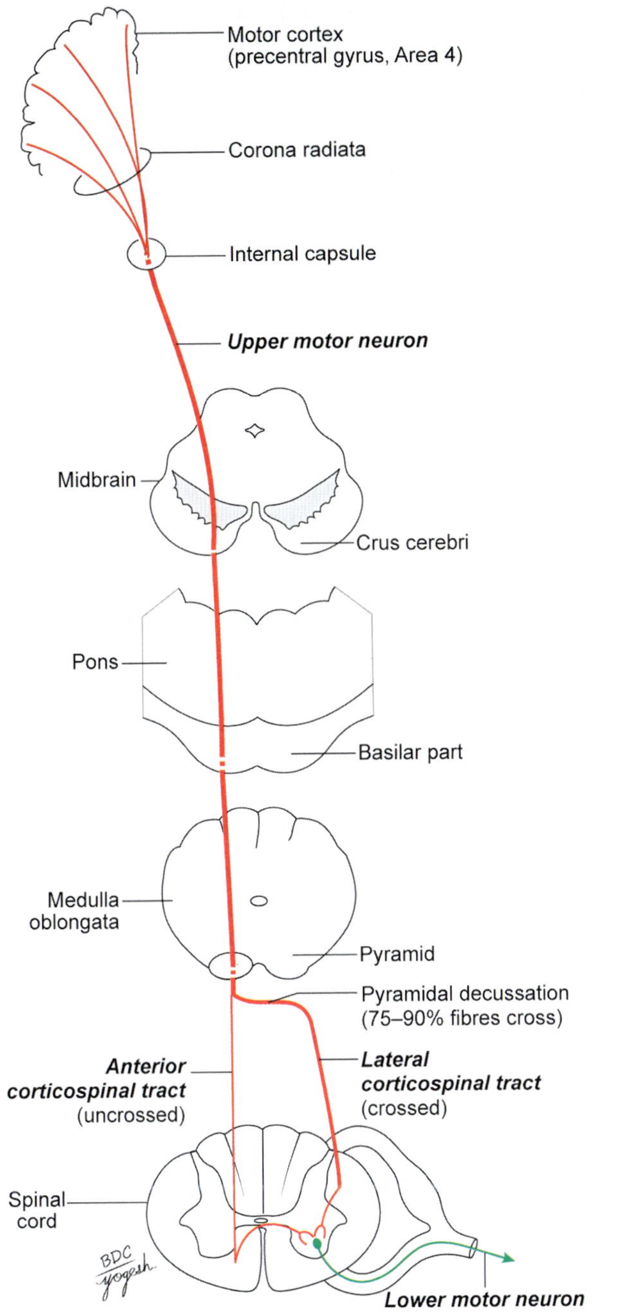

Fig. 5.15: Pyramidal/corticospinal tracts—course of corticospinal fibres

4. *In pons*: These fibres are broken up into number of small bundles by pontine nuclei and transversely running *pontocerebellar fibres* in the basilar part of the pons.
5. *In medulla oblongata*: These fibres converge to form a compact bundle that descends as *pyramid* on each side of the midline. In the lower part of the medulla oblongata, majority of the fibres (75–90%) cross to the opposite side in the *pyramidal decussation* and descends as ***lateral corticospinal* (crossed tract) tract**. Remaining fibres continue as ***ventral corticospinal tract*** [*Reference*: *Grey's Anatomy, 42nd edn*].
6. *In spinal cord*: The lateral corticospinal tract runs in the lateral white column and terminates on the anterior horn cells through interneurons. The ventral corticospinal tract runs in the anterior white column. Its fibres cross to the opposite side in the anterior white commissure of the spinal cord at the level of their termination.

Lower motor neurons

They lie in the *anterior horn of spinal cord*. They receive the impulse from upper motor neurons through interneurons (only 5% upper motor neurons end directly on the lower motor neuron). Axons of lower motor neurons reach the skeletal muscle through the *anterior root of spinal nerves*. They produce contraction of skeletal muscles.

Functional Significance

1. The cerebral cortex controls gross and fine skilled voluntary movements of opposite half of body through anterior horn cells.
2. Influence of this tract is supposed to be facilitatory for flexors and inhibitory for extensors.
3. Anterior corticospinal tract controls voluntary gross movement like walking and running.
4. Corticospinal tract facilitates superficial reflexes and muslce tone.
5. Actions of basal ganglia and cerebellum are mediated by corticospinal tracts.

Extrapyramidal Tracts

These are (Figs 5.16 and 5.17, Table 5.5):

1. Rubrospinal tract
2. Medial reticulospinal tract
3. Lateral reticulospinal tract
4. Olivospinal tract
5. Vestibulospinal tract
6. Tectospinal tract.

Note: The extrapyramidal fibres arise from cortical and subcortical area influence the activity at the anterior horn cell (lower motor neurons). The fibres from cortical centres form synapse with subcortical centre which later send fibres to the spinal cord.

Extrapyramidal pathway: Cortical centres → subcortical centres → spinal cord

Phylogenetically, extrapyramidal system is older than pyramidal system. Extrapyramidal pathway is polysynaptic.

Tectospinal tract (Fig. 5.17): The tract is formed by the axons of neurons lying in the superior colliculus of the midbrain. The fibres cross to the opposite side thus forming *dorsal tegmental decussation* in midbrain. The tract descends through pons, medulla and anterior white column of spinal cord. The fibres terminate on the cells of anterior horn through internuncial neurons. It mediates reflex movements of head and neck in response to visual stimulus.

All these descending tracts control the voluntary movements of skeletal muscles of the body through anterior horn cells directly or through internuncial neurons. The influence is on both alpha and gamma neurons. Gamma neurons also affect alpha neurons through muscle spindles. So, all influences finally reach alpha neurons.

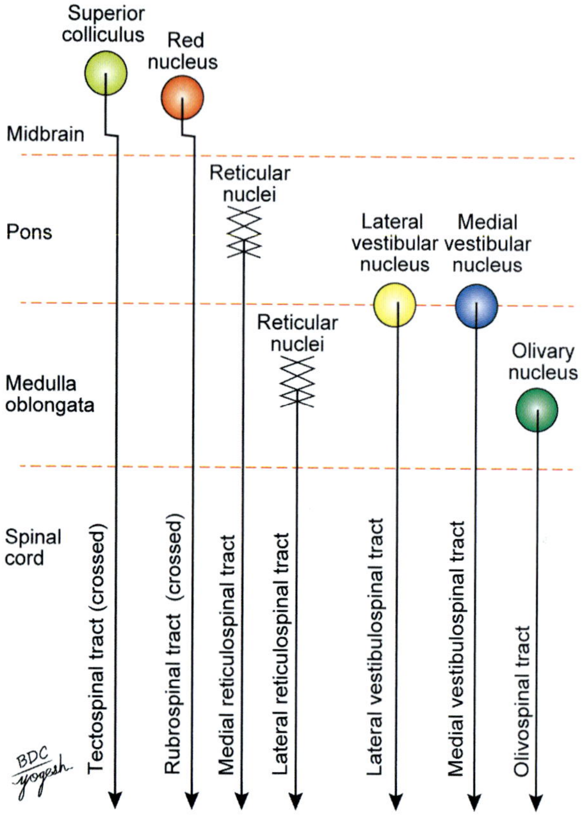

Fig. 5.16: Extrapyramidal tracts

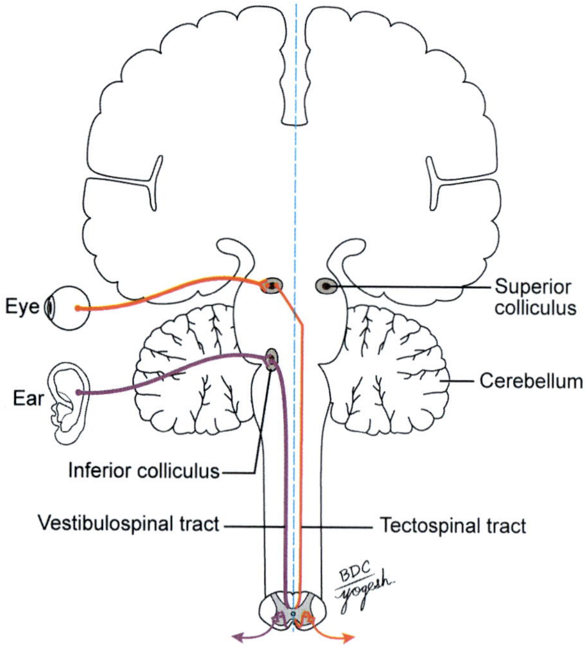

Fig. 5.17: Tectospinal and vestibulospinal tracts

Rubrospinal tract: This tract is formed by the axons of red nucleus, situated in the midbrain. The fibres cross with the fibres of the opposite side in the tegmentum of midbrain; thus constituting the *ventral tegmental decussation*. The tract descends through the pons and medulla oblongata and enters the lateral white column of spinal cord. The fibres terminate by synapsing through internuncial neurons with anterior horn cells (Fig. 5.17). It controls the tone of limb flexor muscles by being excitatory to motor neurons of these muscles.

Medial reticulospinal tract: The medial reticulospinal tract is formed by the fibres from reticular formation in pons and descends to the cervical segments only. It lies in the anterior white column of spinal cord. It has uncrossed fibres (Fig. 5.16). It influences voluntary movement, reflex activity and muscle tone by controlling the activity of both alpha and gamma neurons.

Lateral reticulospinal tract: The lateral reticulospinal tract originates from reticular formation in brainstem (midbrain, pons and medulla oblongata) and descends up to thoracic segments of spinal cord. It has both crossed and uncrossed fibres. It lies in the anterolateral white column of spinal cord. Both the tracts terminate by synapsing with the neurons in lamina VII of the spinal cord.

Vestibulospinal tract (Figs 5.16 and 5.17): The fibres arise from lateral vestibular nucleus lying at pontomedullary junction. The fibres descend uncrossed to spinal cord. This tract is situated in the anterior white column of spinal cord. These fibres synapse with anterior horn cells. It has two types:

a. *Lateral*—controls extensors muscle tone
b. *Medial*—for movement of head.

Olivospinal tract: Its fibres originate from the inferior olivary nucleus in medulla oblongata, descend to spinal cord, lie in the anterolateral column of white matter and synapse with the anterior horn cells. It controls activity of motor neurons in spinal cord.

Pyramidal and extrapyramidal tracts have been compared in Table 5.6.

CLINICAL NEUROANATOMY

Lesions of pyramidal tract: The lesions of pyramidal tract divided into two groups:

1. Lesions of upper motor neuron
2. Lesions of lower motor neuron.

Lesions of upper motor neuron: The lesions cause upper motor neuron paralysis which results into hemiplegia and cranial nerve paralysis based on the location of the lesions as follows:

1. *Lesion of motor cortex and internal capsule*: It results in contralateral hemiplegia and contralateral paralysis of lower face and tongue.
2. *Lesion in midbrain*: It results in contralateral hemiplegia and ipsilateral ocular muscles paralysis supplied by III cranial nerve.
3. *Lesion in pons*: It results in:
   i. Raymond syndrome – contralateral hemiplegia and ipsilateral paralysis of lateral rectus (supplied by cranial nerve VI)
   ii. Millard-Gubler syndrome – crossed facial paralysis
4. *Lesion in medulla oblongata* → crossed hypoglossal paralysis
5. *Lesion in spinal cord* → Brown-Séquard syndrome.

TABLE 5.6: Comparison of pyramidal and extrapyramidal tracts

Pyramidal tracts	*Extrapyramidal tracts*
Recent in evolution	Older in evolution
These comprise only cortico-spinal and corticonuclear tracts	These comprise olivospinal, vestibulospinal, tectospinal, reticulospinal, rubrospinal tracts
Origin from motor cortex	These arise from olivary vestibular, tectum (collicular), reticular and red nuclei
The impulse passes directly to anterior horn cells	Impulse passes by polysynaptic route via cortex, basal ganglia, cerebellum and brainstem
Function is to perform voluntary skilled movement	Control tone and equilibrium. These facilitate/inhibit flexor/extensor reflexes
Injury leads to increased muscle tone and loss of motor activity	Injury leads to increased muscle tone with clasp knife rigidity

Features of upper motor lesions: The lesions of upper motor neurons produce the following effects:

1. *Spastic paralysis*: The lower neurons get hyper stimulated by extrapyramidal fibres after losing control of pyramidal fibres. These hyper stimulated LMN cause hypertonia or spasticity of muscle and exaggerated tendon reflexes.
2. *Positive Babinski sign*: On scratching skin of the foot along the lateral aspect of the sole with a blunt object, the great toe undergoes dorsiflexion and other toes fan outward. This is called positive Babinski's sign.
3. Absence of abdominal and cremasteric reflex.

Lesion of lower motor neurons: It involves:

1. Lesions of motor nuclei of cranial nerve
2. Lesions of anterior horn cells of spinal cord
3. Lesions of ventral root or spinal nerves.

It results in:

1. Flaccid type of muscle paralysis with loss of muscle tone
2. Muscle wasting (atrophy)
3. Loss of all reflexes
4. Absence of Babinski's sign.

- The differences between upper and lower motor neuron paralysis are listed in Table 5.7.

ASCENDING TRACTS

The ascending tracts carry the sensory input to the central nervous system. They carry the following sensations:

1. Pain and temperature sensation
2. Fine touch and conscious proprioception
3. Unconscious proprioception.

The ascending tracts include:

1. Lateral spinothalamic tract
2. Anterior spinothalamic tract
3. Fasciculus gracilis (medially)

TABLE 5.7: Differences between upper and lower motor neuron paralysis

Feature	*UMN lesion*	*LMN lesion*
Lesion	Above the anterior horn cells of spinal cord and cranial nerve nuclei	Lesion of anterior horn cells of spinal cord and cranial nerve nuclei
Paralysis	Spastic paralysis	Flaccid paralysis
Muscle tone	Increased	Decreased
Extent of paralysis	Widespread	Localized
Deep tendon reflexes	Increased	Absent
Superficial reflexes	Absent	Absent
Babinski's sign	Extensor (upgoing toe)	Normal or absent
Muscle wasting	Late	Usually present
Muscle clonus	Present	Absent

4. Fasciculus cuneatus (laterally)
5. Dorsal or posterior spinocerebellar tract
6. Ventral or anterior spinocerebellar tract
7. Spino-olivary tract
8. Spinotectal tract.

General Arrangements of Sensory Pathway

The sensory pathways connect sensory receptors with cerebral cortex. Each sensory pathway consists of multiple neurons which are called first order, second order, and third order neurons.

First order neurons: These are located in dorsal root ganglia of spinal nerves and ganglia of cranial nerves. They are pseudounipolar neurons. These neurons have two processes:

1. Peripheral process that carries signal from receptors.
2. Central process that enters the central nervous system and transfers the signal to the second order neurons.

Second order neurons: They are located within the grey matter of spinal cord and brainstem. Axons of most of the second order neurons cross to opposite side and then ascend upward. Some of the primary order neurons transfer the signals to motor neurons (anterior horn cells) to generate the reflexes.

Third order neurons: They are present in ventral postero-lateral nucleus of thalamus. Their axons transfer the signals to sensory area of the cerebral cortex.

Lateral Spinothalamic Tract

The lateral spinothalamic tract carries *pain and temperature* sensations from opposite side of the body (Fig. 5.18).

Receptors:

For pain: Free nerve endings

For temperature:

- End bulbs of Krause for cold
- End bulbs of Ruffini for warmth.

Location in spinal cord: Lateral white column.

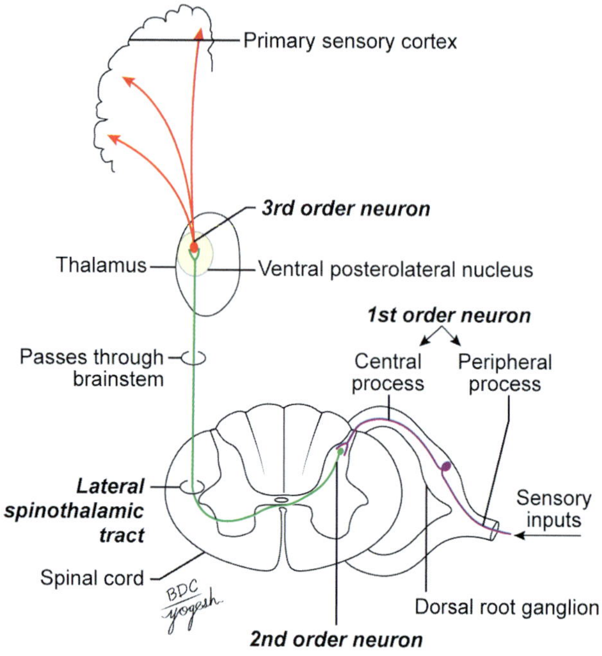

Fig. 5.18: Lateral spinothalamic tract

Composition/Pathway

It consists of three order neurons: First order, second order, and third order neurons.

1. ***First-order neurons:*** These are pseudounipolar neurons of the dorsal root ganglia of spinal cord that has:
   a. *Peripheral processes* that carry pain and temperature sensations through the spinal nerve and its dorsal root.
   b. *Central processes* that enter the spinal cord through the lateral division of dorsal root of spinal nerve.

   These fibres ascend upward for one or two segments as *dorsolateral tract of Lissauer* (at the tip of dorsal horn). They relay in posterior horn by synapsing with neurons of *substantia gelatinosa*.
2. ***Second-order neurons:*** The cells of dorsal horn form the second order neurons. Their axon cross to the opposite side in anterior white commissure and ascends upward in the opposite white column as lateral spinothalamic tract. They ascend as *spinal lemniscus* in brainstem. They terminate in the ventral posterolateral nucleus (VPL) of thalamus.
3. ***Third-order neurons:*** These are neurons of ventral posterolateral nucleus (VPL) of thalamus. Their axons project to the *primary sensory cortex* of the cerebral hemisphere. These fibres pass through the posterior limb of the internal capsule.

Note: In the lateral spinothalamic tract, pain fibres are located anteriorly, while temperature fibres are located posteriorly. The fibres are arranged superficial to deep as sacral, lumbar, thoracic, and cervical. The fibres of lateral spinothalamic tract form *spinal lemniscus* in the brainstem. Pain and perhaps temperature reach consciousness at thalamic level and emotional responses are elicited. Precise source, severity, quantity of pain and temperature stimuli, the cerebral cortex play an important role.

CLINICAL NEUROANATOMY

- *Unilateral lesion of lateral spinothalamic tract* → complete loss of pain and temperature sensations on the opposite side of the body.
- ***Cordotomy*** *for pain relief*: Cordotomy is a surgical procedure. In this procedure lateral spinothalamic tract is severed (incised) to relieve intractable pain.
  Anatomical basis: The fibres carrying pain lie on the lateral side in lateral spinothalamic tract (in lateral white column).
- ***Syringomyelia***: In syringomyelia, crossing fibres of lateral spinothalamic tract are compressed that cause bilateral loss of pain and temperature sensation below the level of lesion.

Anterior Spinothalamic Tract

It carries the following sensations from opposite side of the body (Fig. 5.19):
- Crude touch
- Pressure.

Receptors:
- Hair follicle ending, free nerve ending – for crude touch
- Pacinian corpuscles – for pressure.

Location in spinal cord: Anterior white column.

Composition/Pathway

It consists of three order neurons: First, second, and third.

First order neurons: These are pseudounipolar neurons of the spinal cord that has:

a. *Peripheral processes* that carry the sensation through the spinal nerve and its dorsal root.

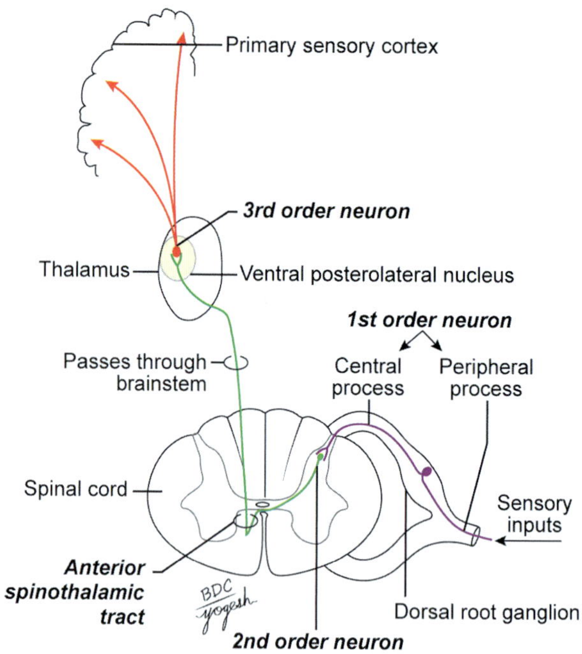

Fig. 5.19: Anterior spinothalamic tract

b. *Central processes* are highly myelinated. They enter the spinal cord through medial division of the dorsal root of spinal nerve. On entering the spinal cord, they ascend one to two segments in a dorsolateral tract of Lissauer. They relay at the cells of substantia gelatinosa.

Second order neurons: They are located in the dorsal horn of spinal cord (in the substantia gelatinosa) their axons cross the midline in the anterior white commissure to reach the contralateral anterior white column. Then they ascend upward as anterior spinothalamic tract just in front of anterior horn. They ascend as *spinal lemniscus* in brainstem. These neurons relay in the ventral posterolateral nucleus (VPL) of the thalamus.

Third order neurons: These are neurons of ventral posterolateral nucleus (VPL) of thalamus. Their axons project to the *primary sensory cortex* of the cerebral hemisphere. These fibres pass through the posterior limb of the internal capsule.

CLINICAL NEUROANATOMY

- *Lesion of anterior spinothalamic tract* → little or no loss of tactile, touch and pressure sensations as these are also transmitted by fasciculus gracilis and cuneatus.
- ***Dissociation anaesthesia***: It indicates the loss of pain and temperature sensations without affecting touch sensation.

  Anatomical basis: In syringomyelia, it affects the second order neurons that cross the midline. They are as follows:
  - Fibres of lateral spinothalamic tract – loss of pain and temperature sensations
  - Fibres of anterior spinothalamic tract – no or little loss of touch sensation as it is carried by uncrossed dorsal white column tract, fasciculus gracilis and cuneatus.

Note: ***Jacket type anaesthesia*** for pain and temperature: In syringomyelia, there is compression of crossing fibres of lateral spinothalamic tract (carry pain and temperature) at the level of lesion. It causes loss of pain and temperature sensations at the level of lesion, but not above and below the lesion. This produces a jacket-type of anaesthesia for pain and temperature.

Tract of Goll and Tract of Burdach

Synonym: Fasciculus gracilis and fasciculus cuneatus (Fig. 5.20).

They carry the following sensations from opposite side of the body:

- Fine touch, two-point discrimination
- Vibration
- *Conscious proprioception*: Joint sense, stereognosis, conscious kinesthesia.

Location: Posterior white column.

Receptors:

- Meissner's corpuscles – for fine touch
- Pacinian corpuscles and free nerve endings – for vibration and proprioception.

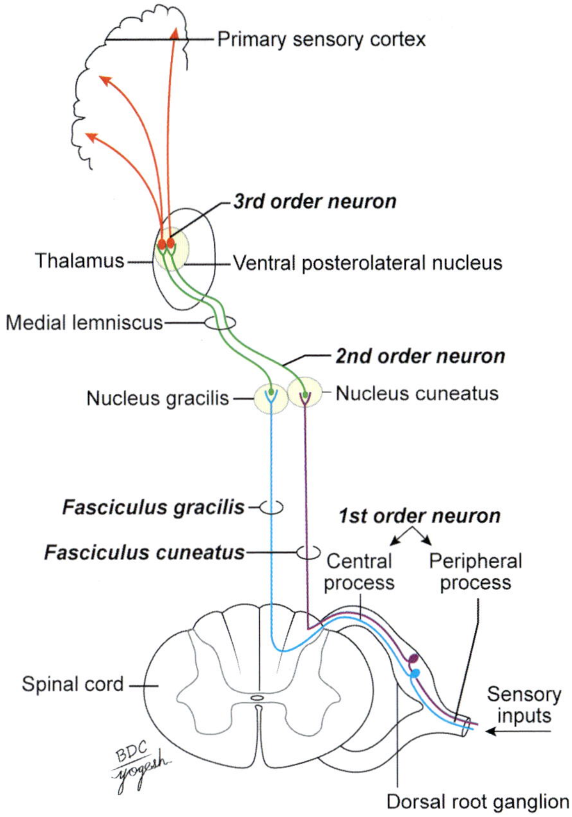

Fig. 5.20: Fasciculus gracillis and fasciculus cuneatus

Composition/Pathway

First order neurons: These are pseudounipolar neurons of the spinal cord that has:

a. *Peripheral processes* that carry the sensation through the spinal nerve and its dorsal root.

b. *Central processes* are thickly myelinated. They enter the spinal cord through median division of the spinal roots of spinal nerves.

Then they ascend upward in the posterior column as follows:

Fasciculus gracilis – fibres from coccygeal, sacral, lumbar, and lower thoracic regions form fasciculus gracilis.

Fasciculus cuneatus – fibres from upper thoracic and cervical regions form fasciculus cuneatus.

Arrangements of fibre lateral to medial: Cervical, thoracic, lumbar, and sacral fibres.

Fasciculus gracilis terminates at the nucleus gracilis and fasciculus cuneatus at the nucleus cuneatus.

Note: Fasciculus gracilis lies medial to the fasciculus cuneatus in the posterior white column. They are separated from each other by posterointermediate sulcus and septum. The fibres in the spinal cord which enter in the coccygeal and lower sacral region are thrust medially by fibres which enter at higher levels (Figs 5.20 and 5.21).

Second order neurons: The neurons of nuclei gracilis and cuneatus form second order neurons. Their axons curve ventromedially as *internal arcuate fibres* which decussate (cross) to the opposite side and ascend upward as ***medial lemniscus***. These nuclei lie on the posterior aspect of medulla oblongata. Then medial

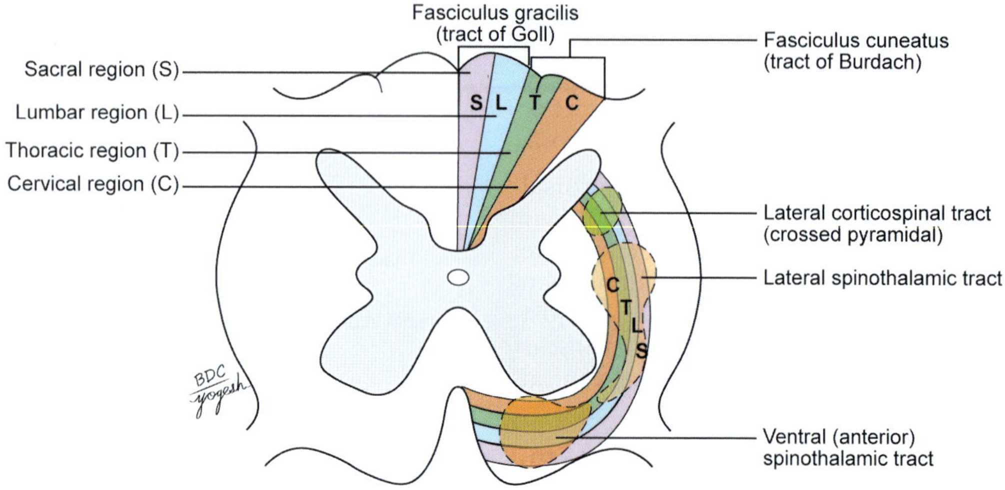

Fig. 5.21: Somatotopic lamination of tracts in the spinal cord

lemniscus ascends in pons and midbrain to terminate in *ventral posterolateral nucleus of thalamus*.

Third order neurons: They are located in VPL nucleus thalamus. Their axons ascend through the posterior limb of internal capsule and terminate in the sensory cortex of cerebral hemisphere.

CLINICAL NEUROANATOMY

- Unilateral lesion of posterior white column → results in loss of the discriminatory touch, sense of position, and vibration sensations below the level of lesion and on the side of lesion.
- ***Tabes dorsalis***: In syphilis, the posterior white column undergoes degenerative changes. These are called tabes dorsalis. It results in loss of position, vibration, and two-point discrimination sensations.
- ***Romberg's sign***: In positive Romberg's sign, the patient falls if he stands with feet together and eyes closed. It may occur due to damage to tract of Goll and Burdach (loss of position sense).

Spinocerebellar Tracts

The spinocerebellar tracts carry the unconscious proprioception to the cerebellum. They form afferent fibres of reflex arc involving cerebellum for maintenance of posture and coordination of movement.

Receptors: Stretch receptor of muscle spindle and Golgi tendon organ for unconscious proprioception.

Composition/Pathway

The spinocerebellar tract consists of two neurons arrangement. The spinocerebellar tracts include (Fig. 5.22 and Table 5.8):

1. Dorsal spinocerebellar tract
2. Ventral spinocerebellar tract
3. Cuneocerebellar tract
4. Rostral spinocerebellar tract.

Posterior (Dorsal) Spinocerebellar Tract

First order neurons: They are pseudounipolar neurons of dorsal root ganglion. Their central processes enter the spinal cord and relay in Clarke's column.

Second order neurons: They are located *in nucleus dorsalis* (*Clarke's column*). Their axons pass to the dorsolateral part of lateral white column of same side and ascend as dorsal tract of spinocerebellar tract.

They ascend to medulla oblongata where they enter *inferior cerebellar peduncle* and terminates in the ipsilateral cerebellar cortex (vermis).

Anterior (Ventral) Spinocerebellar Tract

First order neurons: The location and course of first order neurons are similar to dorsal spinocerebellar tract.

Second order neurons: They are located in laminae V–VII of lumbosacral segments of spinal cord. Their axons mostly decussate (cross) and ascend as anterior or ventral spinocerebellar tracts in the anterolateral part of lateral white column. They ascend to midbrain and enter the cerebellum through *superior cerebellar peduncle*. They decussate in the cerebellum and terminate in the cerebellum cortex (vermis).

Cuneocerebellar Tract

First order neuron: They are located in the dorsal root ganglion. Their central processes enter the spinal cord at C2 to T5 level and ascend in fasciculus cuneatus in posterior white column. They terminate in internal or *accessory cuneate nucleus*. It is similar to nucleus dorsalis of Clarke which is present in the thoracic region.

Second order neurons: They are located in the accessory cuneate nucleus. Their axons join the restiform body or *inferior cerebellar peduncle* and relay in the ipsilateral cerebral cortex.

Note: Clarke's column is not present above C8 level, hence ventral and dorsal spinocerebellar tracts are replaced by cuneocerebellar tract which carries unconscious proprioception from the neck, upper limb and upper part of the trunk.

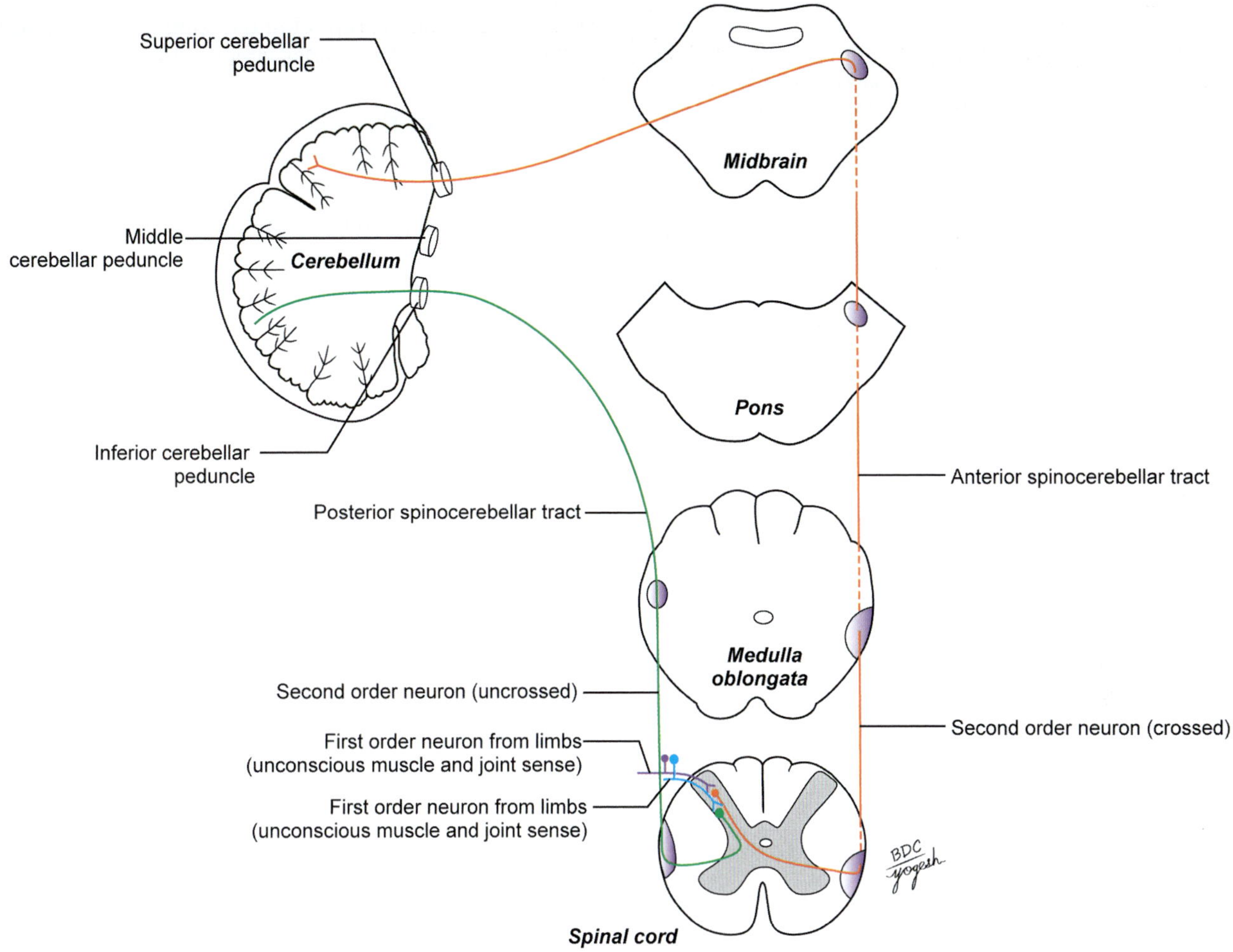

Fig. 5.22: Pathway of posterior and anterior spinocerebellar tracts

TABLE 5.8: Spinocerebellar tracts

Tract	*First order neuron*	*Second order neuron*	*Termination*	*Functions*
Dorsal or posterior spinocerebellar tract (C8 to L3)	Cells of dorsal root ganglion	Cells of dorsal nucleus (Clark's column)	Ipsilateral cerebellar vermis	• Proprioception from ipsilateral trunk and lower limb • Coordination of movements of lower limb • Maintenance of posture
Ventral or anterior spinocerebellar tract (C8–L3)	Cells of dorsal root ganglion	Dorsal horn cells	Ipsilateral cerebellar vermis	• Proprioception from ipsilateral trunk and lower limb • Same as above
Cuneocerebellar (C2 to T5)	Dorsal root ganglion	Accessory cuneate nucleus	Ipsilateral cerebellar vermis	Proprioception from ipsilateral neck and upper limb
Rostral spinocerebellar (C4–C8)	Dorsal root ganglion	Dorsal horn cells	Cerebellum	Proprioception from ipsilateral head and upper limb

Rostral Spinocerebellar Tract

First order neurons: These are the dorsal horn cells (C4–C8) that give information of unconscious proprioception of head and upper limb. Their central processes terminate in the lamina VII of dorsal horn.

Second order neurons: They are located in *lamina VII of dorsal horn at C4 to C8 level*. Their axons ascend as rostral spinocerebellar tract along with ventral spinocerebellar tract. They enter the cerebellum mostly through *inferior cerebellar peduncle* (few through superior cerebellar peduncle) and terminate in cerebellar cortex.

INTERSEGMENTAL TRACTS

These are formed of fibres connecting various segments of spinal cord. These are present in anterior, posterior and lateral columns of white matter adjacent to the grey matter of spinal cord. Tract of Lissauer is also an intersegmental tract.

Competency:

AN57.5 Describe the anatomical basis of clinical conditions affecting the grey and white matter of spinal cord (Brown-Séquard syndrome, poliomyelitis, amyotrophic lateral sclerosis or motor neuron disease, syringomyelia, hereditary sensory neuropathy, subacute combined degeneration, transverse myelitis, paraplegia).

CLINICAL NEUROANATOMY

Amyotrophic lateral sclerosis: It is a degenerative disease which is caused due to damage of the cells in the ventral horn. The clinical features involve weakness, atrophy of muscles of hands and arms and later extending to the lower limb.

Subacute combined degeneration: The posterior and lateral funiculi are degenerated bilaterally and it is caused due to deficiency of intrinsic factor which helps in absorption of vitamin B12. The symptoms include upper motor neuron lesion with loss of position and vibratory sensation of lower limbs.

Syringomyelia (central spinal cord syndrome): There is formation of cavities around the central canal usually in the lower cervical region. Its features are:

1. Bilateral loss of pain and temperature occurs due to injury to the decussating fibres of lateral spinothalamic fibres (Fig. 5.23).
2. Bilateral loss of touch occurs due to injury to anterior spinothalamic tract.

Anatomical basis:

1. As the decussation of lateral and anterior spinothalamic tracts occurs at different levels, there is dissociated sensory loss.
2. As this disease occurs in lower cervical and upper thoracic regions, there is problem in both the upper limbs and front of chest.
3. Syringomyelia disrupts the crossing fibres of anterolateral system. The medial lemniscal system is spared.

Brown-Séquard syndrome: This is caused due to ***hemisection of the spinal cord***. Figure 5.24 shows various features of hemisection on the left side.

Below the level of lesion:

1. Ipsilateral upper motor neuron paralysis caused by pyramidal tract damage.
2. Ipsilateral loss of conscious proprioceptive sensations caused due to damage to posterior white column.
3. Contralateral loss of pain and temperature and touch caused due to damage to lateral spinothalamic and anterior spinothalamic tracts.

At the level of lesion:

1. Ipsilateral lower motor neuron paralysis caused due to damage to ventral nerve roots.
2. Ipsilateral anaesthesia over the skin of the segment due to injury to the dorsal nerve roots.

Above the level: Ipsilateral hyperaesthesia above the level of lesion due to irritation of dorsal nerve roots.

Complete transaction of spinal cord: In severe injury, there may be complete transaction of spinal cord. The clinical features are grouped into two phases:

1. ***Stage of spinal shock:*** Immediately after complete transection of the spinal cord, the stage of spinal shock begins. It lasts for first three weeks of injury. It is characterised by:
   - Flaccid paralysis of all muscles
   - Loss of all superficial and deep reflexes below the level of injury.
   - Retention of urine due to loss of relaxation of internal sphincter of urinary bladder and flaccid paralysis of detrusor muscle.

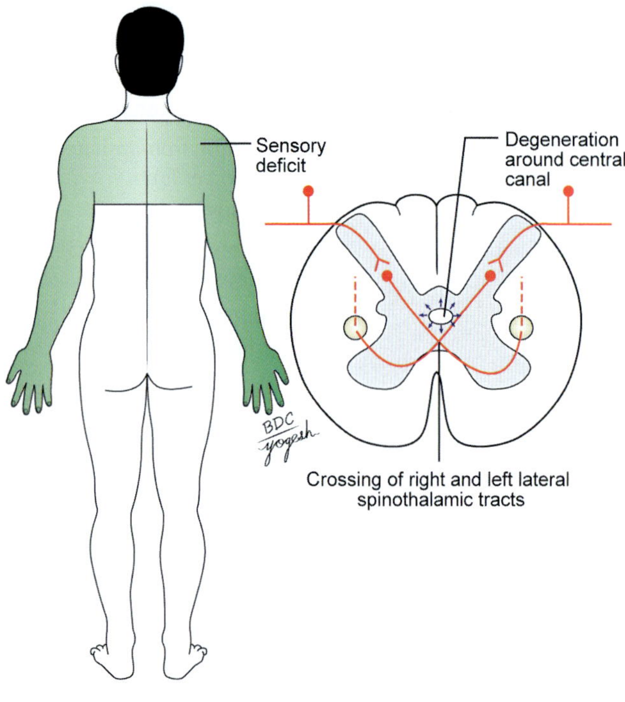

Fig. 5.23: Syringomyelia (central spinal cord syndrome)

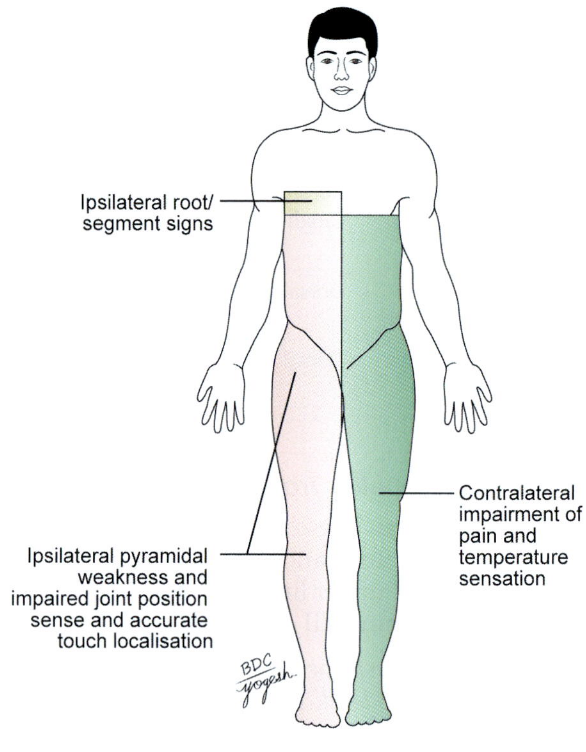

Fig. 5.24: Brown-Séquard syndrome

- Retention of faeces due to non-relaxation of external anal sphincter.
- Retention incontinence – that is urine will accumulate until the pressure is high enough to force the urine through the sphincter.

2. ***Recovery phase:*** After the recovery from the shock, the muscle activity reappears. This phase is characterised by:
   - Upper motor neuron, paralysis (spastic) will appear below the level of the lesion as follows:
     - Lesion above C5 spinal segment → respiratory failure due to paralysis of phrenic nerve.
     - Lesion between C2 to T1 → quadriplegia (paralysis of all 4 limbs).
     - Lesion below T1 segments → paraplegia (paralysis of both lower limb).
     - Automatic emptying of urinary bladder and bowel, that is, involuntary emptying at short interval after their sufficient distention.

BLOOD SUPPLY OF SPINAL CORD

Arterial Supply

The spinal cord is supplied by:

1. Anterior spinal artery
2. Posterior spinal arteries (right and left)
3. Spinal branches of vertebral, deep cervical, posterior intercostal, lumbar, and lateral sacral arteries (Fig. 5.25).

Anterior Spinal Artery

Two spinal branches (right and left) arise from the vertebral arteries, arise in front of upper part of medulla oblongata. These branches unite to form a single anterior spinal artery that descends in anterior median fissures of the spinal cord.

Branches: Anterior spinal artery gives:

Central branches – pass through the anterior median fissure into the substance of spinal cord.

Vasa corona (arteriae coronae) – pass along the outer surface of spinal cord and form plexus within the pia mater.

Distribution: Anterior spinal artery supplies:

- Anterior and lateral horn
- Base of posterior horn
- Anterior white column
- Part of lateral white column.

Posterior Spinal Arteries

They arise from vertebral or inferior cerebellar artery. Each posterior spinal artery divides into two longitudinal branches. One descends in front, and another descends behind the dorsal root.

Branches: They give small branches that penetrate and serve the spinal cord.

Distribution: They supply:

- Posterior horn except its base
- Posterior white column
- Peripheral part of lateral white column.

Radicular Arteries

The anterior and posterior spinal arteries are small vessels that cannot sufficiently supply the entire length of spinal cord, especially lower part. Hence, these arteries are reinforced by segmental branches of vertebral, deep cervical, posterior intercostal, lumbar, and lateral sacral arteries. These spinal branches enter the vertebral canal through corresponding *intervertebral foramen* and divides into *anterior and posterior radicular arteries* which reach the spinal cord along the anterior and posterior root of spinal nerves. Radicular arteries reinforce the anterior and posterior spinal arteries.

Arteria Radicularis Magna *(Artery of Adamkiewicz)*

It is the largest radicular artery; usually it lies at T11 segment of spinal cord.

Venous Drainage

The venous blood is drained from the spinal cord by six longitudinal venous channels as follows (Fig. 5.26):

- *Anteromedian longitudinal venous channel* – lies along the anterior median fissure.

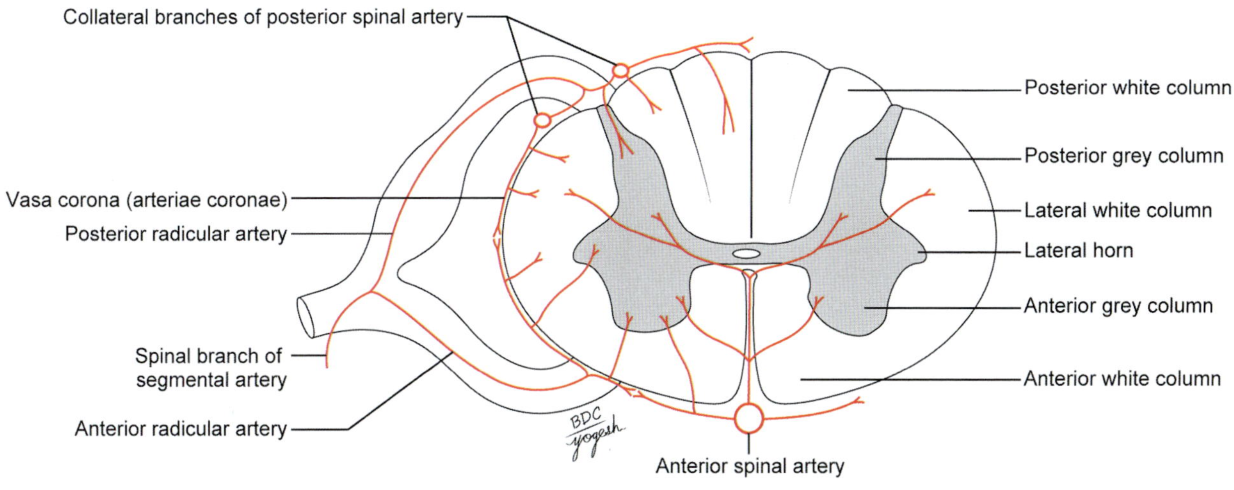

Fig. 5.25: Arterial supply of spinal cord

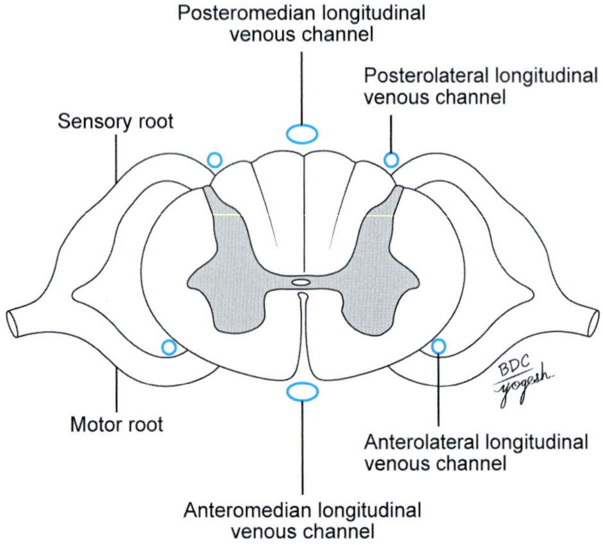

Fig. 5.26: Venous drainage of the spinal cord

- *Posteromedial longitudinal venous channel* – lies along the posterior median sulcus.
- *Pair of anterolateral longitudinal venous channels* – one on each side, behind the ventral root.
- *Pair of posterolateral longitudinal venous channels* – one on each side, behind dorsal nerve root.

These veins lie in the pia matter. They drain into the *internal vertebral venous plexus* and the veins which leave through intervertebral foramen and open into adjacent vertebral, posterior intercostal, lumbar and lateral sacral veins.

CLINICAL NEUROANATOMY

1. ***Transverse myelitis*** is an inflammatory condition affecting both sides of a segment of the spinal cord, leading to sudden weakness, sensory alterations, and loss of bladder or bowel control. It can result from infections, autoimmune disorders, or multiple sclerosis, causing nerve damage and disrupting communication between the brain and the body.
2. ***Subacute combined degeneration*** is a neurological disorder caused by vitamin B12 deficiency, leading to degeneration of the spinal cord's dorsal and lateral columns. It presents with symptoms like weakness, numbness, and impaired coordination. If untreated, it can progress to severe neurological damage, including paralysis, sensory loss, and cognitive changes.
3. ***Hereditary sensory neuropathy*** is a group of genetic disorders that affect sensory nerves, leading to loss of pain, temperature, and touch sensations. Symptoms include numbness, ulcers, and unrecognized injuries, particularly in the hands and feet.
4. ***Amyotrophic lateral sclerosis*** or ***motor neuron disease*** is a progressive neurodegenerative disease affecting motor neurons in the brain and spinal cord. It leads to muscle weakness, paralysis, and loss of voluntary movement, while cognitive function typically remains intact. It gradually impairs breathing and swallowing, ultimately resulting in severe disability and respiratory failure.

Facts to Remember

- Length of spinal cord is 45 cm in adult males.
- Spinal cord ends at L3 vertebra at birth and lower border of L1 or upper border of L2 vertebra in adults.
- Lateral horn is only present in T1–L2 and S2–S4 segments of spinal cord.
- Sympathetic fibres (white ramus communicans) start from lateral horn → ventral root → trunk of spinal nerve → ventral primary ramus → sympathetic ganglion (Fig. 3.7).
- Poliovirus affects the neurons of anterior horn cells of the spinal cord. Polio drops as a vaccine has eradicated the dreadful disease.
- The hemisection of the spinal cord produces Brown-Séquard syndrome.
- Compete transection of spinal cord shows two phases: Stage of spinal shock for first three week and stage of recovery after three weeks.

BDC's Anatomy *e*-book

1. Neuronal columns of grey matter of spinal cord
2. Arrangement of pyramidal tract fibres
3. Extrapyramidal centres
4. Pathway for pain and temperature from head region
5. Proprioception from head
6. Unilateral/partial spinal cord lesion
7. Further reading
8. Viva voce questions

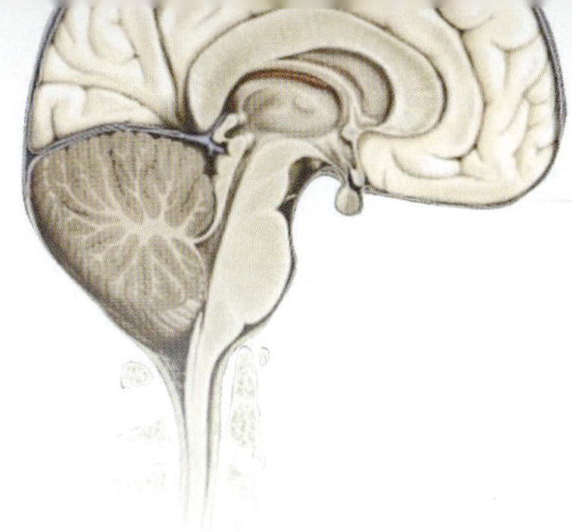

Chapter

6

Cranial Nerves

There are 12 pairs of cranial nerves as follows:
I: Olfactory
II: Optic
III: Oculomotor
IV: Trochlear
V: Trigeminal
VI: Abducent
VII: Facial
VIII: Vestibulocochlear
IX: Glossopharyngeal
X: Vagus
XI: Accessory
XII: Hypoglossal.

Attachment of the nerves to brain is as follows (Fig. 6.1):
I, II to the forebrain.
III, IV to midbrain.
V, VI, VII, VIII to the pons.
IX, X, XI, XII to the medulla oblongata.

Note: During early stages of development, the wall of the neural tube is made up of three layers: inner ependymal layer, middle mantle layer, and the outer marginal layer. The mantle layer represents grey matter and the marginal layer represents the white matter. Soon the mantle layer differentiates into a dorsal alar lamina (sensory) and a ventral basal lamina (motor), the two are partially separated internally by the sulcus limitans.

In the brainstem, the alar and basal laminae of the neural tube come to lie in the same ventral plane because of stretching of the roof plate (dorsal wall) of neural tube by pontine flexure. Further, the grey matter forms separate longitudinal functional columns, where the motor columns (from basal lamina) are medial and the sensory columns (from alar lamina) are lateral in position.

Competency:
AN62.1 Enumerate cranial nerve nuclei with its functional component.

FUNCTIONAL COMPONENTS OF CRANIAL NERVES

The functional component is a part of cranial nerve that performs a specific function, such as:
a. Motor or efferent component and
b. Sensory or afferent component.

These are further classified according to function as follows (Figs 6.2):

Efferent (motor) components (Table 6.1)
1. *General somatic efferent* (*GSE*): They supply striated muscles of head that are not originated from pharyngeal arches.
2. *Special visceral efferent* (*SVE*) or branchial efferent: They supply striated muscles of pharyngeal arches, trapezius, and sternocleidomastoid muscle.
3. *General visceral efferent* (*GVE*) are preganglionic parasympathetic fibres. They supply glands, smooth muscles of viscera and vessels.

Afferent (sensory) components (Table 6.2)
1. *General visceral afferent* (*GVA*): They carry visceral sensation via vagus nerve.
2. *Special visceral afferent* (*SVA*): They carry taste sensation.
3. *General somatic afferent* (*GSA*): They carry proprioception, tactile sensation from face and oral, nasal, and pharyngeal mucosa via trigeminal nerve.
4. *Special somatic afferent* (*SSA*): They carry auditory and vestibular impulse.

Each cranial nerve may carry fibres of one or more components. For example, trochlear nerve carry fibres of somatic efferent column and it supplies muscles developed from cranial somites.

NUCLEI OF CRANIAL NERVES

General Somatic Efferent (GSE) Nuclei (Fig. 6.3)

These nuclei supply skeletal muscle of somatic origin.
1. ***Oculomotor nucleus*** is situated in the midbrain at the level of the superior colliculus. Its fibres enter the oculomotor nerve and supply 5 extrinsic muscles of the eyeball except the lateral rectus and the superior oblique.
2. ***Trochlear nucleus*** is situated in the midbrain at the level of the inferior colliculus. It supplies only the superior oblique muscle through the trochlear nerve.
3. ***Abducent nucleus*** is situated in the lower part of the pons. It supplies only the lateral rectus muscle through the abducent nerve.

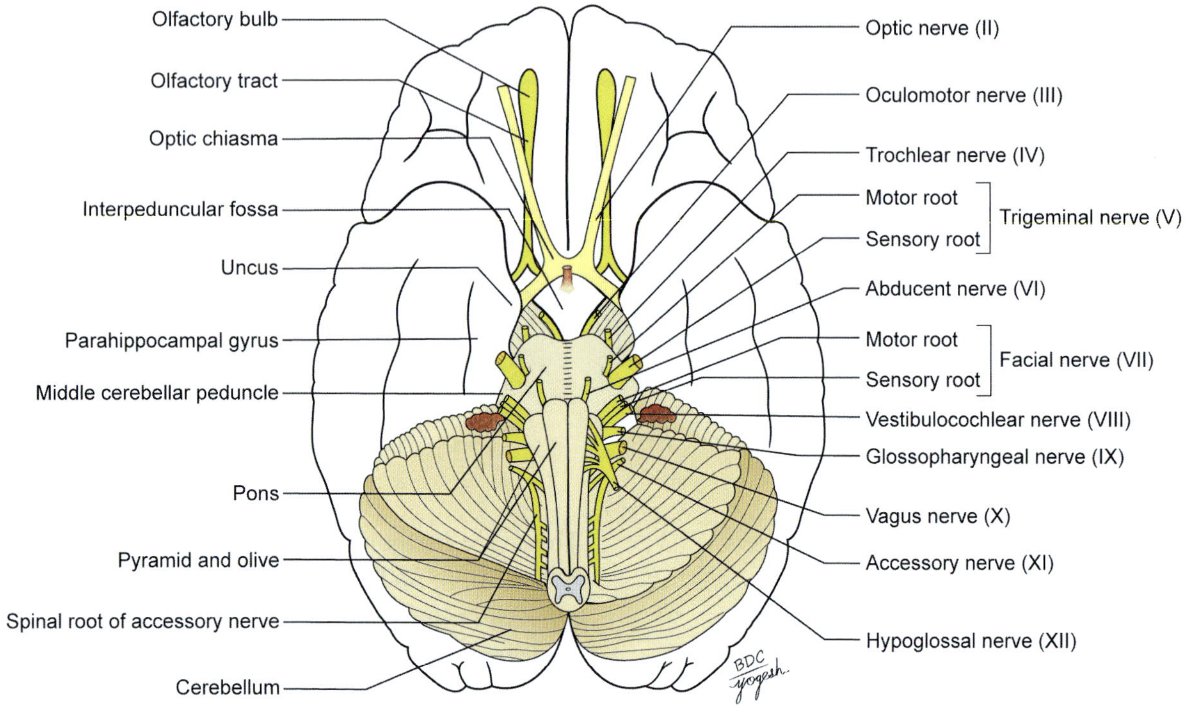

Fig. 6.1: Attachment of cranial nerves to the base of brain

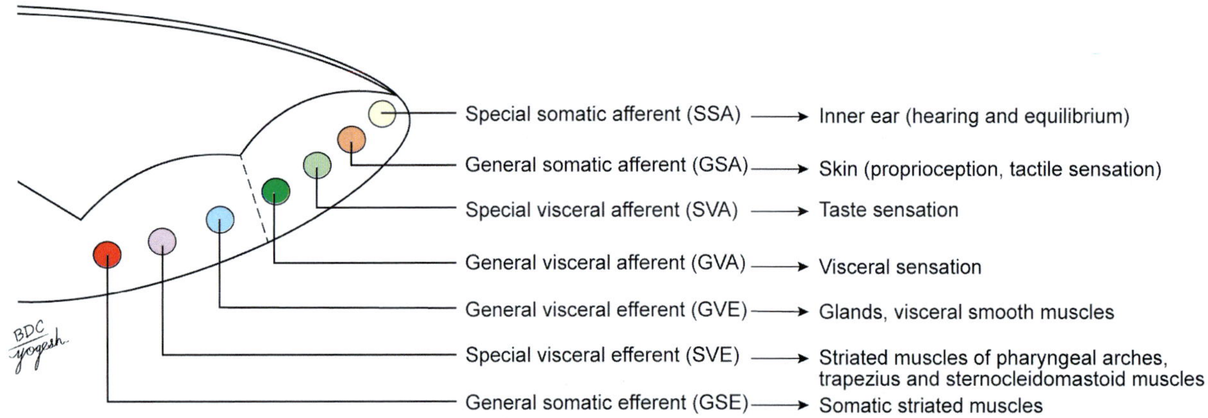

Fig. 6.2: Transverse section of an embryonic brainstem showing the arrangement of functional/nuclear columns of cranial nerve nuclei

TABLE 6.1: Cranial nerve nuclei: Efferent column

	GSE	*SVE*	*GVE*
Functions	Striated muscles of head	Striated muscles of pharyngeal arches	Parasympathetic fibres
Midbrain	Oculomotor nucleus Trochlear nucleus	—	Edinger-Westphal nucleus
Pons	Abducent nucleus	Motor nucleus of Vth nerve and facial nerve	Superior salivatory nucleus Lacrimatory nucleus
Medulla oblongata	Hypoglossal nucleus	Nucleus ambiguus	Inferior salivatory nucleus Dorsal nucleus of vagus

TABLE 6.2: Cranial nerve nuclei: Afferent column (NTS: Nucleus tractus solitarious)

	GVA	*SVA*	*GSA*	*SSA*
Functions	Visceral sensation	Taste sensation	Proprioception Tactile sensation from head	Auditory and vestibular impulses
Midbrain	—	—	Mesencephalic nucleus of Vth nerve	—
Pons	NTS	NTS (for facial nerve)	Main sensory nucleus of Vth nerve	Vestibular and cochlear nuclei
Medulla oblongata	NTS	NTS (for IXth, Xth nerves)	Spinal nucleus of Vth nerve	—

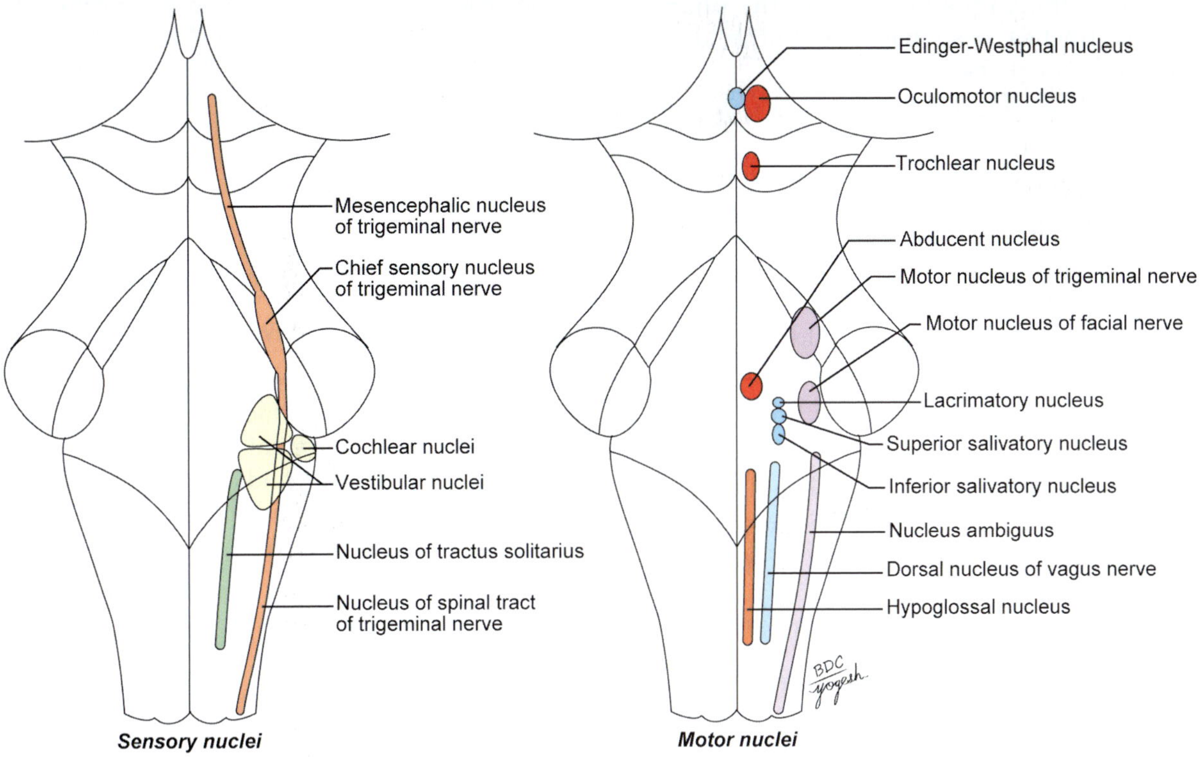

Fig. 6.3: Surface projection of cranial nerve nuclei on the dorsal aspect of the brainstem

4. ***Hypoglossal nucleus*** lies in the medulla. It is elongated and extends into both the open and closed parts of the medulla. It supplies seven out of eight muscles of the tongue through the hypoglossal nerve.

Special Visceral Efferent/Branchial Efferent Nuclei (Fig. 6.3)

These nuclei supply striated muscles derived from the branchial arches.

1. ***Motor nucleus of the trigeminal nerve*** lies in the upper part of the pons. It supplies the muscles of mastication through the mandibular nerve.
2. ***Nucleus of the facial nerve*** lies in the lower part of the pons. It supplies the various muscles innervated by the facial nerve.
3. ***Nucleus ambiguus*** lies in the medulla. It forms an elongated column lying in both the open and closed parts of the medulla. It supplies:
   a. Stylopharyngeus muscle through the glossopharyngeal nerve; and
   b. Muscles of the soft palate, the pharynx and the larynx through the vagus nerve and the cranial part of the accessory nerve.

General Visceral Efferent Nuclei (Fig. 6.3)

These nuclei give origin to preganglionic neurons that relay in a peripheral autonomic ganglion. Postganglionic fibres arising in the ganglion supply smooth muscles or glands.

1. ***Edinger-Westphal nucleus*** lies in the midbrain in close relation to the oculomotor nucleus. Its fibres pass through the oculomotor nerve to the ciliary ganglion to supply the sphincter pupillae and the ciliaris muscles.
2. ***Lacrimatory nucleus*** lies near the salivatory nuclei (in the lower pons). It gives off fibres that pass through the facial nerve and its branch, the greater petrosal nerve to relay in the pterygopalatine ganglion and supply the lacrimal, nasal, palatal and pharyngeal glands.
3. ***Superior salivatory nucleus*** lies in the lower part of the pons. It sends fibres through the facial nerve and its chorda tympani branch to the submandibular ganglion for supply of the submandibular, sublingual salivary glands and glands in the oral cavity.
4. ***Inferior salivatory nucleus*** lies in the lower part of the pons just below the superior nucleus. It sends fibres through the glossopharyngeal nerve to the otic ganglion for supply of the parotid gland.
5. ***Dorsal nucleus of the vagus*** is a long column extending into the open and closed parts of the medulla. It gives off fibres that pass through the vagus nerve to be distributed to thoracic and abdominal viscera (the ganglia concerned are present in the walls of the viscera supplied).

General Visceral Afferent Nucleus and Special Visceral Afferent Nucleus (Fig. 6.3)

The only nucleus in this category is the ***nucleus of solitary tract*** or tractus solitarius. It lies in the medulla and extends into both its closed and open parts.

Its lower part receives *general visceral sensations* as follows:

a. Through the glossopharyngeal nerve from the tonsil, pharynx, posterior part of the tongue, carotid body and carotid sinus.

b. Through the vagus nerve from the pharynx, larynx, trachea, oesophagus and other thoracic and abdominal viscera.

Its upper part also receives *sensations of taste* (special visceral afferent) as follows:

a. From the anterior two-thirds of the tongue, and the palate except circumvallate papillae through the facial (VII) nerve in its superior part.
b. From the posterior one-third of the tongue through the glossopharyngeal nerve (IX) including the circumvallate papillae in its middle part.
c. From the posteriormost part of the tongue and from the epiglottis through the vagus (X) nerve in its inferior part.

General Somatic Afferent Nuclei (Fig. 6.3)

These are all related to the trigeminal nerve.

1. *Main or superior sensory nucleus of the trigeminal nerve* lies in the upper part of the pons.
2. ***Spinal nucleus of the trigeminal nerve*** descends from the main nucleus into the medulla. It reaches the upper two segments of the spinal cord.
   Its parts are:
   a. Pars caudalis which receives impulses of pain, temperature from forehead
   b. Pars interpolaris, which receives impulses from cheek
   c. Pars oralis, which receives impulses from around mouth.
3. ***Mesencephalic nucleus of the trigeminal nerve*** extends upwards from the main sensory nucleus into the midbrain. It is the only example of primary sensory neuron whose cell bodies are within CNS.
   These nuclei receive the following fibres:
   a. Exteroceptive sensations (touch, pain, temperature) from the skin of the face, through the trigeminal nerve; and from a part of the skin of the auricle through the vagus (auricular branch) and through the facial nerve.
   b. Proprioceptive sensations from muscles of mastication reach the mesencephalic nucleus through the trigeminal nerve. The nucleus is also believed to receive proprioceptive fibres from the ocular, facial and lingual muscles, teeth and temporomandibular joint.

Special Somatic Afferent Nuclei (Fig. 6.3)

1. ***Cochlear nuclei*** (dorsal and ventral) that receive impulses of hearing through the cochlear nerve.
2. ***Vestibular nuclei*** (superior, spinal, medial and lateral) that receive fibres from the semicircular canals, the utricle and the saccule through the vestibular nerve.

Note:

Muscles of facial expression of lower quarter of the face are supplied only from contralateral motor cortex.

The muscles of upper face are supplied both from ipsilateral and contralateral motor cortices.

Cranial part of nucleus ambiguus gives fibres to IX, X and cranial root of XI nerve. The caudal part of this nucleus gives fibres to spinal root of XI nerve.

The genioglossus muscle of the tongue receives fibres from contralateral motor cortex only. Rest of the muscles of the tongue receive fibres from both ipsilateral and contralateral motor cortices.

Competency:
AN63.3 Describe the olfactory, visual, auditory and gustatory pathways.

FIRST CRANIAL NERVE

OLFACTORY (SMELL) PATHWAY

It belongs to special visceral afferent column. Olfactory sensation is carried by olfactory system which consists of the following components:

1. Olfactory epithelium and olfactory nerves
2. Olfactory bulb, tract and striae
3. Olfactory areas of cerebrum.

Olfactory Epithelium and Olfactory Nerves

The ***olfactory epithelium*** lines the upper one-third of nasal cavity. It consists of three types of cells (Plate 6.1):

1. *Olfactory receptor cells* (16–20 million in man): These are modified bipolar neurons that receive smell sensation. These cells serve both as receptors as well as the first order neurons in the olfactory pathway.
2. *Supporting cells.*
3. *Basal cells* that can generate the olfactory receptor cells (neurons).

Axons of receptor cells are nonmyelinated. They form about 20 bundles of ***olfactory nerves***. These nerves pass through the cribriform plate of ethmoid to enter the anterior cranial fossa. They terminate in the olfactory bulb.

Olfactory Bulb, Tract, and Striae (Fig. 6.4)

1. ***Olfactory bulb*** is a small oval mass of grey matter situated above the cribriform plate of ethmoid. It has outer *cortical zone* with *olfactory glomeruli* and inner *medullary zones* of nerve fibres.
2. ***Olfactory glomeruli*** consist of mitral cells, tufted cells, stellate cells, periglomerular cells, and axons of olfactory receptor cells.
3. ***Olfactory tract***: The olfactory bulb continues posteriorly as olfactory tract. The posterior end of olfactory tract forms a flat *olfactory trigone.*
4. ***Olfactory striae***: The olfactory tract divides into medial, intermediate, and lateral olfactory striae.
5. ***Anterior olfactory nucleus*** is a group of neurons situated at the junction of olfactory bulb and tract.
6. ***Medial olfactory stria*** continues in paraterminal gyrus which lies in front of lamina terminalis.
7. ***Lateral olfactory stria*** runs laterally and continues into *limen insulae*. It turns medially to form gyrus semilunaris (periamygdaloid area).
8. ***Intermediate olfactory stria*** is occasionally present. It ends as olfactory tubercle in the anterior perforated substance.
9. ***Medial*** **and** ***lateral olfactory gyri*** are thin layers of grey matter that cover the medial and lateral olfactory stria.

Plate 6.1: Olfactory mucosa

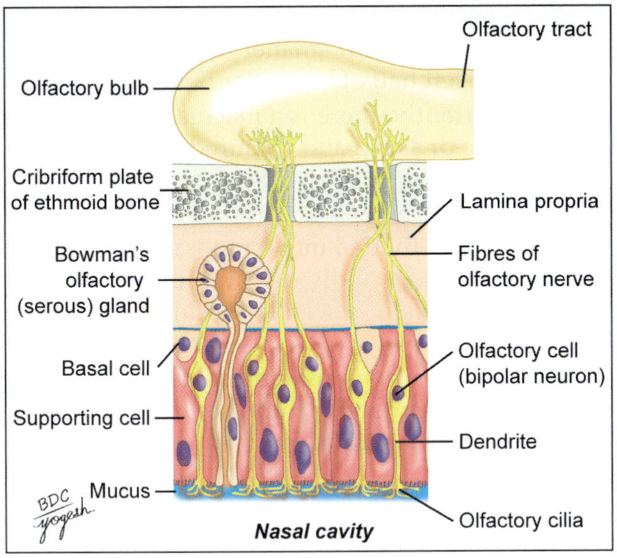

Olfactory Areas

1. ***Primary olfactory area*** is responsible for reception and perception of smell. It includes lateral olfactory gyrus, gyrus ambiens, gyrus semilunaris, limen insulae, uncus and dorsomedial part of amygdaloid body.
2. ***Secondary olfactory area (entorhinal area)*** performs the olfactory association. It includes the anterior part of parahippocampal gyrus. It is called area 28. Fibres arising in the primary olfactory cortex go to the secondary olfactory cortex and tertiary olfactory cortex in posterior part of orbitofrontal cortex.

Note:

Smell is perceived in both the primary and secondary olfactory areas.

Some impulses from uncus travel via medial forebrain bundle and reticular formation to dorsal nucleus of vagus and salivatory nuclei in medulla oblongata, where these may increase or decrease gastric secretion according to type of smell.

Olfactory afferent pathway comprises only two neurons. The fibres reach the cerebral cortex without synapsing in any of the thalamic nuclei.

CLINICAL NEUROANATOMY

- ***Anosmia:*** Loss of olfactory fibres with ageing. Allergic rhinitis causes temporary olfactory impairment.
- Sense of smell is tested separately in each nostril.
- *Head injury:* Olfactory bulbs may be torn away from olfactory nerves as these pass through fractured cribriform plate of ethmoid leading to anosmia. Such a fracture may also cause CSF rhinorrhoea, i.e. CSF leakage through the nose.
- Abscess of frontal lobe of brain or meningioma in the anterior cranial fossa may press on the olfactory bulb or olfactory tract resulting in anosmia.

SECOND CRANIAL NERVE

The optic nerve is the 2nd cranial nerve. It is purely sensory and a nerve of sight or vision. It emerges from the eyeball, about 3 to 4 mm nasal to its posterior pole. It runs backwards and medially to enter the optic canal. Finally, it enters the middle cranial fossa and unite with opposite nerve to form optic chiasma.

Length: The optic nerve is 4 cm long.

Note: Human vision is binocular, though one sees with both the eyes, the inverted images formed are seen as one and straight only. Human vision is stereoscopic, i.e. one sees height, width and thickness of the object. Human vision is coloured, one sees different colours put up by nature.

Parts

It has the following courses:

1. Intraorbital: 25 mm
2. Intracanalicular: 5 mm
3. Intracranial: 10 mm.

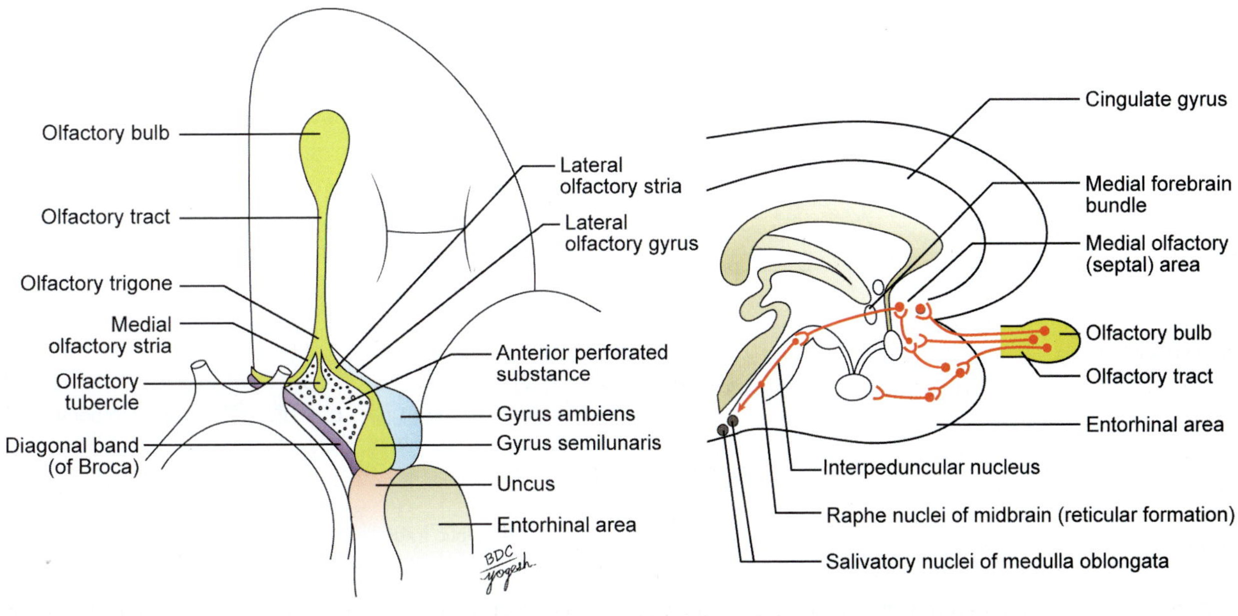

Fig. 6.4: Components of olfactory pathway (inferior view of brain)

Peculiarities of Optic Nerve

1. The optic nerve is not a true cranial nerve.
2. It is an extension of diencephalon during embryonic life.
3. It consists of 2nd order sensory neurons.
4. It consists of fibres myelinated by oligodendrocytes (instead of Schwann cells).
5. It is surrounded by meninges.
6. Its fibre cannot regenerate if damaged.

Functional Component

Special somatic afferent fibres: Optic nerve carries sense of sight from eye.

Course and Relations

Beginning: The ganglion cells of retina give rise to the fibres of optic nerve. These fibres converge toward the optic disc at the posterior pole of the eyeball. These fibres pierce the retina, choroid and sclera and emerge from the eyeball as optic nerve.

Course: The optic nerve pass posteromedially in the orbit and enters the middle cranial fossa through optic canal.

Termination: Both the optic nerves join to form optic chiasma in the middle cranial fossa.

VISUAL PATHWAY

Field of Vision

It includes four fields—upper temporal, lower temporal, upper nasal and lower nasal. Nasal fields are smaller than the temporal fields. Larger right temporal and smaller right nasal fields of vision fuse to form right part of ***binocular field***. Left halves of field of vision, i.e. larger temporal half and smaller nasal half of left field of vision form left half of binocular field (Figs 6.5a to d).

Most importantly, there is a macular vision which is the most acute or sharp and coloured vision.

Retina

The retina is also divided into temporal and nasal parts and each is further subdivided into upper and lower parts. Temporal field is seen by nasal hemiretina and vice versa.

The 1st order neurons are represented by the ***bipolar cells of retina***. They receive impulses from the rods and cones present in the retina.

Optic Nerve

Optic nerve is made up of axons of ***ganglion cells of the retina*** which form the 2nd order neurons. In a strict sense, the optic nerve is not a peripheral nerve because its fibres have no neurilemmal sheaths. It is a tract. Its fibres have no power of regeneration.

Optic Chiasma

In the chiasma, the nasal fibres (i.e. fibres of the optic nerve arising in the nasal, or medial half of the retina) including those from the nasal half of the macula, cross the midline and enter the opposite optic tract. The temporal (lateral) fibres pass through the chiasma to enter the optic tract of the same side.

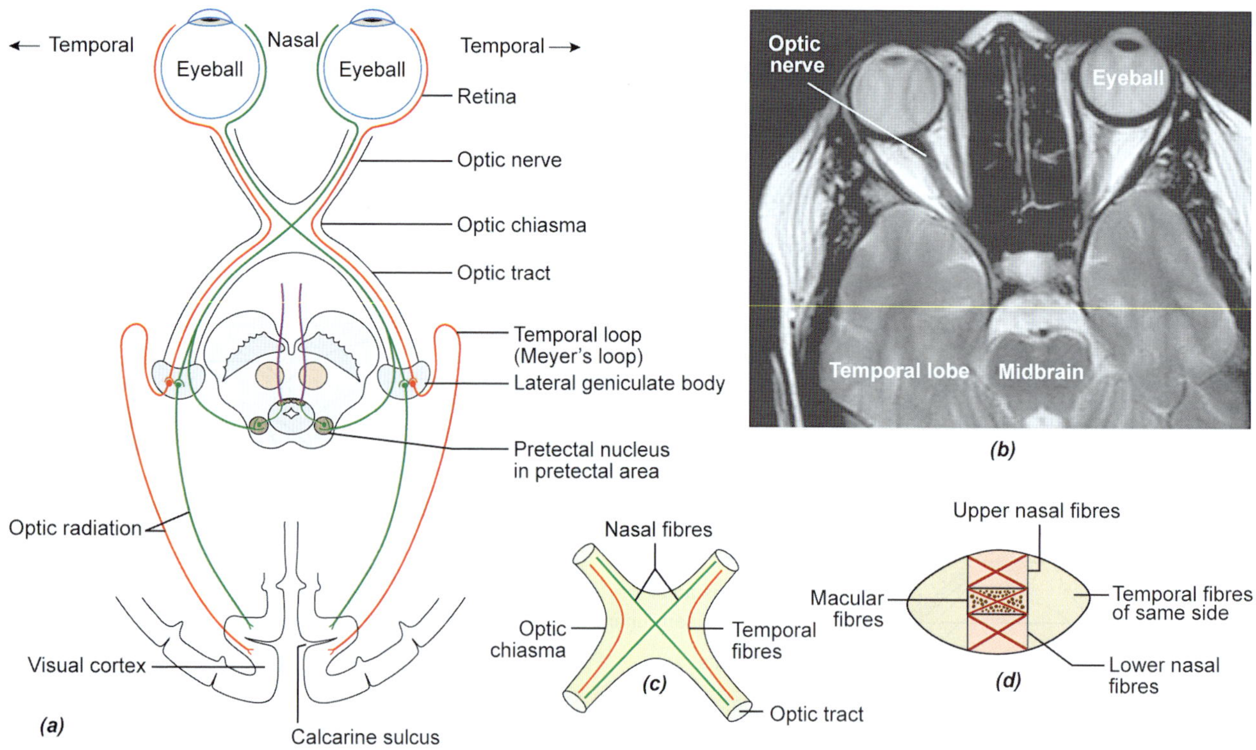

Figs 6.5a to d: (a) Visual pathways showing binocular vision, (b) MRI showing optic nerve, (c) superior view of fibres in optic chiasma, and (d) sectional view of fibres in optic chiasma

Optic Tract

Each optic tract winds round the cerebral peduncle of the midbrain. Near the lateral geniculate body, it divides into ***lateral and medial roots***. The lateral root is thick and terminates in the lateral geniculate body. A few of its fibres pass to the superior colliculus, the pretectal nucleus and the hypothalamus. The medial root is believed to contain the supraoptic commissural fibres.

Each optic tract contains temporal fibres of retina of the same side and nasal fibres of the opposite side.

Lateral Geniculate Body

Lateral geniculate body receives the lateral root of the optic tract. Medially, it is connected to the superior colliculus, and laterally, it gives rise to the optic radiation.

The cells in this body are arranged in six layers which form the third order neurons.

Layers 2, 3, 5 receive ipsilateral fibres, and layers 1, 4, 6 receive contralateral fibres.

Optic Radiation (Geniculocalcarine Tract)

Optic radiation begins from the lateral geniculate body, passes through the retrolentiform part of internal capsule, and ends in the visual cortex.

Visual Cortex

The optic radiation terminates in the striate area where the colour, size, shape, motion, illumination and transparency are appreciated separately. Objects are identified by integration of these perceptions with past experience stored in the parastriate and peristriate areas 18 and 19.

The area of the visual cortex that receives impulses from the macula is relatively much larger than the part related to the rest of the retina.

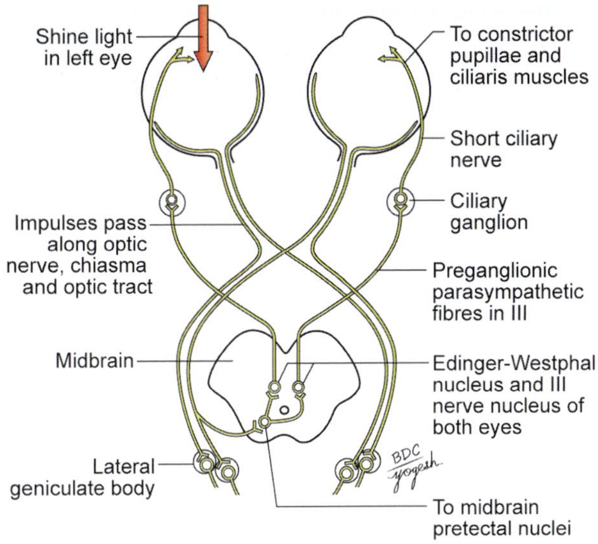

Fig. 6.6: Pupillary light and consensual light reflex

Flowchart 6.1: Pupillary light reflex

Shining of torch light in left eye
↓
Optic nerve
↓
Optic chiasma
↓
Optic tract
↓
A few fibres go to pretectal nucleus of same and even opposite side
↓
Edinger-Westphal nuclei of both sides
↓
III nerve nuclei of both sides
↓
Branch to inferior oblique; relay in ciliary ganglion
↓
Short ciliary nerves of both sides
↓
Sphincter pupillae muscle of both eyes constrict
↓
Both pupils constrict

CLINICAL NEUROANATOMY

- ***Reflexes:*** These are:
  1. Pupillary light and consensual light reflex (Fig. 6.6 and Flowchart 6.1)
  2. Dilation of pupil (Flowchart 6.2)
  3. Accommodation reflex (Fig. 6.7 and Flowchart 6.3)
  4. Corneal/conjunctival reflex (Fig. 6.8 and Flowchart 6.4)
  5. Visual body reflex (Fig. 6.9 and Flowchart 6.5).
- Lesion in retina leads to scotoma, that is certain points may become blind spots.
- Loss of vision in one-half (left or right) of visual field is called ***hemianopia***. If the defect is in same halves of both eyes, it is called ***homonymous hemianopia***. If defect is in different halves, it is called ***heteronymous hemianopia***.
- Optic nerve damage results in complete blindness of that eye (Fig. 6.10).
- Optic chiasma lesion, if central will lead to ***bitemporal hemianopia***, but if peripheral on both sides will lead to ***binasal hemianopia*** (Fig. 6.10).
- Complete destruction of optic tract, lateral geniculate body, optic radiation or visual cortex of one side results in loss of the opposite half of field of vision.
- A lesion on the right optic tract leads to ***left homonymous hemianopia*** (left half of field of vision).
- ***Papilloedema:*** Results due to increased intracranial pressure. It leads to swelling of optic disc due to blockage of tributaries of the retinal veins.
- ***Optic neuritis:*** Lesion of optic nerve that results in decrease of visual acuity. Optic disc appears pale

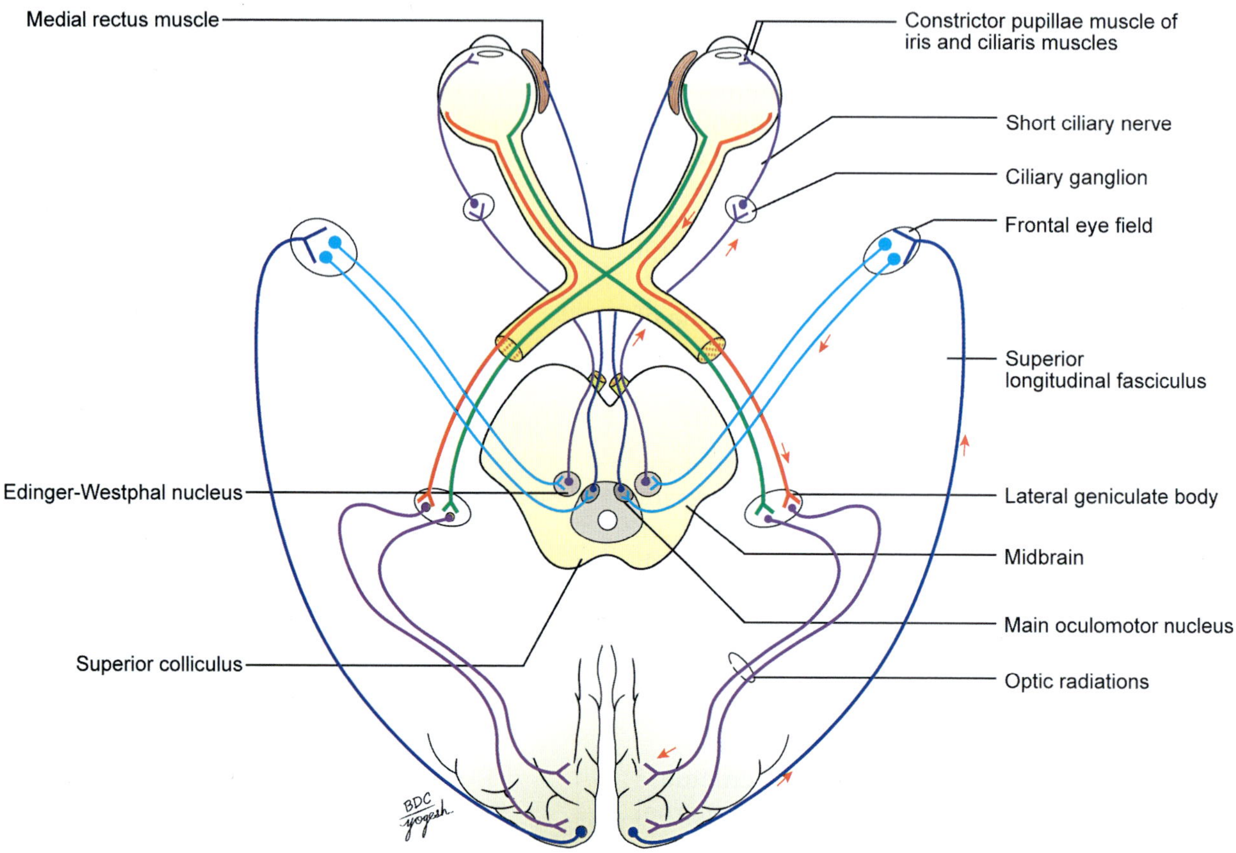

Fig. 6.7: Accommodation reflex

Flowchart 6.2: Dilation of pupil

Hypothalamus
↓
Brainstem
↓
Spinal cord with lateral horn (thoracic segments)
↓
T1–T4 roots
↓
Superior cervical ganglion
↓ Relay
Fibres pass along internal carotid artery
↓
Ophthalmic artery
↓
Long ciliary artery
↓
Branch to ciliary ganglion
↓ No relay
Dilator pupillae

Flowchart 6.3: Accommodation reflex

Read a film magazine (near object)
↓
Optic nerve
↓
Optic chiasma
↓
Optic tract
↓
Lateral geniculate body
↓
Optic radiation
↓
Occipital cortex
↓
Superior longitudinal fasciculus
↓
Medial frontal gyrus (frontal eye field)
↓
III nerve nuclei
↓
III nerve and Edinger-Westphal nuclei of both sides
↓

- Some fibres go to medial recti which result in medial convergence of the eyes
- Nerve to inferior oblique
  ↓
  Branch to ciliary ganglia
  ↓ Relay
  Short ciliary nerves
  ↓
  Constrictor pupillae and ciliaris

and smaller. Methyl alcohol is a usual toxic chemical leading to blindness.

- ***Argyll Robertson pupil:*** In this condition, the accommodation reflex is present but the light reflex is absent. The pretectal area is affected.
- ***Foster Kennedy syndrome*** – tumour at the base of frontal lobe resulting in compression of nerve.

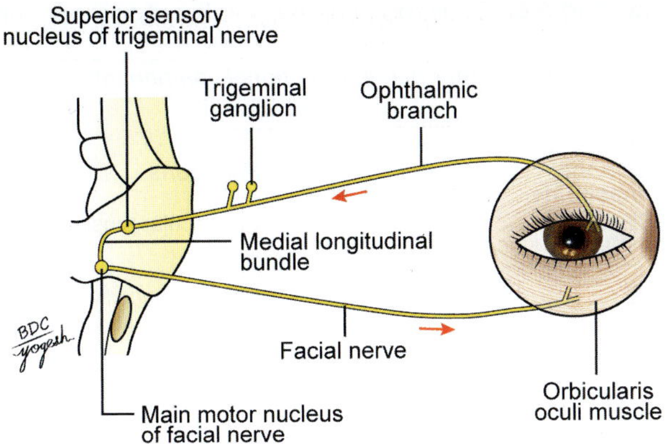

Fig. 6.8: Corneal/conjunctival reflex

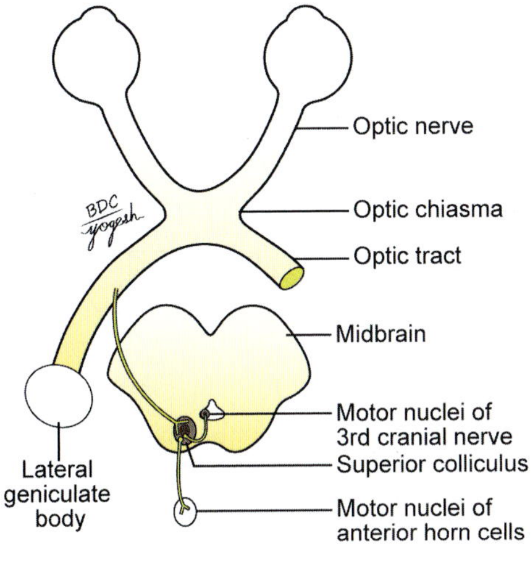

Fig. 6.9: Visual body reflex

Flowchart 6.4: Corneal/conjunctival reflex

Touching of cornea or conjunctiva

↓

Ophthalmic nerve

↓

Superior sensory nucleus of V

↓

Medial longitudinal bundle

↓

Motor nucleus of VII

↓

Orbicularis oculi constricts

Flowchart 6.5: Visual body reflex

Retina

↓

Optic nerve

↓

Optic chiasma

↓

Optic tract

↓

Superior colliculus

↓ Motor nuclei of cranial nerves for movements of head and neck

↓ Anterior horn cells of spinal cord for movements of body

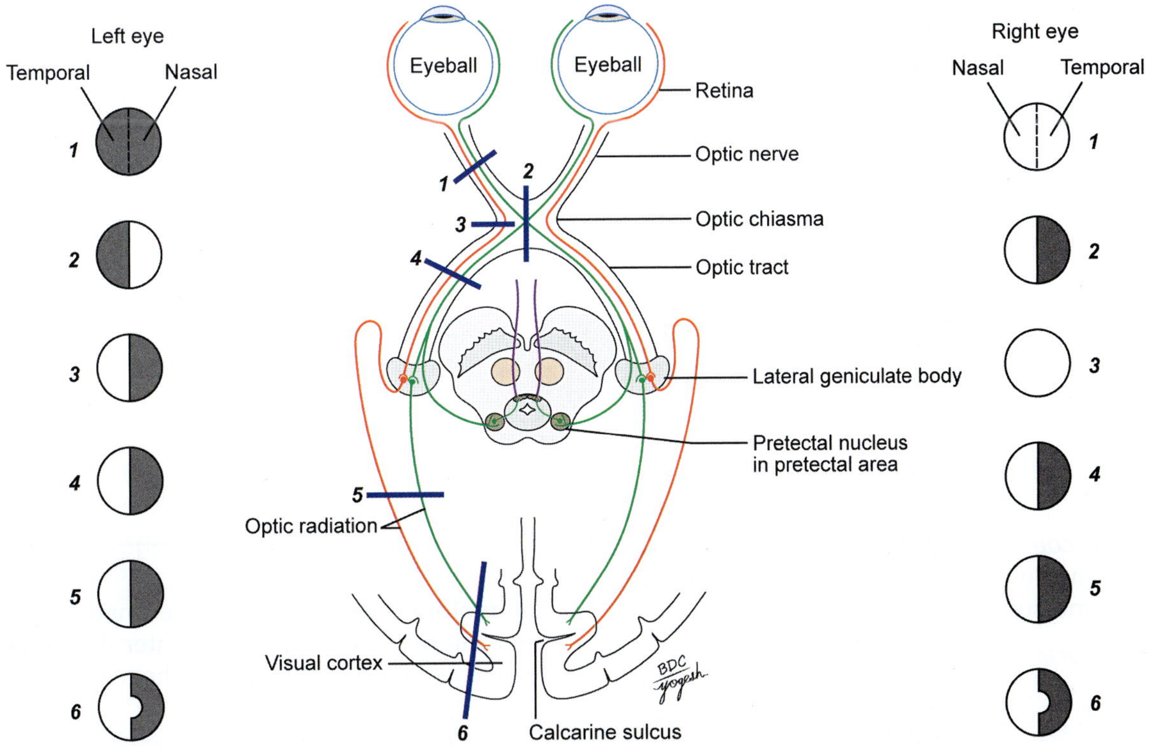

Fig. 6.10: Field defects associated with lesion of visual pathway: (1) Blindness of left eye; (2) Bitemporal hemianopia; (3) Left nasal hemianopia; (4) Right homonymous hemianopia with macular involvement; (5) Right homonymous hemianopia; (6) Right homonymous hemianopia with macular sparing

THIRD CRANIAL NERVE (OCULOMOTOR NERVE)

Oculomotor nerve is the 3rd cranial nerve. It is distributed to the extraocular as well as the intraocular muscles. Since it is a somatic motor nerve, it is in series with the IV, VI and XII cranial nerves, and also with the ventral root of spinal nerves (Flowchart 6.6).

Functional Components

1. *General somatic efferent fibres (GSE)* arise from the *motor nucleus of oculomotor nerve* – for the extraocular muscles of eyeball (Fig. 6.11).
2. *General visceral efferent (GVE)* or *parasympathetic fibres* arise from the *Edinger-Westphal nucleus*. They supply sphincter pupillae and ciliary muscles – for contraction of pupil and accommodation.
3. *General somatic afferent column (GSA)* carries proprioceptive fibres from the extraocular muscles to mesencephalic nucleus of V.

Nucleus

The ***oculomotor nucleus*** is situated in the ventromedial part of central grey matter of midbrain at the level of superior colliculus (Flowchart 6.7). Ventrolaterally, it is closely related to the medial longitudinal bundle.

The nucleus is connected:

a. To the *pyramidal tracts of both sides* which form the supranuclear pathway of the nerve.
b. To the *pretectal nuclei* of both sides for the light reflex.
c. To the *4th, 6th and 8th nerve nuclei* by *medial longitudinal bundle* for coordination of the eye movements.
d. To the *tectobulbar tract* for visuoprotective reflexes.
e. To mesencephalic nucleus of trigeminal nerve.

Origin of Nerve

The oculomotor nerve arises as a single trunk which emerges through a sulcus on the medial side of crus cerebri (midbrain).

Course and Distribution

The course of the oculomotor nerve is divided into three segments (Figs 6.12 and 6.13):

1. Intraneuronal course
2. Intracranial course
3. Orbital course.

Intraneuronal course: The fibres of oculomotor nerve arise from the nucleus and traverse through tegmentum, red nucleus, and substantia nigra (in midbrain).

Intracranial course: The nerve arises from the oculomotor sulcus on the medial aspect of the cerebral peduncle of the *midbrain*. It traverses forwards in the *interpeduncular fossa*, in between the posterior cerebral and superior cerebellar arteries. It *enters the roof of cavernous sinus* and runs in the lateral wall of sinus, superior to the trochlear nerve. In the anterior part of cavernous sinus, the oculomotor nerve divides into the smaller superior and larger inferior divisions which enter the orbit through the *superior orbital fissure* within the tendinous ring.

In the orbit

Superior division: It passes forwards and upward lateral to the optic nerve. It supplies superior rectus and pierces this muscle to reach and supply the *levator palpebrae superioris* muscle.

Flowchart 6.6: Oculomotor nerve: functional components

Oculomotor nerve: Functional components

Cranial nerve III

Functional components	*Nuclei*	*Functions*
GSE	Motor nucleus of oculomotor nerve	Extraocular muscles
GVE	Edinger-Westphal nucleus	Sphincter pupillae Ciliary muscle
GSA	Mesencephalic nucleus of trigeminal nerve	Proprioceptive sensation from extraocular muscles

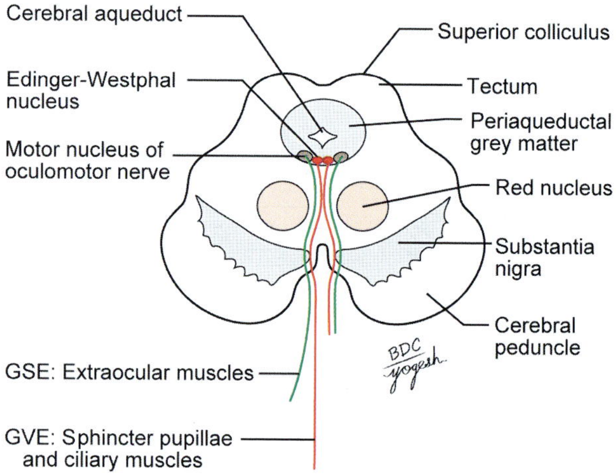

Fig. 6.11: Third cranial nerve and its nucleus

Flowchart 6.7: Oculomotor nerve

Oculomotor nerve

Origin	*Course*	*Branches*
Arises from midbrain from medial side of crus cerebri	Intraneuronal Traverses through tegmentum, red nucleus, substantia nigra Intracranial Passes through interpeduncular fossa, roof and lateral wall of cavernous sinus Enters the orbit through superior orbital fissure	Superior division - Superior rectus - Levator palpebrae superioris Inferior division - Medial rectus - Inferior rectus - Inferior oblique ↓ Branch to ciliary ganglion ↓ Ciliary muscle Sphincter pupillae

Clinical integration: Lesion of oculomotor nerve → ptosis, downward and outward gaze, dilated and fixed pupil, loss of accommodation, diplopia, proptosis

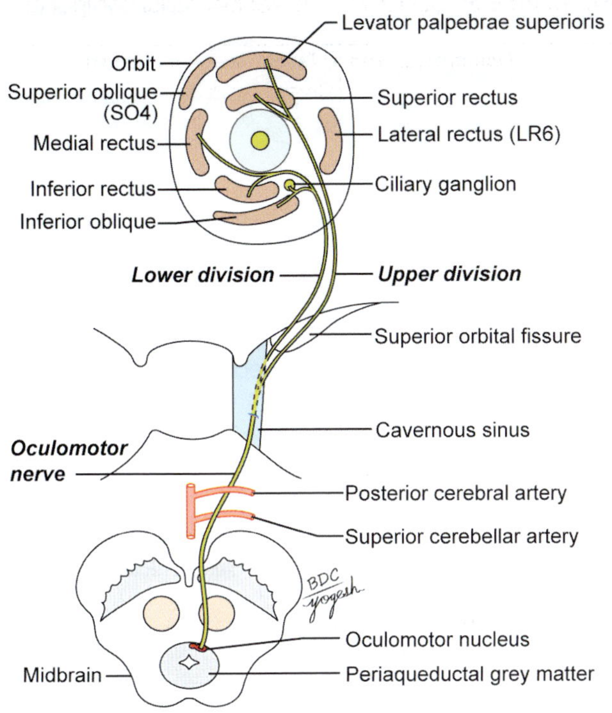

Fig. 6.12: The origin, course and the distribution of oculomotor nerve

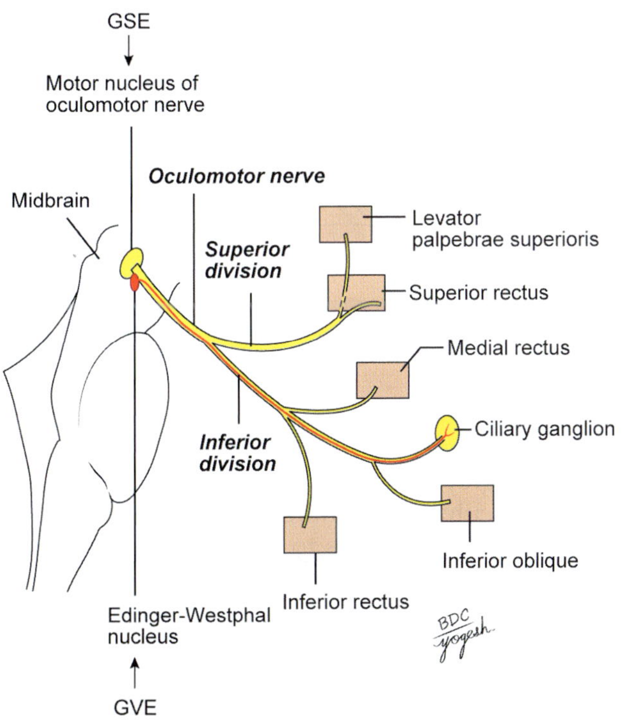

Fig. 6.13: Oculomotor nerve (schematic representation)

Inferior division: It divides into three branches to supply

1. Medial rectus
2. Inferior rectus
3. Inferior oblique.

The branch to the inferior oblique provides a communicating branch to the *ciliary ganglion*.

Competency:

AN31.5 Explain the anatomical basis of oculomotor, trochlear and abducent nerve palsies along with strabismus.

CLINICAL NEUROANATOMY

- The damage to the oculomotor nerve may be caused by compression by aneurysm of posterior cerebral or posterior communicating arteries or internal carotid artery. Complete or total damage to oculomotor nerve results into (Fig. 6.14):
  1. *Ptosis* or drooping of the of the upper eyelid ← due to paralysis of levator palpebrae superioris.
  2. *Downward and outward gaze* (*previous concept: Lateral strabismus or squint*) ← due to unopposed actions of lateral rectus and superior oblique.
  3. *Dilated and fixed pupil* ← due to paralysis of the sphincter pupillae and ciliary muscles.
  4. *Loss of accommodation* ← due to paralysis of sphincter pupillae and ciliary muscles.
  5. *Diplopia* ← due to paralysis of inferior oblique, inferior rectus, and medial rectus muscles.
  6. *Proptosis* ← due to paralysis of extraocular muscles.
- ***Weber syndrome*** (*superior alternating hemiplegia*): A midbrain lesion causing contralateral hemiplegia and ipsilateral paralysis of the third nerve is known as *Weber's syndrome*.
  1. Oculomotor nerve → lower motor neuron paralysis of extraocular muscles of same side.
  2. Crus cerebri (pyramidal fibres) → upper motor neurons paralysis of opposite side of the body.
- ***Supranuclear paralysis of the 3rd nerve*** causes loss of conjugate movement of the eyes.
- ***Compression of III nerve****:* Compression of III nerve due to extradural haematoma causes dilatation of pupil. Parasympathetic fibres lying superficial get affected first. Pupil dilates on affected side and there is little response to light.
- *Aneurysm of posterior cerebral or superior cerebellar artery:* Aneurysm of any of these two arteries may compress III nerve as it passes between them.

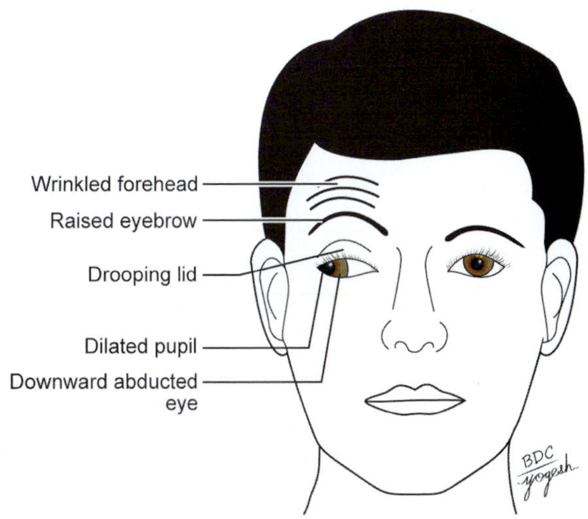

Fig. 6.14: Paralysis of right oculomotor nerve

FOURTH CRANIAL NERVE (TROCHLEAR NERVE)

Trochlear nerve supplies only the superior oblique muscle of the eyeball (Flowchart 6.8 and Fig. 6.15). It is the only cranial nerve which emerges on the dorsal aspect of the brainstem.

Functional Components

1. *General somatic efferent (GSE) fibres* arise from the *trochlear nucleus* in the midbrain at the level of inferior colliculus and it supplies the superior oblique muscle of the eyeball.
2. *General somatic afferent fibres (GSA)* fibres carry proprioception from the superior oblique muscle to the *mesencephalic nucleus of the trigeminal nerve.*

Peculiarities of Trochlear Nerve

1. It is the thinnest cranial nerve.
2. It supplies only one muscle – superior oblique.
3. It is the only cranial nerve that emerges on the dorsal aspect of the brain.
4. It is only cranial nerve whose fibres decussate in the brainstem before it emerges.
5. Its nucleus receives only the ipsilateral corticonuclear fibres.

Nucleus

The ***trochlear nucleus*** is situated in the ventromedial part of the central grey matter of midbrain at the level of inferior colliculus. Ventrally, it is closely related to the medial longitudinal bundle.

The connections of the nucleus are similar to those of the oculomotor nucleus, except for the pretectal nuclei.

Origin of Nerve

The trochlear nerve emerges on the dorsal aspect of the *midbrain,* one on either side of frenulum veli.

Course and Distribution

The course of the trochlear nerve is divided into the following parts (Fig. 6.16):

1. Intraneural course
2. Intracranial course
3. Orbital course.

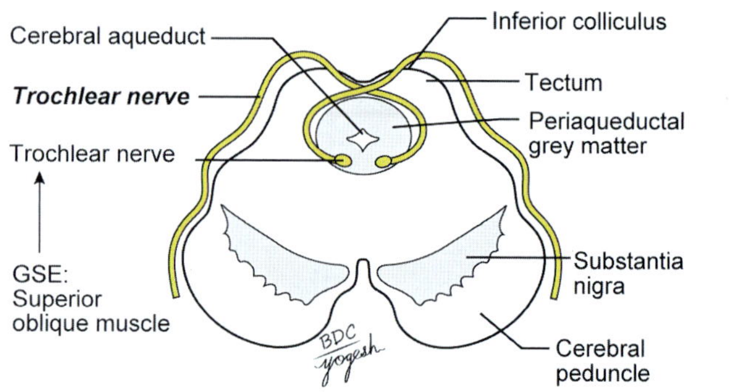

Fig. 6.15: Emerging fibres of trochlear nerves with their nuclei

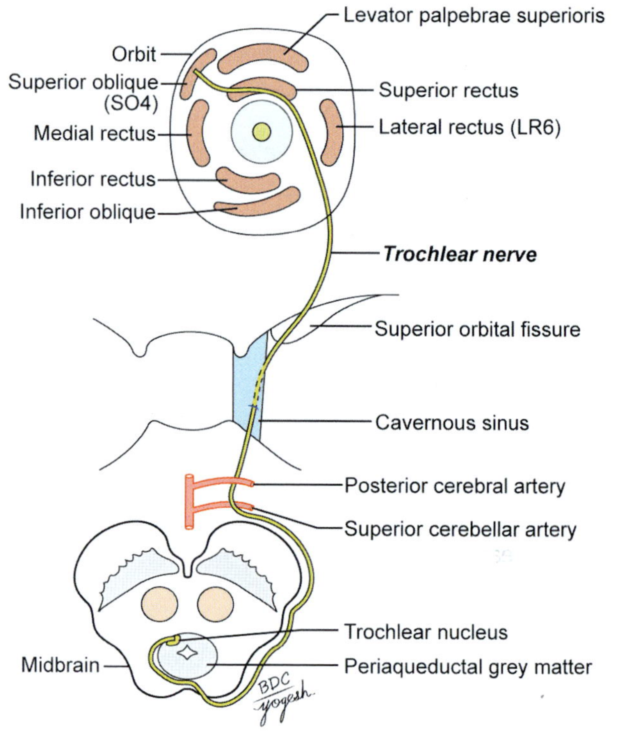

Fig. 6.16: The origin, course and the distribution of the trochlear nerve

Intraneural course: The fibres of trochlear nerve begin from the *trochlear nucleus* which located in the periaqueductal grey matter of the *midbrain* at the level of inferior colliculus. These fibres pass backwards around the grey matter and cross to opposite side behind the periaqueductal grey matter.

Flowchart 6.8: Trochlear nerve (CN IV)

Trochlear nerve (CN IV)

Functional components	***Nuclei***	***Functions***	***Origin***	***Course***	***Branches***
GSE	Trochlear nucleus	Superior oblique muscle	From dorsal aspect of midbrain	Intraneuronal - Passes backward, crosses to opposite side Intracranial - Winds around midbrain, superior cerebellar peduncle and crus cerebri - Runs in lateral wall of cavernous sinus Enters orbit through superior orbital fissure	Supplies superior oblique muscle
GSA	Mesencephalic nucleus of trigeminal nerve	Proprioception from superior oblique muscle			

Clinical integration: Lesion of trochlear nerve → extorsion eyeball weakness of downward gaze, diplopia

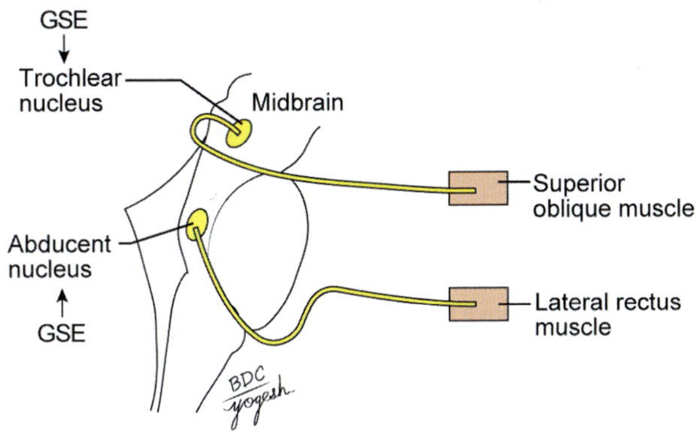

Fig. 6.17: Trochlear and abducent nerve (schematic representation)

Intracranial course: The nerve emerges on the dorsal aspect of the midbrain, one on either side of frenulum veli. Then, it winds around the superior cerebellar peduncle and cerebral peduncle, just above the pons. It passes forwards between the posterior cerebral and superior cerebellar arteries. It pierces the roof of cavernous sinus and runs forwards in its lateral wall between oculomotor and ophthalmic nerves.

Orbital course: Trochlear nerve enters the orbit through the *superior orbital fissure*, superolateral to the tendinous ring. It runs medially and forwards above the levator palpebrae superioris to enter the orbital surface of superior oblique muscle.

Branch

The trochlear nerve supplies only one muscle – *superior oblique muscle* (Fig. 6.17).

CLINICAL NEUROANATOMY

- The trochlear nerve lesion causes paralysis of the superior oblique muscle. It produces two effects as follows:
  1. *Extorsion* of eyeball and weakness of downward gaze
  2. *Diplopia* (double vision) on looking downward.
- Due to these effects, the patient faces difficulty while going downstairs or reading newspaper. To avoid diplopia, the patient tilts the head forwards and to the unaffected side.

SIXTH CRANIAL NERVE (ABDUCENT NERVE)

Abducent nerve supplies the lateral rectus muscle of the eyeball (Figs 6.18, 6.19 and Flowchart 6.9). It has a long intradural course.

Functional Components

1. *General somatic efferent* (GSE) fibres arise from *abducent nucleus* in the pons and supply the lateral rectus muscle of the eyeball.
2. *General somatic afferent* (GSA) fibres carry proprioception from the lateral rectus muscle to the *mesencephalic nucleus of trigeminal nerve*.

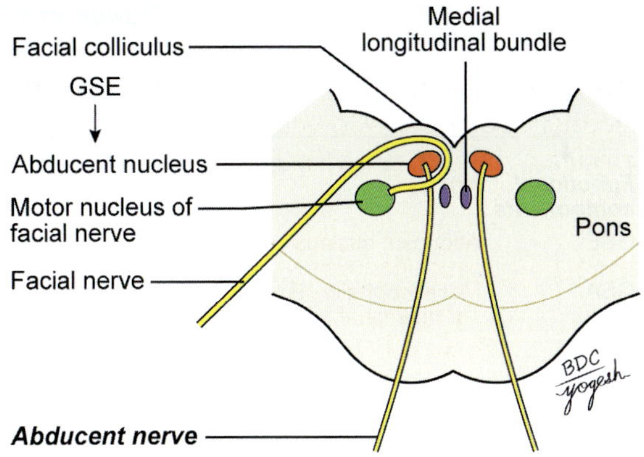

Fig. 6.18: VI nerve with its nucleus. It includes unusual course of VII nerve

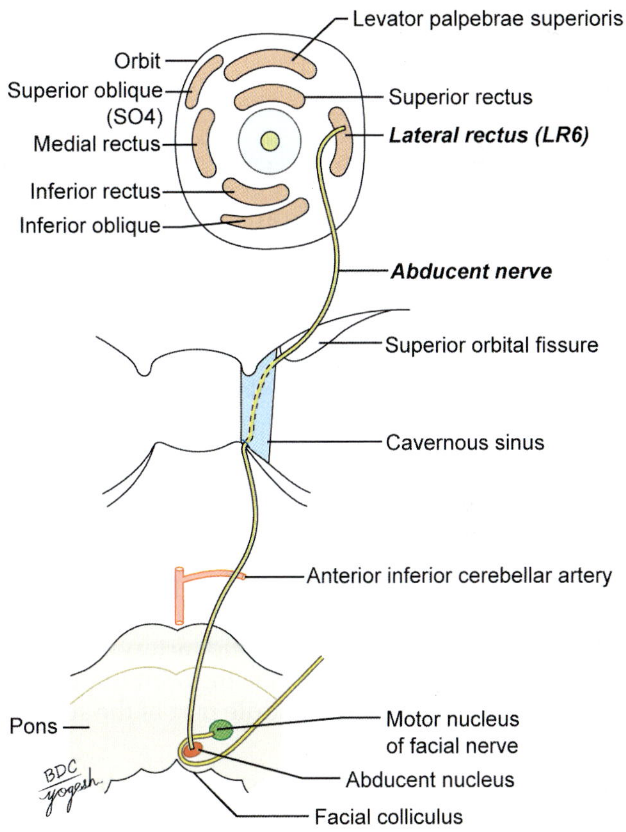

Fig. 6.19: The origin, course and distribution of the abducent nerve

Nucleus

Abducent nucleus is situated in the upper part of the floor of fourth ventricle in the lower pons, beneath the facial colliculus. Ventromedially, it is closely related to the medial longitudinal bundle. Connections of the nucleus are similar to those of the third nerve, except for the pretectal nuclei.

Origin of Nerve

The abducent nerve is attached to the brainstem between the lower border of pons and upper end of medulla (at the pontomedullary junction). Here, the nerve lies medial to the facial 7th nerve.

Flowchart 6.9: Abducent nerve (CN VI)

Abducent nerve (CN VI)

- ***Functional components***
  - GSE
  - GSA
- ***Nuclei***
  - Abducent nucleus
  - Mesencephalic nucleus of trigeminal nerve
- ***Functions***
  - Lateral rectus
  - Proprioception from lateral rectus
- ***Origin***
  - From pontomedullary junction
- ***Course***
  - Intraneuronal
    - passes through trapezoid body and basilar part of pons
  - Intracranial
    - Emerges above pyramid
    - Runs upward and turns sharply forward across the petrous part of temporal bone
    - Traverses through cavernous sinus
  - Enters orbit through superior orbital fissure
- ***Branches***
  - Supplies lateral rectus muscle

Clinical integration: Lesion of abducent nerve→ inability to abduct the eye, exotropia, diplopia on looking toward affected side.

Course and Distribution

The course of abducent nerve is divided into three parts:

1. Intraneuronal course
2. Intracranial course
3. Intraorbital course.

Intraneuronal course: The nucleus of abducent nerve is located in the pons, in the floor of 4th ventricle deep to the facial colliculus. The fibres arising from the nucleus run ventrally and downwards through the trapezoid body and basilar part of the pons.

Intracranial course: Abducent nerve has the longest intracranial course. It emerges at the pontomedullary junction, just at the upper border of pyramid of the medulla. Then, the nerve runs upward, forward and laterally in front of pons and dorsal to the anterior inferior cerebellar artery. Abducent nerve pierces the dura mater lateral to the dorsal sellae to enter the cavernous sinus. Here, the nerve takes sharp forwards turn across the upper border of petrous part of temporal bone. The nerve traverses the cavernous sinus, at first lateral to the internal carotid artery and then inferolateral to the artery. It enters the orbit through the tendinous ring, through the middle part of the superior orbital fissure.

Intraorbital course: In the orbit, the nerve lies below the two divisions of oculomotor nerve and nasociliary nerve. Then the nerve runs forwards and laterally over the ocular surface of the lateral rectus muscle and supplies this muscle.

Branch

The abducent nerve supplies only 1 muscle – lateral rectus.

CLINICAL NEUROANATOMY

- ***Lesions of abducent nerve:*** The abducent nerve is damaged commonly in the increased intracranial pressure due to the following reasons:
  1. Long intracranial course
  2. Sharp bending over the sharp upper border of petrous temporal bone.

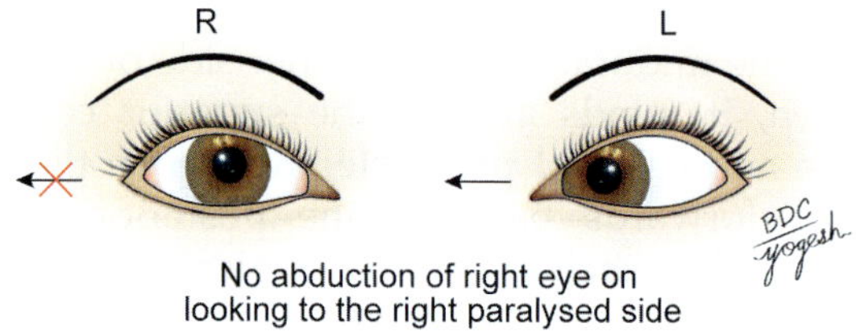

Fig. 6.20: Paralysis of right sixth nerve

  3. Due to these reasons, the abducent nerve is stretched due to the descent of brainstem in the increased intracranial pressure.

Effects of lesions: The paralysis of abducent nerve results in the paralysis of the lateral rectus muscle which causes (Fig. 6.20):

1. Inability to abduct the eye
2. Exotropia (convergent squint) due to unopposed action of the medial rectus
3. Diplopia on looking toward the affected side.

FIFTH CRANIAL NERVE (TRIGEMINAL NERVE)

The fifth cranial nerve (trigeminal nerve) is the largest cranial nerve. It comprises three branches, two of which are purely sensory and third, the largest branch is mixed nerve. Trigeminal nerve is the nerve of first brachial arch (Fig. 6.21 and Flowchart 6.10).

Functional Components and Nuclei

1. *Special visceral efferent* (*SVE*) *fibres* from *motor nucleus of trigeminal nerve* (located in upper part of pons). They supply the muscle of first pharyngeal arch.
2. *General somatic afferent* (*GSA*) *fibres* terminate in three nuclei:
   a. *Spinal nucleus of Vth nerve*: It extends from pons to second cervical spinal segment. It receives pain and temperature sensation from most of the face.
   b. *Principal sensory nucleus of Vth nerve*: It lies in dorsolateral region of tegmentum of upper part of the pons. It receives touch and pressure sensations from face and head.

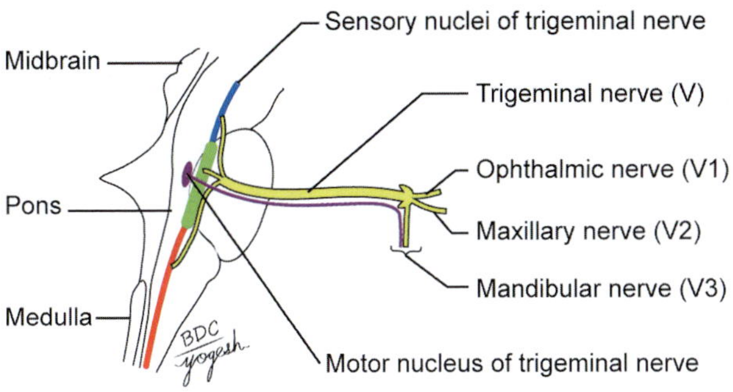

Fig. 6.21: Nuclei of trigeminal nerve

Flowchart 6.10: Functional components and nuclei of trigeminal nerve

Functional components and nuclei of trigeminal nerve

- ***Special visceral efferent (SVE)***
  - Motor nucleus of Vth nerve
  - Supplies the muscles of 1st pharyngeal arch
- ***General somatic afferent (GSA)***
  - ***Spinal nucleus of Vth nerve***: Pain and temperature sensations of face
  - ***Principal sensory nucleus***: Touch and pressure sensations from face and head
  - ***Mesencephalic nucleus***: Proprioceptive impulses from muscles of mastication, TMJ, teeth

c. *Mesencephalic nucleus of Vth nerve*: It lies in the periaqueductal grey matter in the midbrain. It receives proprioceptive impulses from muscles of mastication, temporomandibular joint and teeth.

Origin of Nerve

The trigeminal nerve arises by two roots from the pons at its junction with the middle cerebellar peduncle. The roots are:

1. Large, lateral sensory root
2. Smaller, medial motor root.

Course and Distribution

The trigeminal nerve runs forwards and laterally over the apex of petrous part of temporal bone to enter the middle cranial fossa. It forms the enlargement called *trigeminal ganglion*.

Branches:

1. Ophthalmic nerve
2. Maxillary nerve
3. Mandibular nerve.

Ganglia Related to Trigeminal Nerve

Four peripheral parasympathetic ganglia are topographically related to trigeminal nerve:

1. *Ciliary ganglion* related to occulomotor nerve (branch to inferior oblique muscle)
2. *Pterygopalatine ganglion* is related to maxillary nerve
3. *Otic ganglion* related to mandibular nerve
4. *Submandibular ganglion* is related to lingual branch of mandibular nerve.

Ophthalmic Nerve Division (Sensory)

The ophthalmic (V1) nerve is the smallest branch of trigeminal nerve (others are maxillary and mandibular nerves). The ophthalmic nerve is purely *sensory* nerve (Figs 6.22 a and b). It arises from the anterolateral aspect of trigeminal ganglion in the middle cranial fossa. Then the nerve enters the lateral wall of the cavernous sinus and runs forwards below the trochlear nerve and above the maxillary nerve. In the lateral wall of cavernous sinus, the ophthalmic nerve divides into three terminal branches: Lacrimal, frontal, and nasociliary (*Mnemonic*: LFN). All the branches enter the orbit through the superior orbital fissure.

Branches of Ophthalmic Nerve

1. Frontal nerve:
   a. Supratrochlear: Upper eyelid, conjunctiva and lower part of forehead
   b. Supraorbital: Frontal air sinus, upper eyelid, forehead and scalp till vertex
2. Nasociliary nerve:
   a. Branch to ciliary ganglion
   b. 2–3 long ciliary nerves: Sensory to eyeball
   c. Posterior ethmoidal: Sphenoidal air sinus, posterior ethmoidal air sinuses
   d. Intratrochlear: Both eyelids, side of nose and lacrimal sac
   e. Anterior ethmoidal:
      - Middle and anterior ethmoidal sinuses
      - Medial internal nasal
      - Lateral internal nasal
      - External nasal: Skin of ala of vestibule and tip of nose.
3. Lacrimal nerve:
   a. Branch to upper eyelid
   b. Secretomotor fibres to the lacrimal gland.

Maxillary Nerve Division (Sensory)

It is a branch of trigeminal nerve that arises from the trigeminal ganglion. It arises from the trigeminal ganglion, runs forwards in the lateral wall of the cavernous sinus below the ophthalmic nerve. It leaves the middle cranial fossa by passing through the foramen rotundum. Next, the nerve crosses the upper part of pterygopalatine fossa, beyond which it is continued as the *infraorbital nerve*.

Branches of Maxillary Nerve (Fig. 6.23)

In the middle cranial fossa

Meningeal branch.

In the pterygopalatine fossa

1. Ganglionic branches
2. Posterior superior alveolar nerves
3. Zygomatic nerve
   a. Zygomaticotemporal nerve
   b. Zygomaticofacial nerve.

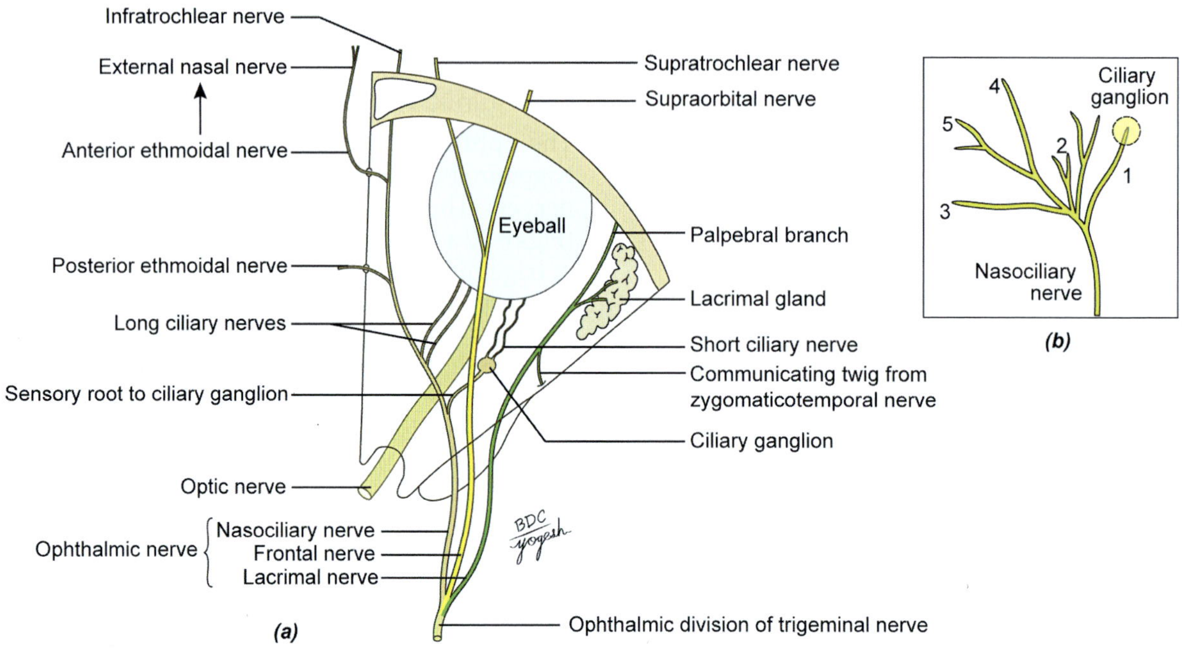

Figs 6.22a and b: (a) Branches and distribution of the ophthalmic nerve and (b) schematic representation (1. Branch to ciliary ganglion, 2. Long ciliary nerves, 3. Posterior ethmoidal nerve, 4. Infratrochlear nerve, 5. Anterior ethmoidal nerve)

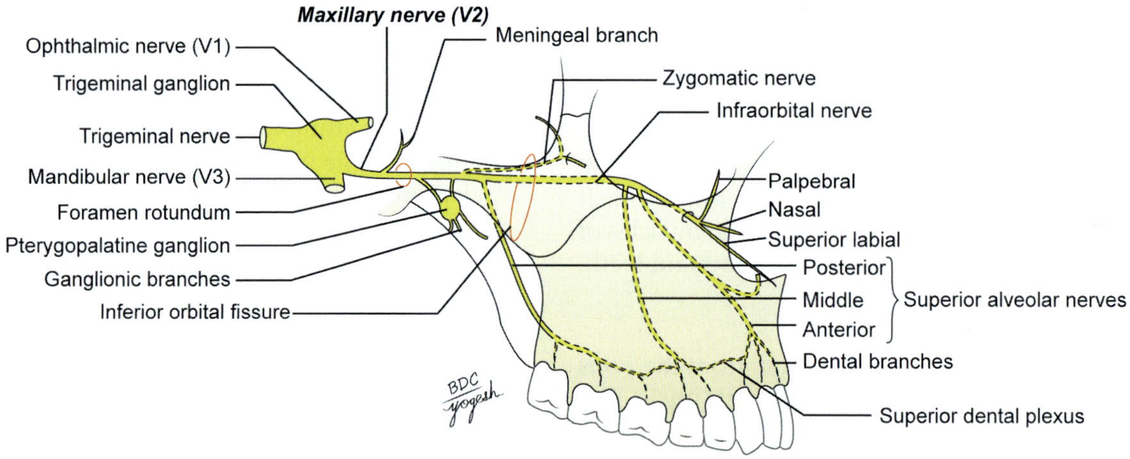

Fig. 6.23: Branches and distribution of the maxillary nerve

Branches through infraorbital nerve

A. *In the infraorbital canal:*

1. Middle superior alveolar nerve
2. Anterior superior alveolar nerve
   a. Dental branches
   b. Nasal branches

B. *On the face:*

1. Palpebral branch
2. Nasal branch
3. Superior labial branch.

Mandibular Nerve Division (Sensory and Motor)

It is the largest branch of trigeminal nerve. It consists of sensory and motor fibres. It is the nerve of 1st pharyngeal arch. The mandibular nerve begins in the middle cranial fossa by two roots: Sensory root from the trigeminal ganglion, and the motor root from the pons. The motor root is smaller, and it lies deep to the trigeminal ganglion and the sensory root.

Both the roots pass downwards through the foramen ovale and unite immediately below the foramen to form the main nerve trunk. The mandibular nerve lies in the infratemporal fossa. Here, it lies on the tensor veli palatini, deep to the lateral pterygoid muscle. To visualize the main trunk, remove the upper head of lateral pterygoid muscle carefully. It divides into a small anterior and large posterior trunk (Fig. 6.24).

Branches of Mandibular Nerve

Branches from main trunk

1. Nervus spinosus (meningeal branch)
2. Nerve to medial pterygoid: It supplies—
   a. Medial pterygoid
   b. Tensor veli palatini
   c. Tensor tympani

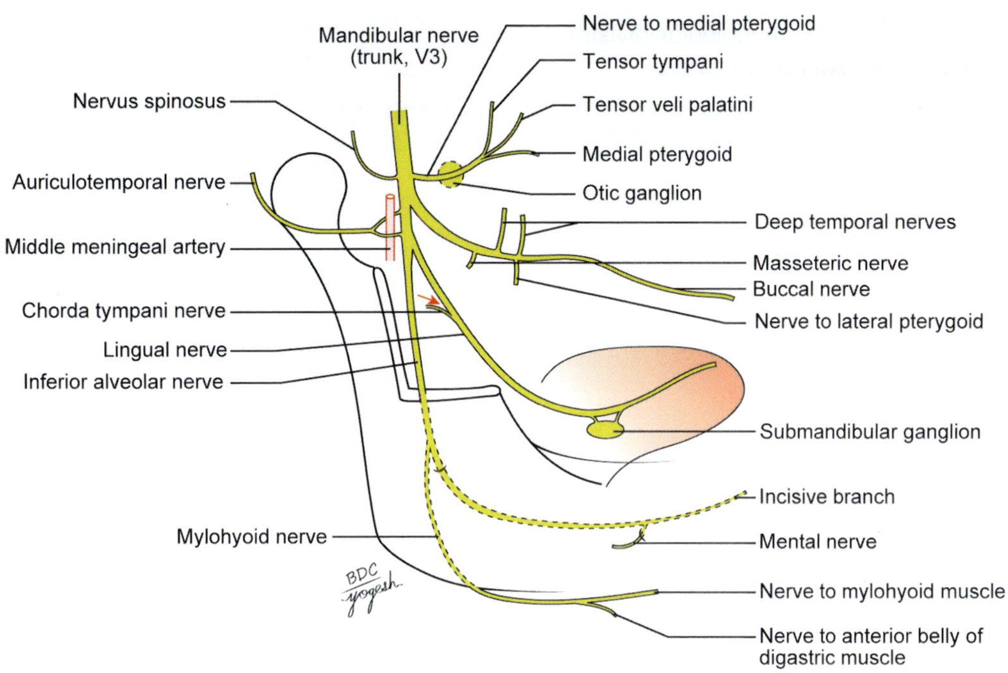

Fig. 6.24: Course and distribution of the mandibular nerve

From anterior division

1. Masseteric nerves – for masseter
2. Deep temporal nerves – for temporalis
3. Nerve to lateral pterygoid
4. Buccal nerve for skin of cheek and buccal mucosa.

From posterior division

1. Auriculotemporal nerve
   a. Auricular branch
   b. Temporal branch
   c. Parasympathetic fibres from otic ganglion
2. Lingual nerve
   a. Sensory to anterior 2/3rd of tongue
   b. Via chorda tympani – carries special sensation (taste) from anterior 2/3rd of tongue and parasympathetic fibres to submandibular and sublingual glands.
3. Inferior alveolar nerve
   a. Mylohyoid nerve – for mylohyoid and anterior belly of digastric
   b. Branches to lower teeth and gum
   c. Mental nerve – to skin of chin, lower lip, gum, and canine and incisor teeth.

CLINICAL NEUROANATOMY

- The separate location of main sensory nucleus and spinal nucleus accounts for ***dissociated sensory loss***, i.e. low pontine or medullary lesion will result in loss of pain and temperature sensation while light sensation is preserved. Low pontine, medullary and cervical lesions produce a characteristic '***onion skin***' distribution of pinprick and temperature loss (Fig. 6.25).

Sensory examination

- An ascending lesion spares the openings of nose and mouth (muzzle area) till last.
- Test with pinprick, temperature and light touch over each side of the whole face.
- The sensations in three branches of V nerve can be tested clinically.

Motor examination

- Look for wasting or thinning of temporalis muscle. There may be 'hollowing out' of the temporal fossa.
- Ask patient to press upper and lower teeth together and feel for temporalis and masseter muscles.
- Ask patient to open the mouth. If pterygoid muscles are weak, the jaw would deviate to weak side as the normal muscles will push the jaw to the weak side.

In injury to

- *Ophthalmic nerve:* There is loss of corneal blink reflex (Fig. 6.26) This reflex is mediated by V1 which is afferent pathway and VII nerve which subserves as efferent pathway.
- *Maxillary nerve:* There is loss of sneeze reflex. This branch is the afferent path of sneeze reflex. Efferent pathway of sneeze reflex is nucleus ambiguus, respiratory centre in medulla oblongata, phrenic nerve nucleus, motor cells of spinal cord for intercostal muscles.
- *Mandibular nerve:* There is loss of jaw jerk reflex (Fig. 6.27). Flaccid paralysis of muscles of mastication in injury of mandibular nerve leading to decrease strength for biting. Hypoacusis, i.e. partial deafness to low-pitched sounds due to paralysis of tensor tympani muscle.

Trigeminal neuralgia

- Pain along the distribution of the nerve which is caused due to local lesion or unknown cause. The principal disease affecting sensory root of V nerve is characterized by attacks of severe pain in the area of distribution of maxillary or mandibular divisions. Maxillary nerve is most frequently involved.

- The trigeminal ganglion harbours the herpes simplex virus causing herpes (shingles) in the distribution of the nerve.

Frey's syndrome

1. Penetrating wounds of parotid gland may damage both auriculotemporal and great auricular nerves.
2. During regeneration, the two nerves join with each other.
3. While eating, drops of perspiration appear on skin over parotid gland.

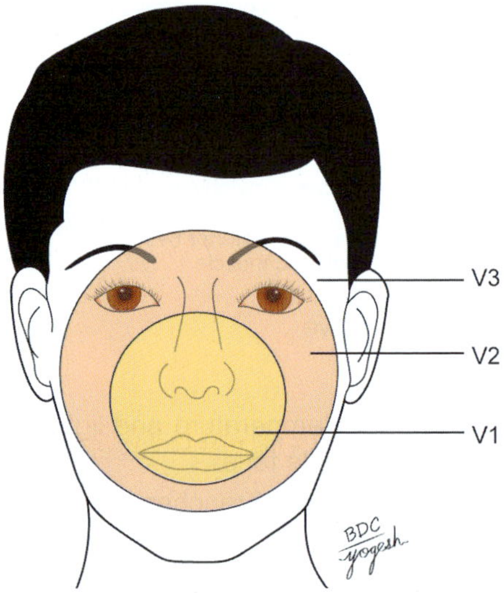

Fig. 6.25: Brainstem lesion of trigeminal nerve (V1: Ophthalmic, V2: Maxillary, V3: Mandibular branches)

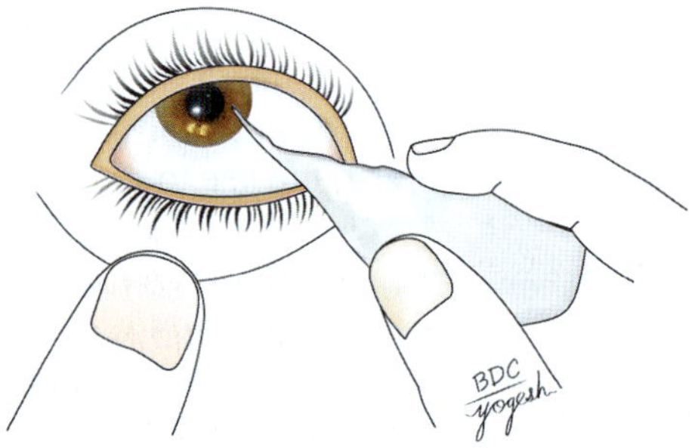

Fig. 6.26: Testing the corneal blink reflex

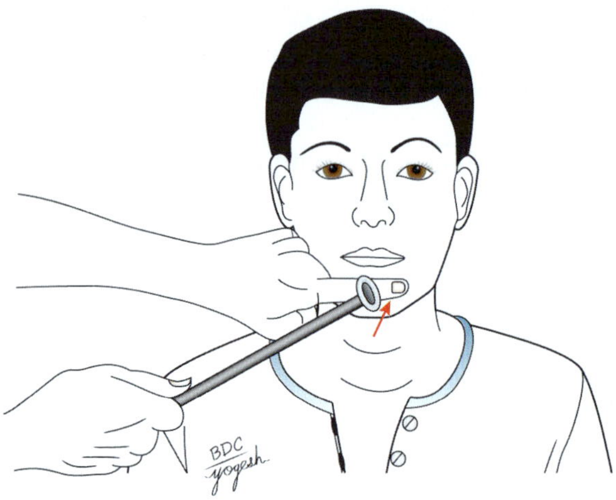

Fig. 6.27: Elicitation of jaw jerk reflex

SEVENTH CRANIAL NERVE (FACIAL NERVE)

Facial nerve is the nerve of the second branchial arch. It supplies mainly the muscles of facial expressions (Figs 6.28 to 6.31 and Flowchart 6.11 and 6.12).

Functional Components

1. *Special visceral efferent* (*SVE*) *fibres* arise from *motor nucleus of facial nerve* and supplies the muscles derived from the 2nd pharyngeal arch.
2. *General visceral efferent* (*GVE*) *fibres* are preganglionic parasympathetic fibres. They arise from lacrimatory and superior salivatory nucleus of pons and relay at the pterygopalatine and submandibular ganglia for lacrimation and salivation, respectively. The postganglionic fibres of the pterygopalatine ganglion supply the lacrimal gland through zygomatic branch of trigeminal nerve. The postganglionic fibres arising from the submandibular ganglion supply the submandibular and sublingual salivary glands.
3. *Special visceral afferent* (*SVA*) *fibres* carry the taste sensations from anterior two-thirds of the tongue except vallate papillae to the upper part of the nucleus of tractus solitarius. The cell bodies of these fibres lie in the geniculate ganglion.
4. *General somatic afferent* (*GSA*) *fibres* have their cell bodies in the geniculate ganglion. The peripheral processes of these cells innervate part of the skin of the external ear, while the central processes terminate in the spinal nucleus of trigeminal nerve.

Note: The motor nucleus of the facial nerve lies deep in the reticular formation of the lower pons. The part of the nucleus that supplies muscles of the upper part of the face receives corticonuclear fibres from the motor cortex of both the right and left sides. In contrast, the part of the nucleus that supplies muscles of the lower part of the face, receives corticonuclear fibres only from the opposite cerebral hemisphere.

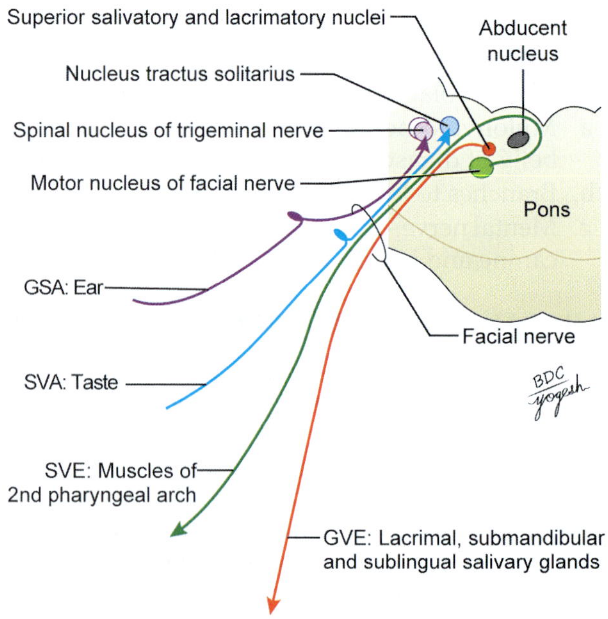

Fig. 6.28: Facial nerve nuclei (transverse section passing through the pons, at the level of facial colliculus)

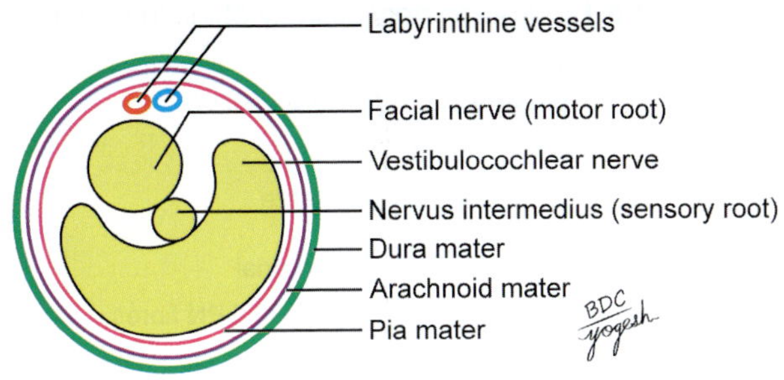

Fig. 6.29: Structures in the left internal acoustic meatus

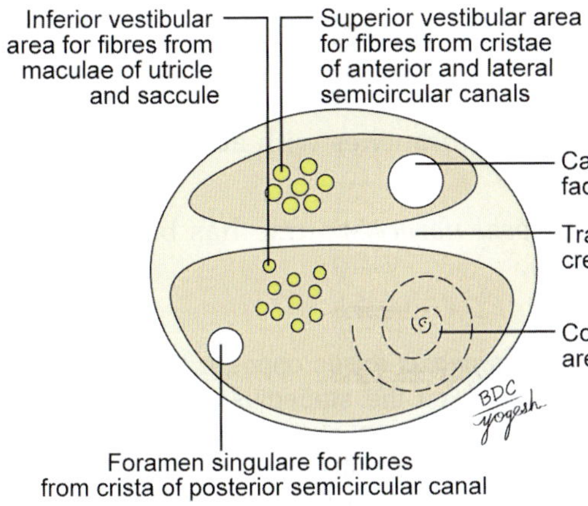

Fig. 6.30: Some features seen on the fundus of the left internal acoustic meatus

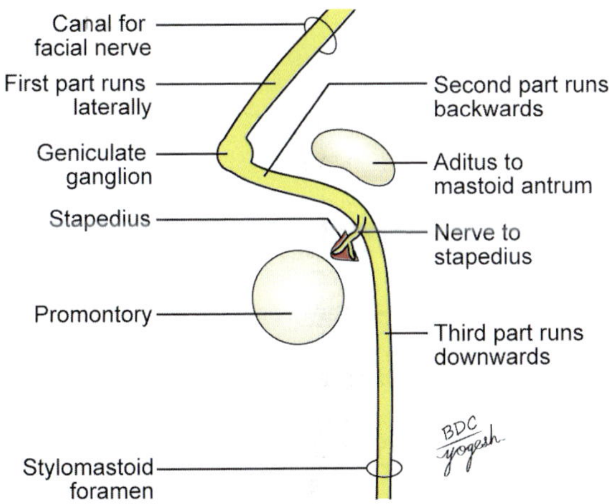

Fig. 6.31: Course of facial nerve

Origin of Nerve

The facial nerve is attached to the brainstem between the lower border of pons and upper end of medulla (at the pontomedullary junction). Here, the nerve lies lateral to abducent nerve and medial to the 8th nerve (Fig. 6.28).

The facial nerve arises by two roots – medial larger motor root and lateral smaller sensory root (***nervus intermedius*** of Weisberg). The roots enter the internal auditory meatus along with vestibulocochlear nerve and labyrinthine vessels. At the lateral end of meatus, two roots unite to form the trunk of the facial nerve.

Flowchart 6.11: Functional components and nuclei of facial nerve

Functional components and nuclei of facial nerve

SVE	***GVE***	***SVA***	***GSA***
Motor nucleus of facial nerve Supplies muscles of 2nd pharyngeal arch	Lacrimatory nucleus ↓ Parasympathetic to lacrimal gland ——— Superior salivatory nucleus ↓ Parasympathetic to submandibular and sublingual glands	Nucleus tractus solitarius Taste sensation from anterior 2/3rd of tongue except vallate papillae	Spinal nucleus of trigeminal nerve for skin of external ear

Flowchart 6.12: Facial nerve: Origin, course and distribution

Facial nerve: Origin, course and distribution

Origin	***Course***	***Branches***
From brainstem at pontomedullary junction 2 roots: - Medial larger motor root - Lateral small nervus intermedius or sensory root	Pontomedullary junction ↓ Internal acoustic meatus ↓ Facial canal (geniculate ganglion) ↓ Stylomastoid foramen ↓ within parotid gland	Greater petrosal nerve: Secretomotor fibres to lacrimal, nasal, palatal glands Nerve to stapedius Chorda tympani nerve: - Parasympathetic to submandibular and sublingual glands - Taste sensation from anterior 2/3rd of tongue except vallate papillae Posterior auricular nerve: To occipitalis, posterior auricular muscles Nerve to posterior belly of digastric and stylohyoid Terminal branches: Temporal, zygomatic, buccal, marginal mandibular and cervical

Course and Relations

1. *In the meatus,* the motor root lies in a groove on the eighth nerve, with the sensory root intervening. Here the seventh and eighth nerves are accompanied by the labyrinthine vessels. At the bottom or fundus of the meatus, the two roots, sensory and motor, fuse to form a single trunk, which lies in the petrous temporal bone (Figs 6.29 and 6.30).
2. Within the canal, the course of the nerve can be divided into three parts by two bends (Fig. 6.31).

The first part is directed laterally above the vestibule; the second part runs backwards in relation to the medial wall of the middle ear, above the promontory. The third part is directed vertically downwards behind the promontory.

The first bend at the junction of the first and second parts is sharp. It lies over the anterosuperior part of the promontory, and is also called the *genu*. The ***geniculate ganglion*** of the nerve is so-called because it lies on the genu. The second bend is gradual, and lies between the promontory and the aditus to the mastoid antrum.

3. The facial nerve leaves the skull by passing through the stylomastoid foramen.
4. In its ***extracranial course***, the facial nerve crosses the lateral side of the base of the styloid process. It enters the posteromedial surface of the parotid gland, and runs forwards through the gland crossing the retromandibular vein and the external carotid artery. Behind the neck of the mandible, it divides into its five terminal branches which emerge along the anterior border of the parotid gland.

Branches and Distribution (Fig. 6.32)

1. Within the bony facial canal:
   a. Greater petrosal nerve
   b. Nerve to the stapedius
   c. Chorda tympani.
2. At its exit from the stylomastoid foramen:
   a. Posterior auricular
   b. Digastric
   c. Stylohyoid.
3. Terminal branches within the parotid gland:
   a. Temporal
   b. Zygomatic
   c. Buccal
   d. Marginal mandibular
   e. Cervical.

Flowchart 6.13: Tracing nerve supply of lacrimal gland

Greater petrosal nerve (GPN)
Joins ↓
Deep petrosal nerve
↓
Nerve of pterygoid canal
↓ Relay of GPN fibres
Postganglionic fibres for lacrimal gland join zygomatic nerve
↓
Pass through communicating branch
↓
Lacrimal nerve
↓
Lacrimal gland

4. Communicating branches with adjacent cranial and spinal nerves.

Greater petrosal nerve—course has been traced in Flowchart 6.13.

Note:

The *nerve to the stapedius* arises opposite the pyramid of the middle ear, and supplies the stapedius muscle. The muscle dampens excessive vibrations of the stapes caused by high-pitched sounds. In paralysis of the muscle, even normal sounds appear too loud and is known as *hyperacusis*.

The ***chorda tympani nerve*** arises in the vertical part of the facial canal about 6 mm above the stylomastoid foramen. It runs upwards and forwards in a bony canal. It enters the middle ear and runs forwards in close relation to the tympanic membrane. It leaves

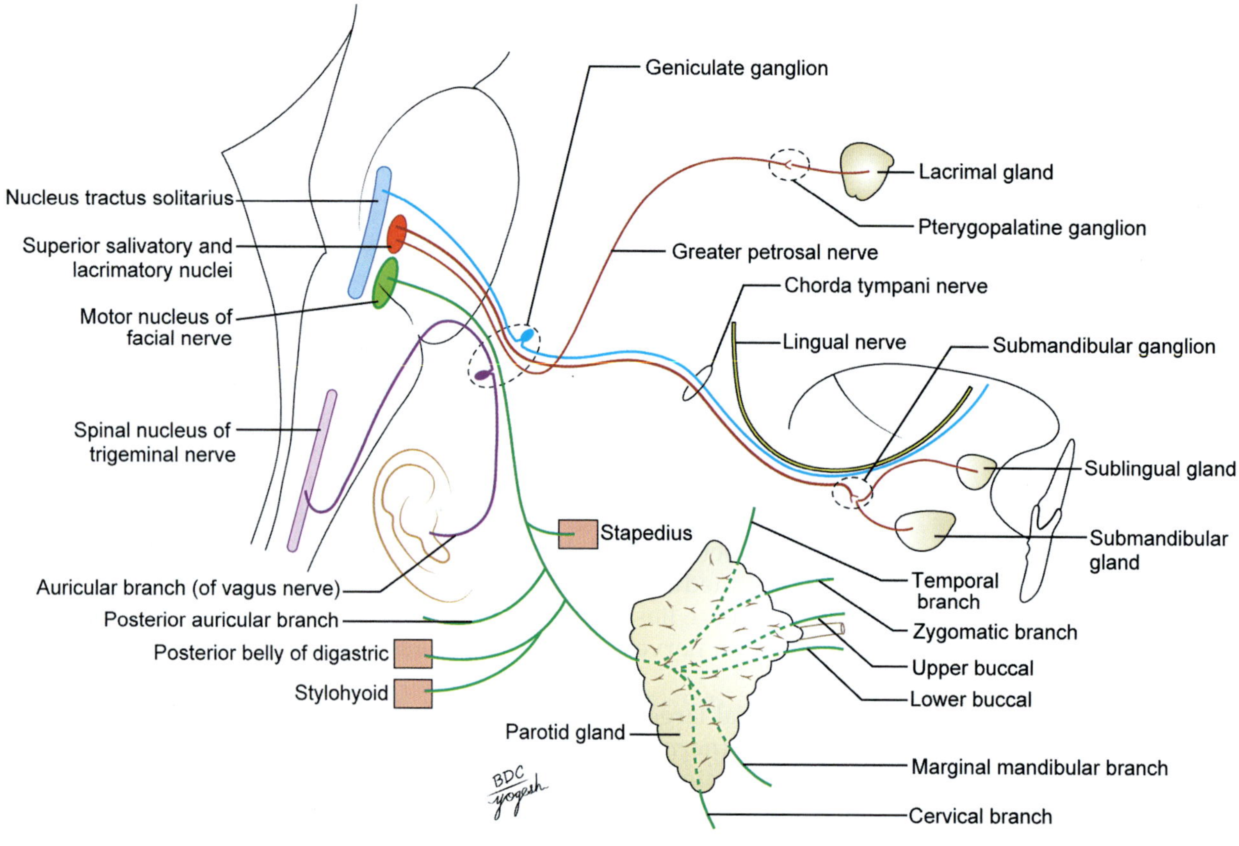

Fig. 6.32: Distribution of functional components of VII nerve

the middle ear by passing through the petrotympanic fissure. It then passes medial to the spine of the sphenoid and enters the infratemporal fossa. Here it joins the lingual nerve through which chorda tympani nerve is distributed. It carries:

a. Preganglionic secretomotor fibres to the submandibular ganglion for supply of the submandibular and sublingual salivary glands.
b. Taste fibres from the anterior two-thirds of the tongue except circumvallate papillae.

The *posterior auricular nerve* arises just below the stylomastoid foramen. It ascends between the mastoid process and the external acoustic meatus, and supplies:

a. Auricularis posterior
b. Occipitalis
c. Intrinsic muscles on the back of auricle.

The *digastric branch* arises close to the previous nerve. It is short and supplies the posterior belly of the digastric.

The *stylohyoid branch* arises with the digastric branch, is long and supplies the stylohyoid muscle.

The *temporal branches* cross the zygomatic arch and supply:

a. Auricularis anterior
b. Auricularis superior
c. Intrinsic muscles on the lateral side of the ear
d. Frontalis
e. Orbicularis oculi
f. Corrugator supercilii.

The *zygomatic branches* run across the zygomatic bone and supply the lower part of orbicularis oculi.

The *buccal branches* are two in number. The upper buccal branch runs above the parotid duct and the lower buccal branch below the duct. They supply muscles in that vicinity especially the buccinator.

The *marginal mandibular branch* runs below the angle of the mandible deep to the platysma. It crosses the body of the mandible and supplies muscles of the lower lip and chin.

The *cervical branch* emerges from the apex of the parotid gland, and runs downwards and forwards in the neck to supply the platysma.

Communicating branches: For effective coordination between the movements of the muscles of the first, second and third branchial arches, the motor nerves of the three arches communicate with each other. The facial nerve also communicates with the sensory nerves distributed over its motor territory.

CLINICAL NEUROANATOMY

- ***Bell's palsy:*** Injury to the facial nerve near or outside the stylomastoid foramen produces Bell's palsy (Fig. 6.33). It is lower motor neuron type of paralysis of muscles of facial expressions. It may be due to viral infection or unknown cause.

  Features: The following features are present on the side of paralysis:

  1. Facial asymmetry due to unopposed action of muscle of unaffected side.
  2. Loss of horizontal wrinkles of forehead due to paralysis of occipitofrontalis muscle.
  3. Inability to close the eye and widening of palpebral fissure due to paralysis of orbicularis oculi.
  4. *Epiphora* (spilling of tears on the face) due to paralysis of orbicularis oculi.
  5. Drooping of angle of mouth toward affected side and drooling of saliva due to paralysis of orbicularis oris.
  6. Inability of whistling and accumulation of food in vestibule of mouth due to paralysis of buccinator.
  7. Loss of nasolabial furrow due to paralysis of levator labii superioris alaeque nasi.

  [***Mnemonics***: ***BELL'S Palsy:*** **B**link reflex abnormal, **E**ar ache, **L**acrimation (deficient), **L**oss of taste in anterior two-thirds of tongue, **S**udden onset, **Palsy** of muscles supplied by VII nerve, all symptoms are ipsilateral]

  Note: The facial muscles of the upper half of the face are controlled by both the cerebral hemispheres. The damage to one cerebral hemisphere or the fibres from it to the nucleus of facial nerve cause *supranuclear palsy of facial nerve*. In this type of paralysis, the muscles of the upper half of the face remain unaffected.

- For clinical testing of the facial nerve, and for different types of facial paralysis—infranuclear.

  Facial nerve palsy in newborn: The mastoid process is absent in newborn and stylomastoid foramen is superficial. Manipulation of baby's head during delivery may damage the VII nerve. This leads to paralysis of facial muscles especially the buccinator, required for sucking the milk.

  Crocodile tears syndrome: Lacrimation during eating occurs due to aberrant regeneration after trauma.

- In case of damage to facial nerve proximal to geniculate ganglia, regenerating fibres for submandibular salivary gland grow in endoneurial sheaths of preganglionic secretomotor fibres supplying the lacrimal gland. That is why patient lacrimates while eating food.

  Ramsay-Hunt syndrome: Involvement of geniculate ganglia by herpes zoster results in this syndrome.

  It shows following symptoms:

  a. Hyperacusis
  b. Loss of lacrimation
  c. Loss of sensation of taste in anterior two-thirds of tongue
  d. Bell's palsy and lack of salivation
  e. Vesicles on the auricle.

Ganglia Related to Facial Nerve

The ganglia associated with the facial nerve are as follows:

1. The ***geniculate ganglion*** is located on the first bend of the facial nerve, in relation to the medial wall of the middle ear. It is a *sensory ganglion*. The taste fibres present in the nerve are peripheral processes of pseudounipolar neurons present in the geniculate ganglion.
2. The ***submandibular ganglion*** is a *parasympathetic ganglion* for relay of secretomotor fibres to the submandibular and sublingual glands. The preganglionic fibres come from the chorda tympani nerve (Table 6.3). It is described in Chapter 7 of *BD Chaurasia's Human Anatomy, Volume 3*.

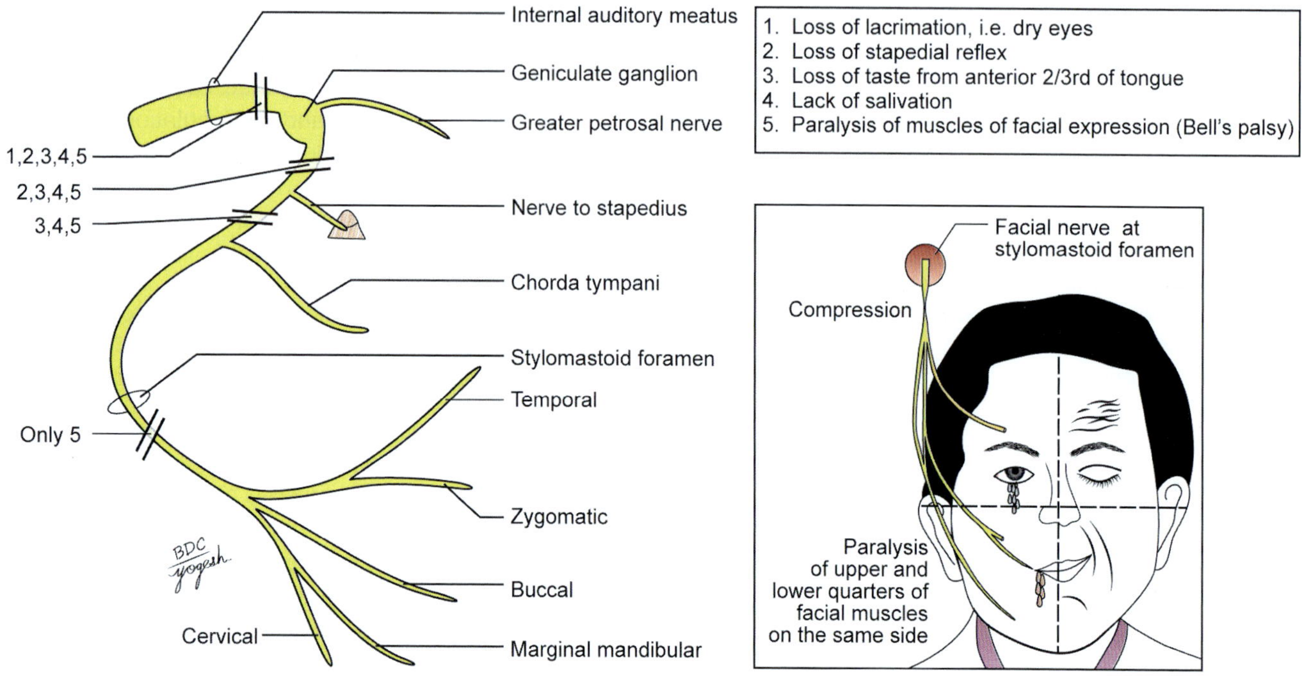

Fig. 6.33: Symptoms according to the level of injury to cranial nerve VII; Inset showing Bell's palsy

TABLE 6.3: Connections of parasympathetic ganglia

Ganglia	*Sensory root*	*Sympathetic root*	*Secretomotor parasympathetic root*	*Motor root*	*Distribution*
Ciliary	From nasociliary nerve	Plexus along ophthalmic artery	Edinger-Westphal nucleus → oculomotor nerve → nerve to inferior oblique	—	Ciliaris muscles Sphincter pupillae
Otic	Branch from auriculotemporal nerve	Plexus along middle meningeal artery	Inferior salivatory nucleus → glossopharyngeal nerve → tympanic branch → tympanic plexus → lesser petrosal nerve	Branch from nerve to medial pterygoid	Secretomotor to parotid gland via auriculotemporal nerve Tensor veli palatini and tensor tympani via nerve to medial pterygoid (unrelayed)
Pterygopalatine	Two branches from maxillary nerve	Deep petrosal from plexus around internal carotid artery	Lacrimatory nucleus → nervus intermedius → facial nerve → geniculate ganglion → greater petrosal nerve + deep petrosal = nerve of pterygoid canal	—	Mucous glands of nose, paranasal sinuses, palate, nasopharynx Some fibres pass through zygomatic nerve → zygomatico nerve temporal nerve → communicating branch to lacrimal nerve → lacrimal gland
Submandibular	Two branches from lingual nerve	Branch from plexus around	Superior salivatory nucleus → facial nerve → chorda tympani facial artery → joins the lingual nerve	—	Submandibular, sublingual and anterior lingual glands

3. The ***pterygopalatine ganglion*** is also a *parasympathetic ganglion*. Secretomotor fibres meant for the lacrimal gland relay in this ganglion. The fibres reach the ganglion from the nerve to the pterygoid canal (Table 6.3). It is described in Chapter 15 of *BD Chaurasia's Human Anatomy, Volume 3*.

EIGHTH CRANIAL NERVE (VESTIBULOCOCHLEAR NERVE)

This nerve comprises hearing and vestibular parts.

Functional Components

Special somatic afferent fibres: They carry sensory information of:
1. Equilibrium to the vestibular nucleus of brainstem.
2. Hearing to the dorsal and ventral cochlear nuclei located in pons.

Ganglion

1. ***Vestibular or Scarpa's ganglion*** is located on the vestibular nerve in the lateral part of the internal acoustic meatus. It consists of bipolar neurons.
2. ***Cochlear or spiral ganglion*** is located in modiolus. It also consists bipolar neurons.

Origin Nerve

Vestibulocochlear nerve is attached to the pontomedullary junction, lateral to the facial nerve.

Course and Relations

Vestibulocochlear nerve emerges at the pontomedullary junction and runs laterally to enter internal acoustic meatus along with facial nerve and labyrinthine vessels.
1. ***Vestibular part*:** As it is sensory nerve, the nerve begins from the macula of utricle, ampullary crests of semicircular canals, and macula of saccule. These fibres are peripheral processes of bipolar neurons of vestibular ganglion. The central processes of these neurons form vestibular nerve. The fibres terminate at the vestibular nuclei of the brainstem.
2. ***Cochlear part*** begins from the organ of Corti. These are the peripheral processes of the bipolar neurons of spiral ganglion. The central processes of these neurons form cochlear nerve which terminates at the ventral and dorsal cochlear nuclei of pons.

Pathway of Hearing (Figs 6.34 to 6.36)

1. The first neurons of the pathway are located in the ***spiral ganglion***. They are ***bipolar***. Their peripheral processes innervate the spiral organ of Corti (Fig. 6.34), while central processes form the cochlear nerve (Fig. 6.35). This nerve terminates in the dorsal and ventral cochlear nuclei.
2. The second neurons lie in the dorsal and ventral cochlear nuclei. Most of the axons arising in these nuclei cross to the opposite side (in the trapezoid body) and terminate in the superior olivary nucleus. (Many fibres end in the nucleus of trapezoid body or of the lateral lemniscus.) Some fibres are uncrossed.
3. The third neurons lie in the superior olivary nucleus. Their axons form the lateral lemniscus and reach the inferior colliculus.
4. The fourth neurons lie in the inferior colliculus. Their axons pass through the inferior brachium to reach the medial geniculate body (Some fibres of lateral lemniscus reach the medial geniculate body without relay in the inferior colliculus).
5. The fifth neurons lie in the medial geniculate body. Their axons form the auditory radiation, which passes through the sublentiform part of the internal capsule to reach the auditory area (Fig. 6.36) in the temporal lobe.

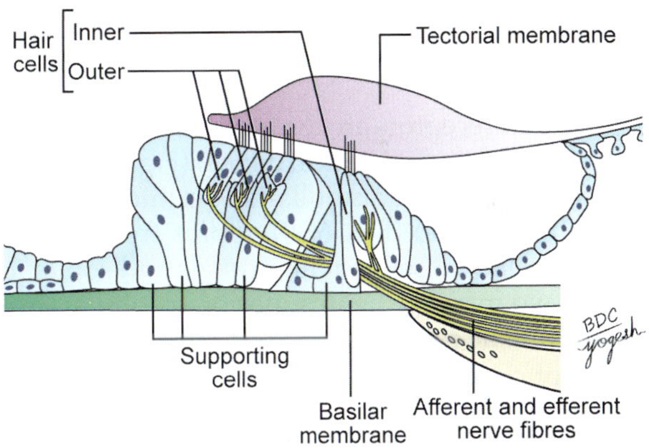

Fig. 6.34: Organ of Corti

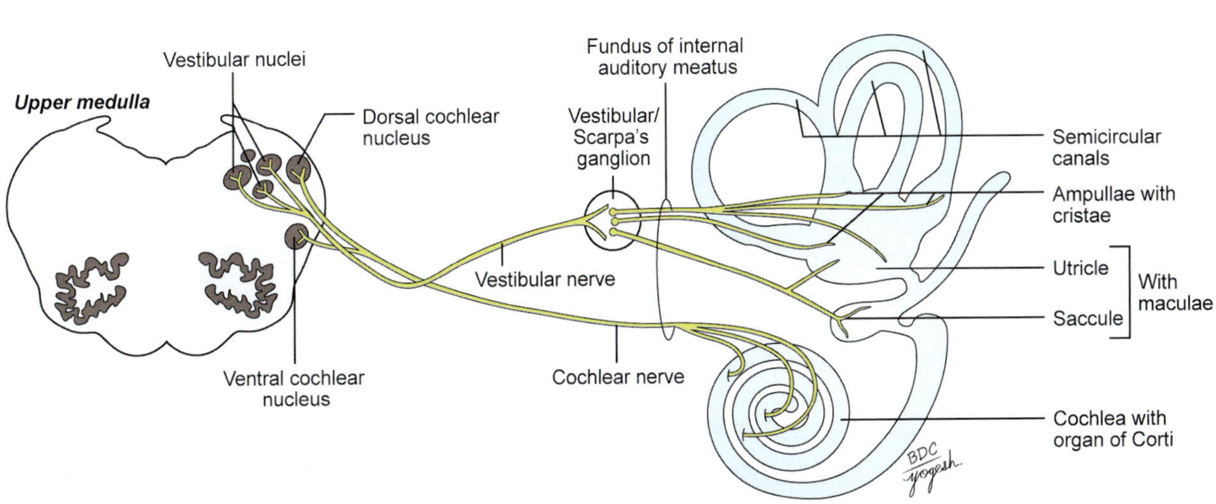

Fig. 6.35: Course of cochlear and vestibular nerves

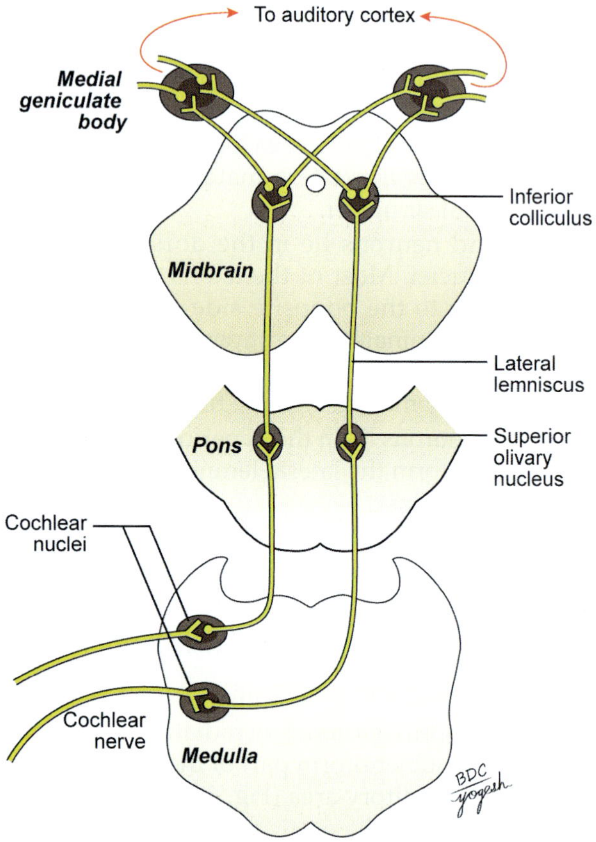

Fig. 6.36: Auditory pathway

Vestibular Pathway

The vestibular receptors are the maculae (Fig. 6.38) of the saccule and utricle (for static balance) (Figs 6.37a and b) and in the crista of the ampullaris of semicircular ducts (for kinetic balance) (Fig. 6.39). Fibres from cristae of anterior and lateral semicircular canals and some fibres from the two maculae lie in superior vestibular area of internal acoustic meatus.

Fibres of crista of posterior semicircular canal lie in foramen singulare.

Most of the fibres from maculae of utricle and saccule lie in inferior vestibular area.

These three nerve divisions are peripheral processes of bipolar neurons of the vestibular ganglion. This ganglion is situated in the internal acoustic meatus. The central processes arising from the neurons of the ganglion form the vestibular nerve which ends in the vestibular nuclei.

The second neurons in the pathway of balance lie in the vestibular nuclei. These nuclei send fibres:

a. To the archicerebellum through the inferior cerebellar peduncle (vestibulocerebellar tract).
b. To the motor nuclei of the brainstem (chiefly of the III, IV, VI and XI nerves) through the medial longitudinal bundle.
c. To the anterior horn cells of the spinal cord through the vestibulospinal tract.
d. Fibres also reach thalamus and premotor cortex of frontal lobe.

Through the vestibular pathway, the impulses arising in the labyrinth can influence the movements of the eyes, the head, the neck and the trunk (Fig. 6.40).

CLINICAL NEUROANATOMY

Deafness: Three types of hearing loss are seen:

1. Conductive deafness is the failure of sound waves to reach the cochlea.
2. Sensorineural deafness is the failure of production or transmission of action potential due to cochlear disease, cochlear nerve disease or defects in cochlear nerve central connections.
3. Cortical deafness is a bilateral or dominant posterior temporal lobe lesion. It results in a failure to understand spoken language even though hearing is preserved.

Vertigo: This is an illusion of rotatory movement due to disturbed orientation of the body in space. The patient feels that the environment is moving. It is due to disease of vestibular nerve.

Tinnitus: It is a sensation of buzzing, ringing, hissing or singing quality. Tinnitus may be unilateral or bilateral; high or low pitch; continuous or intermittent.

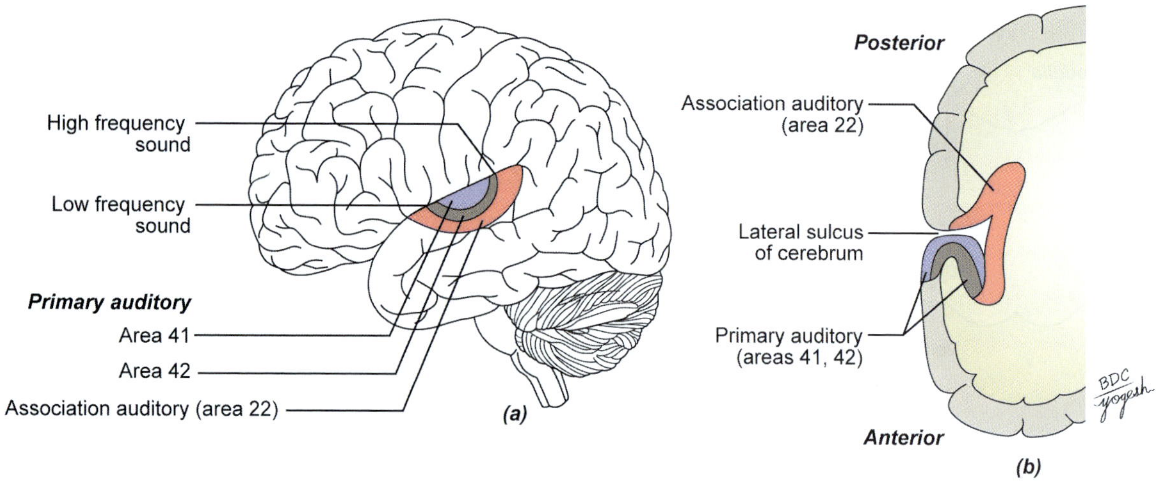

Figs 6.37a and b: Auditory cortex: (a) Posterior ramus of lateral sulcus and (b) depth of lateral sulcus

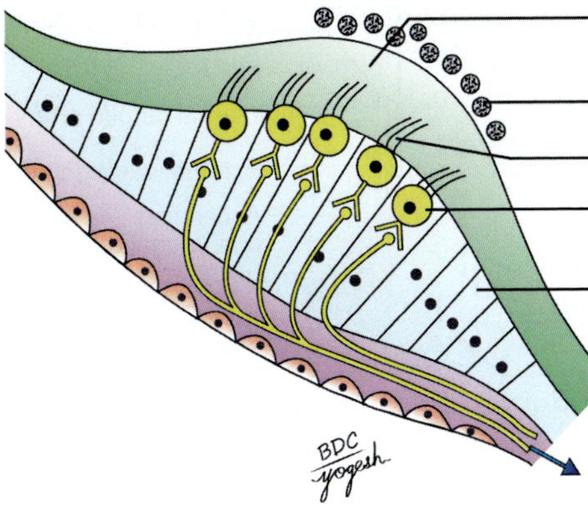

Fig. 6.38: Structure of the macula

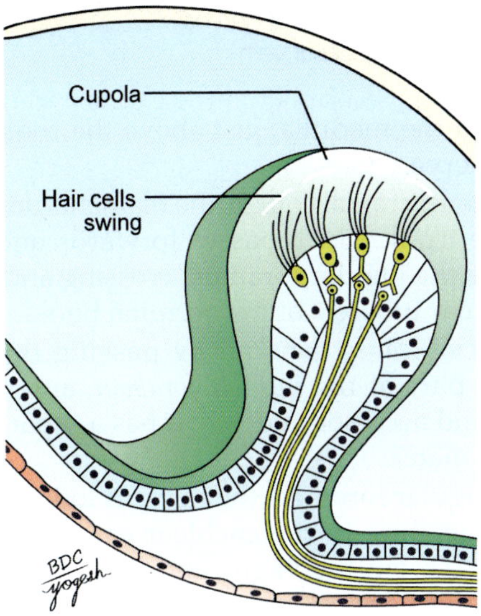

Fig. 6.39: Structure of crista ampullaris

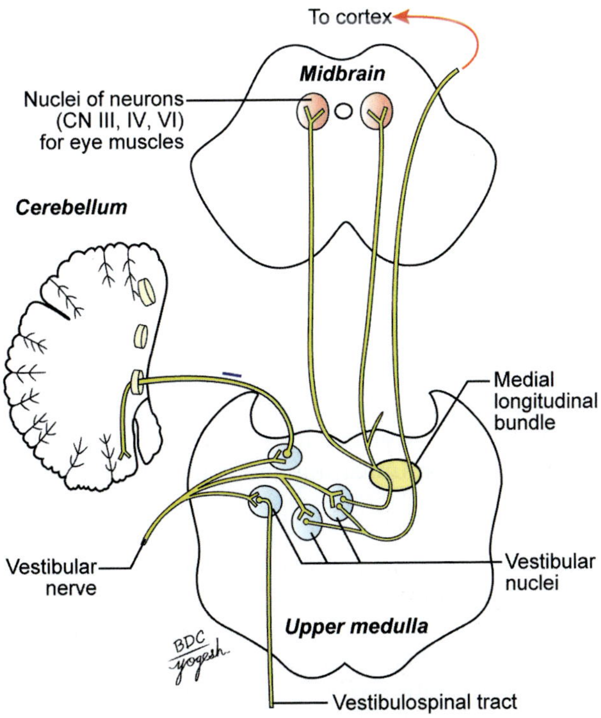

Fig. 6.40: Vestibular pathway

Meniere's syndrome: It is characterised by recurrent attacks of tinnitus, vertigo and hearing loss accompanied by a sensitivity to noises. It affects middle-aged or older persons. In this condition, there is an increase in volume of endolymph.

Acoustic neuroma: It is a slow growing benign tumour of neurolemmal cells. It causes an early loss of hearing.

NINTH CRANIAL NERVE (GLOSSOPHARYNGEAL NERVE)

Glossopharyngeal nerve is the ninth cranial nerve (Fig. 6.41 and Flowchart 6.14). It is the nerve of the third branchial arch.

It is motor to the stylopharyngeus. It is secretomotor to the parotid gland and gustatory to the posterior one-third of the tongue including the circumvallate papillae.

It is sensory to the pharynx, the tonsil, soft palate, the posterior one-third of the tongue, carotid body and carotid sinus.

Functional Components

1. ***Special visceral efferent*** (*SVE*) *fibres* arise from the *nucleus ambiguus*. They supply stylopharyngeus muscle (muscle of 3rd pharyngeal arch).
2. ***General visceral efferent*** (*GVE*) *fibres* arise from the *inferior salivatory nucleus*. These are preganglionic parasympathetic fibres that relay in otic ganglion and supply the parotid gland.
3. ***General visceral afferent*** (*GVA*) *fibres* carry general sensation from pharynx, palate, posterior one-third of tongue, tonsil, carotid body, and carotid sinus. These sensations are carried to the *nucleus tractus solitarius*.
4. ***Special visceral afferent*** (*SVA*) *fibres* carry taste sensation from the posterior one-third of tongue including circumvallate papillae. They carry sensation to the *nucleus tractus solitarius*.
5. ***General somatic afferent*** (*GSA*) *fibres* carry general sensation from middle ear, proprioceptive sensation from stylopharyngeus to the *nucleus of spinal tract of trigeminal nerve*.

Nuclei

The three nuclei in the upper part of medulla are:
1. Nucleus ambiguus (branchiomotor)
2. Inferior salivatory nucleus (parasympathetic)
3. Nucleus of tractus solitarius (gustatory).

Ganglia of Glossopharyngeal Nerve

The glossopharyngeal nerve has two sensory ganglia: Smaller superior and larger inferior ganglion. They contain cell bodies for sensory fibres.

Origin of Nerve

The glossopharyngeal nerve arises by 3–4 rootlets which are attached to the posterolateral sulcus of medulla, just above the rootlets of vagus nerve (Fig. 6.42).

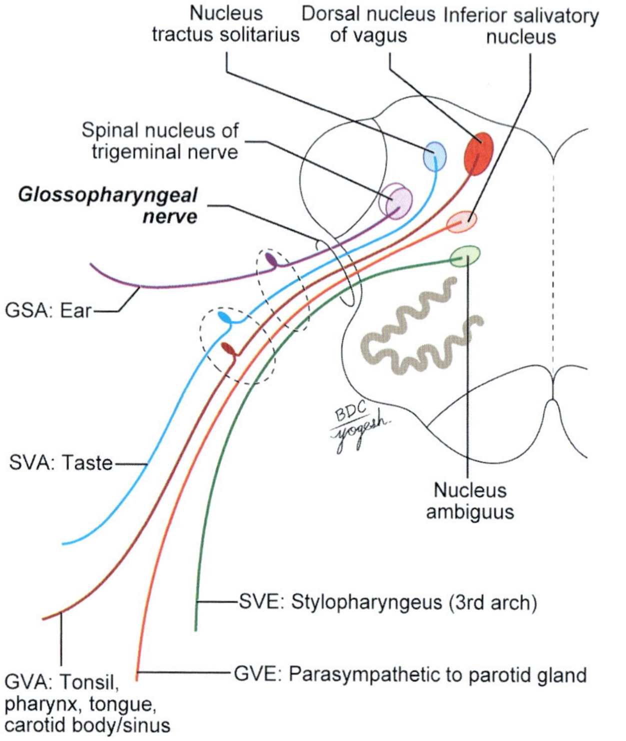

Fig. 6.41: Functional components and nuclei of IX cranial nerve (transverse section passing through the medulla oblongata, superior and inferior ganglia of glossopharyngeal nerve are shown in dotted line)

Flowchart 6.14: Glossopharyngeal (IX) nerve

Glossopharyngeal (IX) nerve

Nerve of 3rd arch

Functional components and nuclei	***Distribution/ branches***	***Clinical integration***
SVE: Nucleus ambiguus for stylopharyngeus GVE: Inferior salivatory nucleus–parasympathetic for parotid gland GVA: Nucleus tractus solitarius: General sensation from pharynx, palate, tongue, tonsil, carotid body and sinus SVA: Nucleus tractus solitarius for taste (posterior 1/3rd of tongue) GSA: Nucleus of spinal tract of V nerve: General sensation from middle ear	Tympanic Carotid Pharyngeal To stylopharyngeus Lingual Auricular	1. Lesion of IX ↓ Absence of gag reflex No taste sensation at posterior 1/3rd of tongue Absence of parotid salivation 2. Glossopharyngeal neuralgia 3. Referred ear pain in pharyngitis

(SVE: Special visceral efferent, GVE: General visceral efferent, GVA: General visceral afferent, SVA: Special visceral afferent, GSA: General somatic afferent)

Course and Relations

1. In **their *intraneural course***, the fibres of the nerve pass forwards and laterally, between the olivary nucleus and the inferior cerebellar peduncle, through the reticular formation of the medulla.
2. At the base of the brain, the nerve is attached by 3 to 4 filaments to the upper part of the posterolateral sulcus of the medulla, just above the rootlets of the vagus nerve.

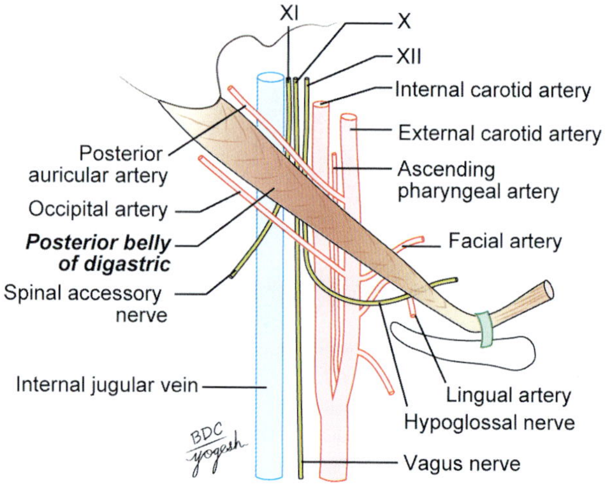

Fig. 6.42: Relation of cranial nerves IX, X, XI, and XII to carotid arteries and internal jugular vein

3. In their intracranial course, the filaments unite to form a single trunk which passes forwards and laterally towards the jugular foramen, crossing and grooving the jugular tubercle of the occipital bone.
4. The nerve *leaves the skull* by passing through the middle part of the *jugular foramen,* anterior to the vagus and accessory nerves. It has a separate sheath of dura mater.
5. In the jugular foramen, the nerve is lodged in a deep groove leading to the cochlear canaliculus, and is separated from the vagus and accessory nerves by the inferior petrosal sinus.

   In its ***extracranial course***, the nerve descends:

   a. Between the internal jugular vein and the internal carotid artery, deep to the styloid process and the muscles attached to it.
   b. It then turns forwards winding round the lateral aspect of the stylopharyngeus, passes between the external and internal carotid arteries, and reaches the side of the pharynx. Here it gives pharyngeal branches.
   c. It enters the submandibular region by passing deep to the hyoglossus, where it breaks up into tonsillar and lingual branches.
6. At the base of skull, ninth nerve presents a superior ganglion and an inferior ganglion. Superior ganglion is a detached part of the inferior ganglion, and gives no branches. The inferior ganglion is larger, occupies notch on the lower border of petrous temporal, and gives out communicating and tympanic branches.

Branches and Distribution (Fig. 6.43)

1. *Tympanic branch*: It carries sensation from the mucous membrane of the tympanic cavity, tympanic membrane, mastoid antrum, mastoid air cells and most of the auditory tube. The preganglionic parasympathetic fibres of tympanic branch (fibres from inferior salivatory nucleus) supply the parotid glands through otic ganglion.

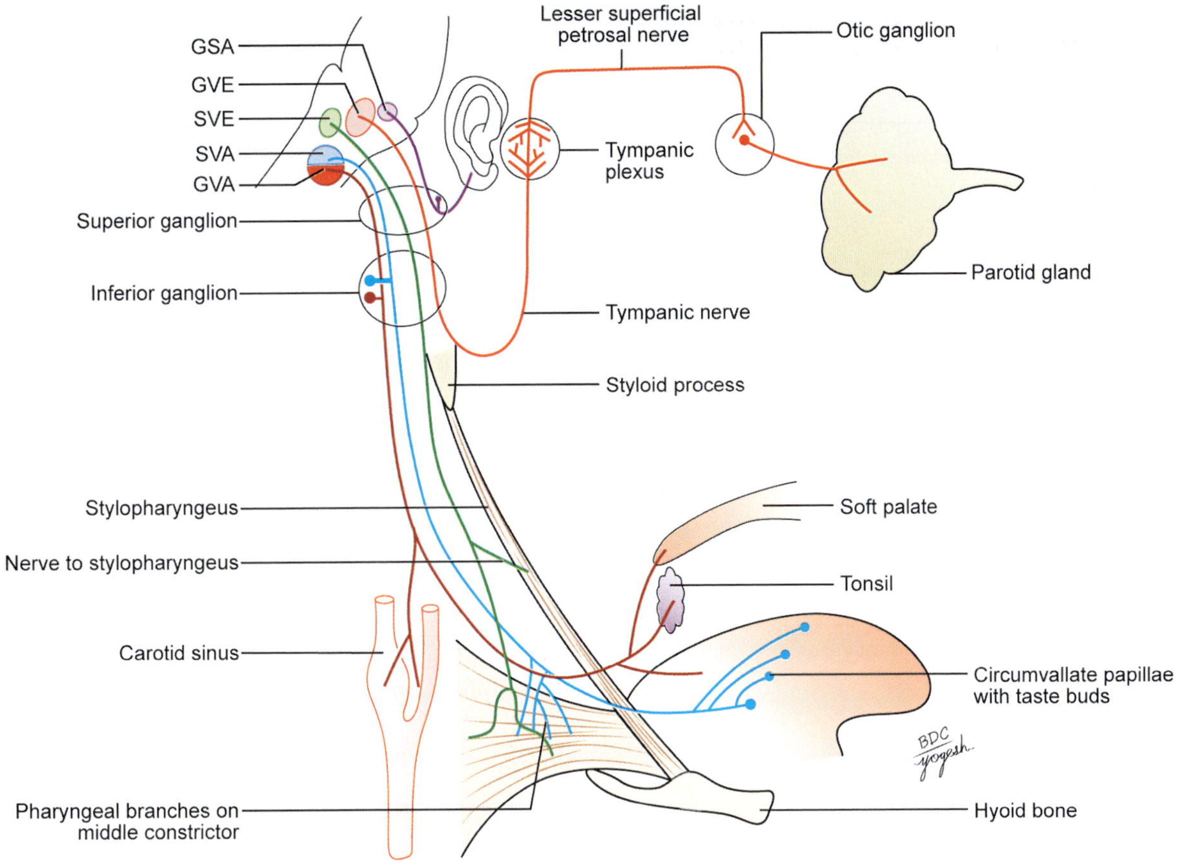

Fig. 6.43: Distribution of functional components of glossopharyngeal nerve

2. *Carotid branch* to the carotid sinus and carotid body.
3. *Pharyngeal branches* from pharyngeal plexus and carry sensation from mucosa of the pharynx.
4. *Muscular branch* to stylopharyngeus muscle (muscle of 3rd pharyngeal arch)
5. *Tonsillar branches* supply palatine tonsil, soft plate, and palatoglossal arches.
6. *Lingual branches* supply the posterior one-third of the tongue and circumvallate papillae and carry both taste and general sensations.
7. *Auricular branch* supplies the pinna of the ear and the external auditory meatus. The cell bodies of these sensory neurons are located in the superior ganglion of the glossopharyngeal nerve.

CLINICAL NEUROANATOMY

- ***Clinical testing** of glossopharyngeal nerve*: It can be tested clinically by:
  1. ***Eliciting gag reflex:*** Normally tickling the posterior wall of pharynx, soft palate or tonsillar fossa, a reflex contraction of pharyngeal muscle occurs. This is called *gag reflex*. It is absent in glossopharyngeal nerve paralysis.
  2. *Testing taste sensation* on the posterior one-third of tongue. It is lost in glossopharyngeal nerve paralysis.
- ***Glossopharyngeal neuralgia:*** It is a short sharp severe attack of pain affecting posterior part of pharynx or tonsillar area.
- ***Lesion of glossopharyngeal nerve*** causes:
  a. Absence of secretions of parotid gland.
  b. Absence of taste from posterior one-third of tongue and the circumvallate papillae.
  c. Loss of pain sensations from tongue, tonsil, pharynx and soft palate.
  d. Gag reflex is absent.
- ***Jugular foramen syndrome*** is due to injury at the jugular foramen resulting in multiple cranial nerve palsies.
- Isolated lesions of the ninth nerve are almost unknown. They are usually accompanied by lesions of the vagus nerve.
- ***Referred pain in pharyngitis:*** The pharyngitis may cause referred pain in the ear as both are supplied by IX nerve. However, in these cases, eustachian catarrh should be excluded.

TENTH CRANIAL NERVE (VAGUS NERVE)

Vagus nerve is the tenth cranial nerve. It is so-called because of its extensive ('vague') course, through the head, the neck, the thorax and the abdomen. The fibres of the cranial root of the accessory nerve are also distributed through it (Fig. 6.44 and Flowchart 6.15).

Functional Components

1. *Special visceral efferent (SVE) fibres*: They supply the palate, pharynx, and larynx. They arise from the *nucleus ambiguus*.

Flowchart 6.15: Vagus nerve

Vagus nerve

- ***Functional components and nuclei***
  - SVE: Nucleus ambiguus for palate, pharynx, larynx
  - GVE: Motor nucleus of vagus: Parasympathetic fibres to thorax and abdomen
  - GVA: Nucleus tractus solitarius, dorsal nucleus of vagus: For general sensation from pharynx, larynx, thorax
  - SVA: Nucleus tractus solitarius: Taste sensation from posteriormost part of tongue, epiglottis
  - GSA: Nucleus of spinal tract of trigeminal nerve: Ear
- ***Branches***
  - ***In head and neck***
    - Meningeal branches
    - Auricular branch
    - Pharyngeal branches
    - Carotid branches
    - Superior laryngeal branch – external and internal laryngeal nerves
    - Right recurrent laryngeal
    - Superior and inferior carotid branches
  - ***In thorax***
    - Left recurrent laryngeal:
      - Cardiac, tracheal, oesophageal branches
      - To inferior constrictor
      - To all intrinsic muscle of larynx except cricothyroid
      - Sensory branch to larynx below vocal cords
    - Pulmonary branches
    - Carotid branch
    - oesophageal branches
  - ***In abdomen***
    - From anterior vagal trunk
      - Hepatic branch
      - Upper gastric branches
      - Greater anterior gastric nerve
    - From posterior vagal trunk
      - Gastric branches
      - Coeliac branch
      - Nerve of Grassi

(SVE: Special visceral efferent, GVE: General visceral efferent, GVA: General visceral afferent, SVA: Special visceral afferent, GSA: General somatic afferent)

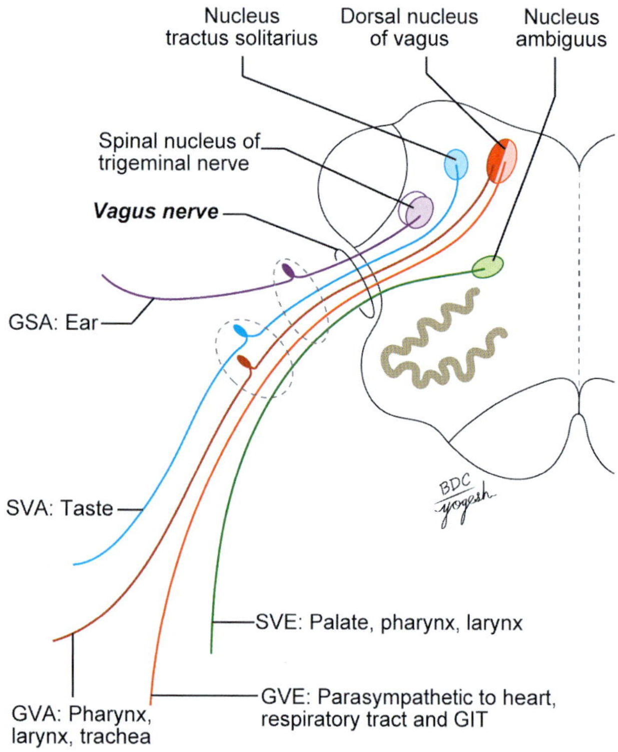

Fig. 6.44: Functional components and nuclei of the vagus nerve (transverse section passing through the medulla oblongata, superior and inferior ganglia of vagus nerve are shown in dotted line)

2. ***General visceral efferent*** (*GVE*) *fibres*: They are preganglionic parasympathetic fibres for thoracic and abdominal viscera. They arise from the dorsal *motor nucleus of vagus*.
3. ***General visceral afferent*** (*GVA*) *fibres*: They carry sensation from pharynx, larynx, oesophagus, carotid body, and from thoracic viscera to the lower part of *nucleus tractus solitarius* and few fibres to the *dorsal nucleus of vagus*.
4. ***Special visceral afferent*** (*SVA*) *fibres*: They carry taste sense from the posterior most part of the tongue and epiglottis to the upper part of *nucleus tractus solitarius*.
5. ***General somatic afferent*** (*GSA*) *fibres*: They carry general sensation from the skin of the external ear to the *spinal nucleus of trigeminal nerve*.

Nuclei

1. *Nucleus ambiguus (branchiomotor):* Mostly a part of the cranial root of accessory nerve; partly of vagus.
2. *Dorsal nucleus of vagus (parasympathetic):* It is a mixed nucleus, being both motor (visceromotor and secretomotor) and sensory (viscerosensory). Its fibres form the main bulk of the nerve.
3. *Nucleus of tractus solitarius (gustatory):* Distributed through internal laryngeal nerve to the taste buds of epiglottis and vallecula.
4. *Nucleus of spinal tract of trigeminal nerve.*

Ganglia of Vagus Nerve

The vagus nerve has two ganglia:

1. ***Smaller superior (jugular) ganglion:*** It lies within the jugular foramen. The superior ganglion contains the cell bodies of pseudounipolar sensory neurons carrying GSA information from the pinna of the ear and external auditory meatus and the dura of the posterior cranial fossa.
2. ***Large inferior ganglion (nodose ganglion):*** It lies just below the jugular foramen. It contains cell bodies of neurons that carry general visceral afferent sensory innervation from the mucosa of the soft palate, pharynx, and larynx, and a minor SVA (taste) sensation from posteriormost part of the tongue and epiglottis.

Note: The cranial root of the accessory nerve (11th nerve) joins the vagus nerve just below the inferior ganglion.

Origin of Vagus Nerve

The vagus nerve arises by about 10 rootlets from the lateral aspect of the medulla between the olive and inferior cerebellar peduncle (Fig. 6.45). These rootlets

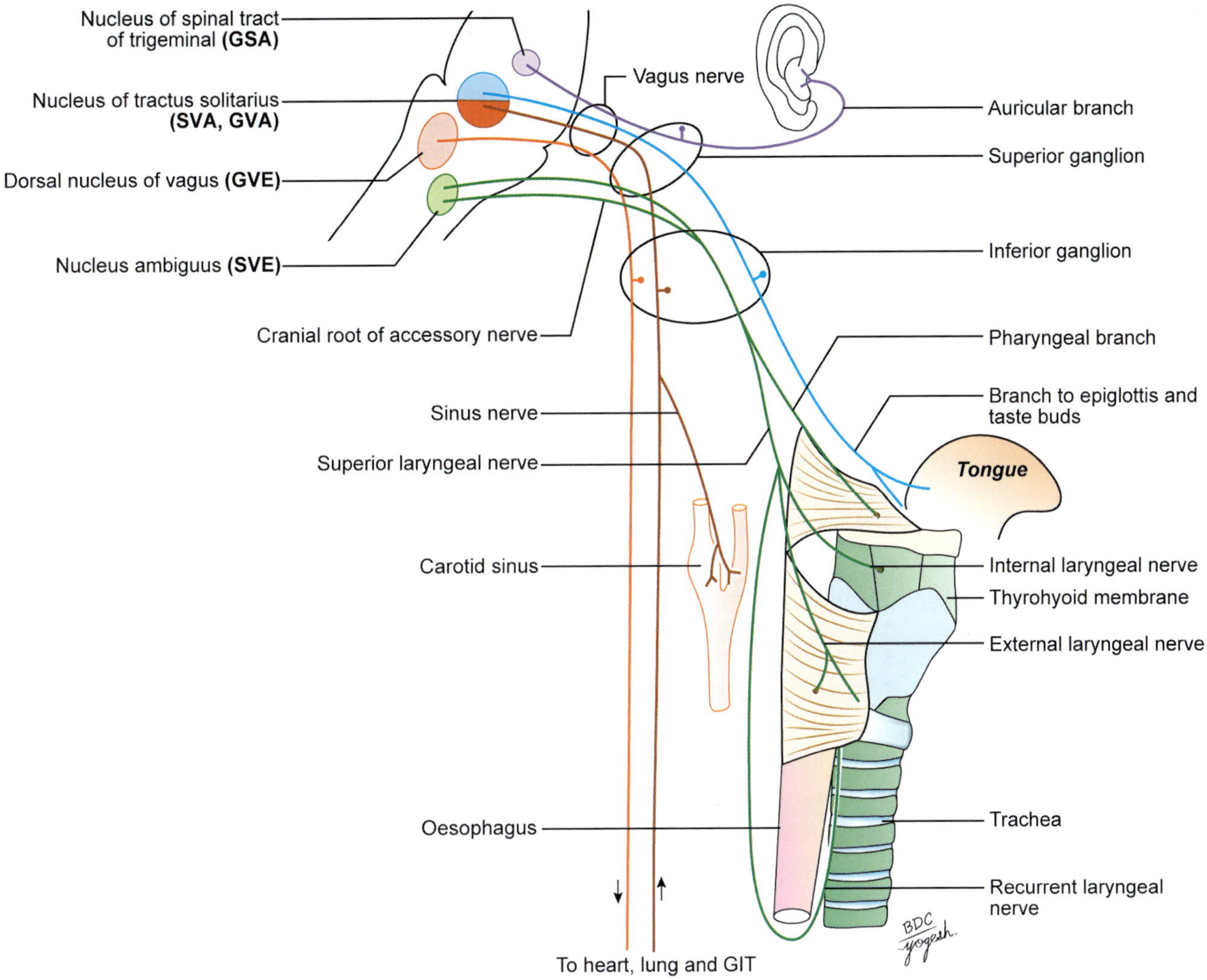

Fig. 6.45: Distribution of functional components of vagus in head and neck

emerge through the posterolateral sulcus of medulla and unite to form a single nerve trunk.

Course and Relations in Head and Neck

1. In the *intracranial course*, fibres run forwards and laterally through the reticular formation of medulla, between the olivary nucleus and inferior cerebellar peduncle.
2. The nerve is attached, by about ten rootlets, to the posterolateral sulcus of medulla.
3. In the intracranial course, the rootlets unite to form a large trunk which passes laterally across the jugular tubercle along with the glossopharyngeal and cranial root of accessory nerves, and reaches the jugular foramen.
4. The nerve *leaves the cranial cavity* by passing through the middle part of the jugular foramen, between the sigmoid and inferior petrosal sinuses. In the foramen, it is joined by the cranial root of the accessory nerve.
5. Leaving the skull, the nerve descends within the carotid sheath, in between the internal jugular vein (laterally), and the internal and common carotid arteries (medially).
6. At the *root of the neck,* the right vagus enters the thorax by crossing the first part of the subclavian artery, and then inclining medially behind the brachiocephalic vessels, to reach the right side of the trachea. The left vagus enters the thorax by passing between the left common carotid and left subclavian arteries, behind the internal jugular and brachiocephalic veins.
7. Vagus bears two ganglia—superior and inferior. The *superior ganglion* is rounded and lies in the jugular foramen. It gives meningeal and auricular branches of vagus, and is connected to glossopharyngeal and accessory nerves and to superior cervical ganglion of sympathetic chain. The *inferior ganglion* is cylindrical (2.5 cm) and lies near the base of skull. It gives pharyngeal, carotid, superior laryngeal branches and is connected to hypoglossal nerve, superior cervical ganglion and the loop between first and second cervical nerves.

Cranial root of XI nerve joins vagus nerve at the inferior ganglion.

Branches in Head and Neck

The branches are listed in Table 6.4.

TABLE 6.4: Branches of vagus nerve

Region	*Branches*
A. In head and neck	
1. From the superior ganglion	• Meningeal branches: Sensory supply to dura mater of the posterior cranial fossa • Auricular branch (Arnold's nerve or Alderman's nerve): Supplies the posterior half of external auditory meatus, outer surface of the tympanic membranes, concha and root of the auricle
2. From inferior ganglion	• Pharyngeal branches: All the muscles of pharynx except stylopharyngeus which is supplied by the glossopharyngeal nerve. All the muscles of soft palate except the tensor veli palatini which is supplied by mandibular nerve • Carotid branches: Sensation from the carotid body and sinus • Superior laryngeal branch – external and internal laryngeal nerves. *Internal laryngeal nerve*: Sensation from mucous membranes of pharynx, epiglottis, vallecula and laryngeal vestibule, mucosa of pyriform fossa aryepiglottic folds, mucosa of larynx up to the vocal folds. *External laryngeal nerve*: Supplies cricothyroid and inferior constrictor of pharynx • Right recurrent laryngeal nerve: Supply—all the intrinsic muscles of larynx except cricothyroid which is supplied by the external laryngeal nerve and mucous membranes of larynx below the vocal folds • Superior and inferior carotid branches
B. In the thorax	
1. Left recurrent laryngeal nerve	• Cardiac, tracheal and oesophageal branches • To inferior constrictor • To all intrinsic muscle of larynx except cricothyroid • Sensory branch to mucous membrane of larynx below the vocal cords
2. Pulmonary branches	Supply the lungs through pulmonary plexuses
3. Carotid branch	Supply the carotid body and carotid sinus
4. Oesophageal branches	Supply oesophagus
5. Cardiac branches	Supply the heart through cardiac plexuses
C. In abdomen	
From anterior vagal trunk	1. Hepatic branch for liver, pylorus, duodenum, and pancreas 2. Upper gastric branches for anterior surface of body and fundus 3. Greater anterior gastric nerve – the main gastric branch, gives fibres to the body and antrum. It ends at incisura angularis in crow's foot pattern 4. Pyloric branch to supply pylorus
From posterior vagal trunk	1. Gastric branches for posterior surface of stomach except pylorus. Its major gastric branch is called greater posterior gastric nerve or posterior nerve of lesser curvature 2. Coeliac branch reaches the coeliac plexus via left gastric artery 3. Nerve of Grassi: For fundus of stomach

Note: The *right recurrent laryngeal nerve* arises from the vagus in front of the right subclavian artery, winds backwards below the artery, and runs upwards and medially behind the subclavian and common carotid arteries to reach the tracheo-oesophageal groove. In the upper part of the groove, it is intimately related to the inferior thyroid artery.

The *left recurrent laryngeal nerve* arises from the vagus in the thorax, as the latter crosses the left side of the arch of the aorta. It loops around the ligamentum arteriosum and reaches the tracheo-oesophageal groove. Its distribution is similar to that of the right nerve. It does not have to pass behind the subclavian and carotid arteries; and usually, it is posterior to the inferior thyroid artery.

CLINICAL NEUROANATOMY

- ***Clinical testing of vagus nerve***: The vagus nerve is tested clinically by comparing the palatal arches on the two sides. On the paralysed side, there is no arching, and the uvula is pulled to the normal side.
- ***Paralysis of the vagus nerve*** produces (Fig. 6.46):
  a. Nasal regurgitation of swallowed liquids
  b. Nasal twang in voice
  c. Hoarseness of voice
  d. Flattening of the palatal arch
  e. Cadaveric position of the vocal cord
  f. Dysphagia.
- ***Aldermen's nerve phenomenon***: Stimulation of auricular area supplied by vagus cause increased appetite. In the Alderman, in ancient Rome, used to stimulate the appetite by dropping cold water behind the ear. This stimulation causes reflex, increased gastric motility and acid secretion.
- ***Irritation of the auricular branch of the vagus*** in the external ear (by ear wax, syringing, etc.) may reflexly cause persistent cough (ear cough), vomiting, or even death due to sudden cardiac inhibition.
- Irritation of the recurrent laryngeal nerve by enlarged lymph nodes in children may also produce a persistent cough.

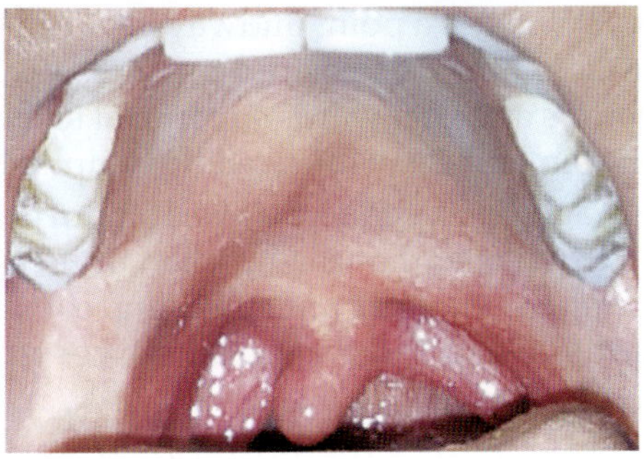

Fig. 6.46: Paralysis of muscles of soft palate on left side

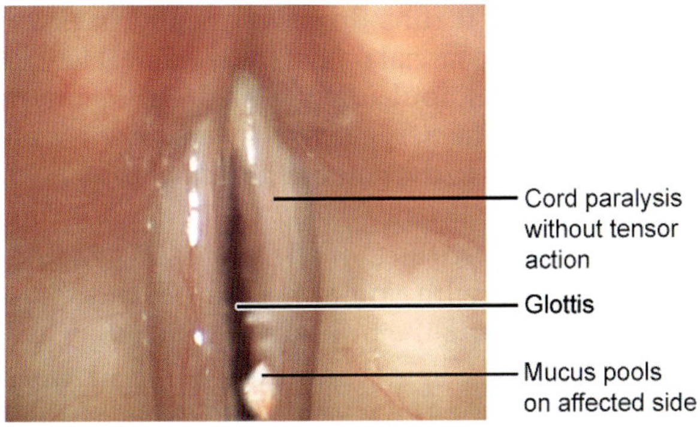

Fig. 6.47: Injury to right recurrent laryngeal nerve

- Some fibres arising in the geniculate ganglion of facial nerve pass into the vagus through communications between the two nerves. They reach the skin of auricle through the auricular branch of vagus. Sometimes a sensory ganglion may have a viral infection (called herpes zoster) and vesicles appear on the area of skin supplied by the ganglion. In herpes zoster of the geniculate ganglion, vesicles appear on the skin of auricle.
- Injury to pharyngeal branch causes dysphagia. Paralysis of muscles of soft palate results in nasal regurgitation of fluids and nasal tone of voice. Lesions of superior laryngeal nerve produces anaesthesia in the upper part of larynx and paralysis of cricothyroid muscle. The voice is weak and gets tired easily.
- Injury to right recurrent laryngeal nerve results in hoarseness and dysphonia due to paralysis of the right vocal cord (Fig. 6.47).
- Paralysis of both vocal cords results in aphonia and inspiratory stridor (high-pitched and harsh respiratory sound). It may occur during thyroid surgery.
- During thyroidectomy, recurrent laryngeal nerve may be injured resulting in fixed and paramedian vocal cords.
- In severe peptic ulcer, ***vagotomy*** is done to relieve the symptoms.

ELEVENTH CRANIAL NERVE (ACCESSORY NERVE)

Accessory nerve is the eleventh cranial nerve. It has two roots—cranial and spinal. The cranial root is assisting the vagus, and is distributed through its branches as vagoaccessory complex. The spinal root has a more independent course (Fig. 6.48 and Flowchart 6.16).

Functional Components

1. ***Special visceral efferent*** (*SVE*) *fibres*: They begins from *nucleus ambiguus*. These are motor fibres for the muscles of soft palate, pharynx, and larynx. They form the cranial root and get distributed through the branches of vagus nerve.
2. ***General somatic efferent*** (*GSE*) *fibres*: They begins from *spinal nucleus of accessory nerve* which extends in the anterior grey column of the spinal cord from C1 and C5 segments. These fibres supply sternocleidomastoid and trapezius.

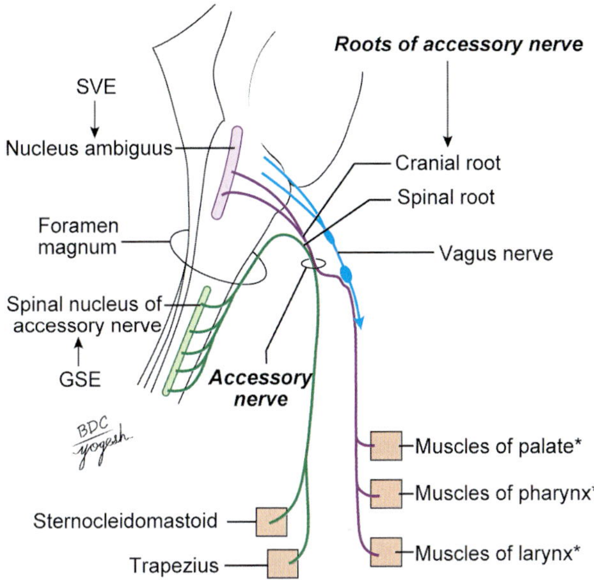

Fig. 6.48: Course and distribution of the accessory nerve (SVE: Special visceral efferent, GSE: General somatic efferent, *: for details about exceptions, refer the text)

Flowchart 6.16: Spinal accessory nerve

Spinal accessory nerve
11th cranial nerve

- ***Roots***
  - Cranial root: Accessory to vagus
  - Spinal root: For SCM and trapezius
- ***Functional components and nuclei***
  - SVE: Nucleus ambiguus, for muscles of palate, pharynx and larynx
  - GSE: Spinal nucleus of accessory nerve: For SCM and trapezius
- ***Surfaces***
  - ***Spinal root***: SCM, Trapezius
  - ***Cranial root***: Muscles of:
    1. Pharynx except stylopharyngeus
    2. Palate except tensor veli palatini
    3. Larynx except mucous membrane below vocal cord

Clinical integration: Test SCM – ask to turn chin to the opposite side,
Trapezius – ask to shrug the shoulder
Torticollis (wry neck)

(SCM: Sternocleidomastoid, GSE: General somatic efferent, SVE: Special visceral efferent)

Origin of Accessory Nerve

1. *Cranial root*: It emerges as 4–5 rootlets from the posterolateral sulcus of the medulla. They join to from a single trunk.
2. *Spinal root*: It arises as a row of filaments from the upper 5 segments of spinal cord between the ventral and dorsal nerve roots. In the vertebral canal, the filaments unite to form a single trunk which ascend in front of the dorsal root and behind the ligamentum denticulatum.

Nuclei

1. The cranial root arises from the lower part of the *nucleus ambiguus*.
2. The spinal root arises from a long *spinal nucleus* situated on the lateral part of anterior grey column of spinal cord, extending from C1 to C5 segments. It is in line with nucleus ambiguus.

Course and Distribution of the Cranial Root (Fig. 6.48)

1. The cranial root emerges in the form of 4 to 5 rootlets which are attached to the posterolateral sulcus of the medulla. Just below, the rootlets soon join together to form a single trunk.
2. It runs laterally with the glossopharyngeal vagus and spinal accessory nerves, crosses the jugular tubercle, and reaches jugular foramen.
3. In the jugular foramen, the cranial root unites for a short distance with the spinal root, and again separates from spinal root as it passes out of the foramen.
4. The cranial root finally fuses with the vagus at its inferior ganglion, and is distributed through the branches of the vagus to the muscles of the palate, the pharynx, the larynx and possibly the heart.

Course and Distribution of the Spinal Root (Fig. 6.48)

1. It arises from the upper five segments of the spinal cord.
2. It emerges in the form of a row of filaments attached to the cord midway between the ventral and dorsal nerve roots.
3. *In the vertebral canal,* the filaments unite to form a single trunk which ascends in front of the dorsal nerve roots and behind the ligamentum denticulatum.
4. The nerve *enters the cranium* through the foramen magnum lying behind the vertebral artery.
5. Within the cranium, the nerve runs upwards and laterally, crosses the jugular tubercle (with the ninth and tenth cranial nerves) and reaches the jugular foramen.
6. The nerve *leaves the skull* through the middle part of the jugular foramen where it fuses with a short length of the cranial root. It soon separates from the latter and passes out of the foramen.
7. In its *extracranial course,* the nerve descends vertically between the internal jugular vein and the internal carotid artery deep to the parotid and to the styloid process. It reaches a point midway between the angle of mandible and the mastoid process. Then it runs downwards and backwards superficial to the internal jugular vein and is surrounded by lymph nodes.

   The nerve pierces the anterior border of the sternocleidomastoid at the junction of its upper one fourth with the lower three-fourths, and communicates with second and third cervical nerves within the muscle.

   The nerve enters the posterior triangle of the neck by emerging through the posterior border of the sternocleidomastoid a little above its middle. In the triangle, it runs downwards and backwards embedded in the fascial roof of the triangle. Here it lies over the levator scapulae. It is related to the superficial lymph nodes. The nerve leaves the posterior triangle by passing deep to the anterior border of the trapezius 5 cm above the clavicle.

   On the deep surface of the trapezius, the nerve communicates with spinal nerves C3 and C4, and ends by supplying the trapezius.
8. ***Distribution:*** The spinal accessory nerve supplies:
   a. The sternocleidomastoid—the chin turning muscle.
   b. The trapezius—the shrugging muscle.

Cervical nerves provide a proprioceptive sensations to these muscles.

CLINICAL NEUROANATOMY

- ***Clinical testing:*** The accessory nerve is tested clinically:
  a. By asking the patient to shrug his shoulders (trapezius) against resistance and comparing the power on the two sides.
  b. By asking the patient to turn the chin to the opposite side (sternocleidomastoid) against resistance and again comparing the power on the two sides.
- ***Paralysis of spinal accessory nerve*:** Lesions of spinal root of accessory nerve cause drooping of the shoulder and inability to turn chin to opposite side.
- Irritation of the nerve during biopsy of enlarged caseous lymph nodes may produce ***torticollis*** or wry neck.
- Supranuclear connections act on the ipsilateral sternocleidomastoid and on the contralateral trapezius. This results in turning of the head away from relevant hemisphere during seizure.
- Spasmodic torticollis—irritation of the nerve resulting in clonic spasm of the sternocleidomastoid and trapezius muscles.

TWELFTH CRANIAL NERVE (HYPOGLOSSAL NERVE)

Hypoglossal nerve is the twelfth cranial nerve. It supplies the muscles of the tongue (Figs 6.50, 6.51 and Flowchart 6.17).

Functional Components/Nuclear Columns

1. ***General somatic efferent** (GSE) fibres*: They arise from the *hypoglossal nucleus* and supply all the intrinsic and extrinsic muscles of tongue except palatoglossus.
2. ***General somatic afferent** (GSA) fibres*: They carry proprioceptive fibres from the muscles of tongue to the *mesencephalic nucleus of trigeminal nerve*.

Hypoglossal Nucleus

The hypoglossal nucleus, 2 cm long, lies in the floor of fourth ventricle beneath the hypoglossal triangle. It is divided into a part for genioglossus and a part for rest of the muscles (Fig. 6.49).

Nucleus for genioglossus muscle receives only contralateral corticonuclear fibres. Nucleus for rest of the lingual muscles receives both ipsilateral and contralateral corticonuclear fibres.

Origin of Hypoglossal Nerve

The hypoglossal nerve arises by 10–15 rootlets on the ventral aspect of the medulla from anterolateral sulcus between pyramid and olive.

Course and Relations

1. In their *intraneural course,* the fibres pass forwards lateral to the medial longitudinal bundle, medial lemniscus and pyramidal tract, and medial to the reticular formation and olivary nucleus.
2. The nerve is attached to the anterolateral sulcus of the medulla, between the pyramid and the olive, by 10 to 15 rootlets (Fig. 6.50).

The rootlets run laterally behind the vertebral artery, and join to form two bundles which pierce the dura mater separately near the hypoglossal canal.

The nerve leaves the skull through the hypoglossal (anterior condylar) canal.

Extracranial Course

1. The nerve first lies deep to the internal jugular vein, but soon inclines between the internal jugular vein and the internal carotid artery, crosses the vagus (laterally), and reaches in front of it.
2. It then descends between the internal jugular vein and the internal carotid artery in front of the vagus, deep to the parotid gland, the styloid process, the posterior belly of the digastric.
3. At the lower border of the posterior belly of the digastric, it curves forwards, crosses the internal and external carotid arteries and the loop of the lingual artery, and passes deep to the posterior belly of the digastric again to enter the submandibular region.
4. The nerve then continues forwards on the hyoglossus and genioglossus, deep to the submandibular gland and the mylohyoid, and enters the substance of the tongue to supply all its intrinsic muscles and most of its extrinsic muscles.

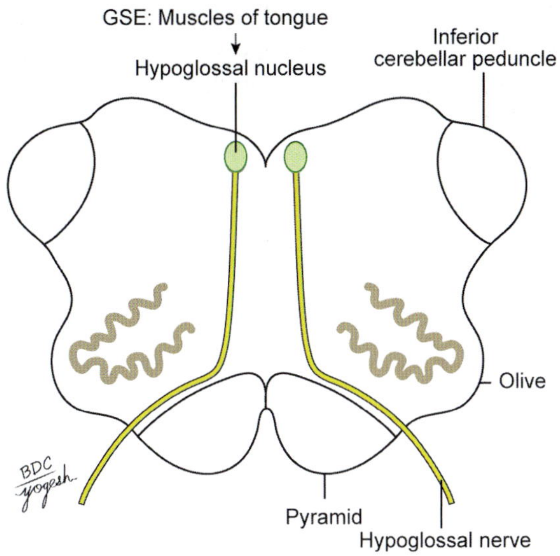

Fig. 6.49: Functional components and nucleus of the hypoglossal nerve (transverse section of the medulla oblongata)

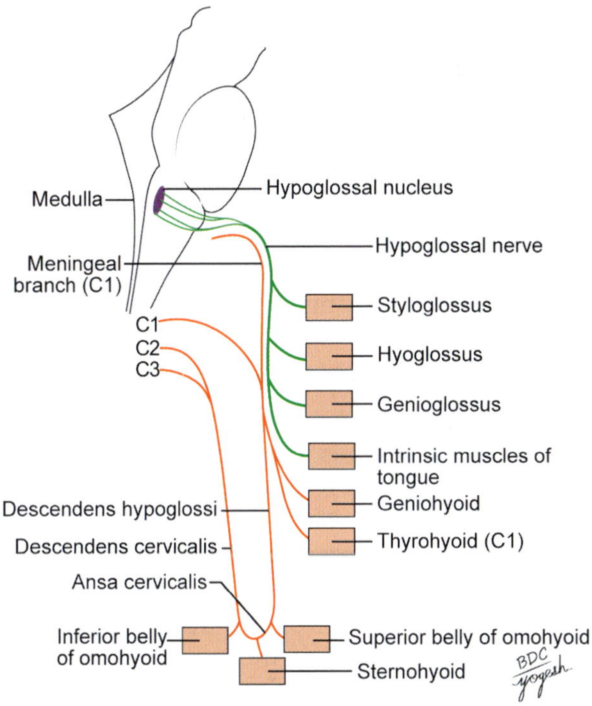

Fig. 6.50: Hypoglossal nerve

Flowchart 6.17: Hypoglossal nerve

Hypoglossal nerve
C1 fibres join hypoglossal nerve

Functional components
- GSE: Hypoglossal nucleus – for muscle of tongue except palatoglossus
- GSA: Mesencephalic nucleus of V – for proprioception from muscles of tongue

Branches
- ***From hypoglossal nerve***: All muscles of tongue except palatoglossus
- ***C1 Fibres***: Meningeal branch; To thyrohyoid; To geniohyoid; Descendens hypoglossi

Clinical integration: Clinical testing – ask to protrude the tongue paralysis of hypoglossal nerve → Tongue deviates to the side of paralysis

(GSE: General somatic efferent, GSA: General somatic afferent)

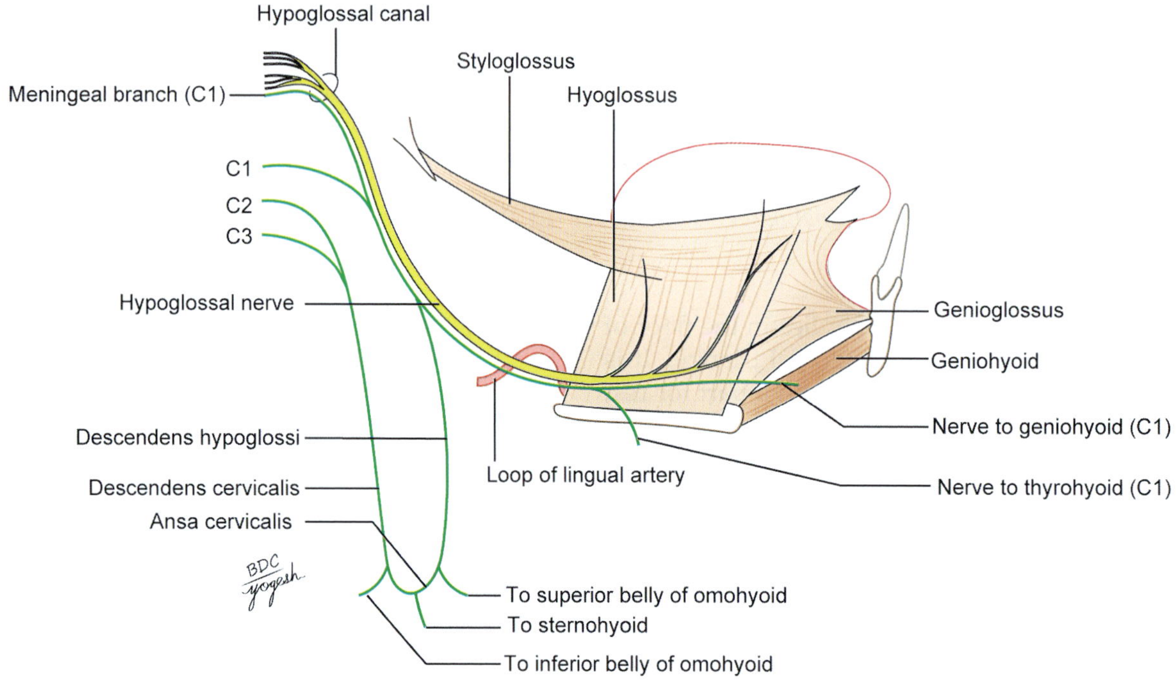

Fig. 6.51: Hypoglossal nerve and ansa cervicalis

Branches and Distribution (Fig. 6.50 and 6.51)

Branches of Hypoglossal Nerve Proper

Branches to supply all the intrinsic and extrinsic muscles of tongue except palatoglossus which is supplied by cranial part of accessory nerve through the vagus nerve.

Branches of Hypoglossal Nerve Containing C1 Fibres

The hypoglossal nerve is joined by fibres of C1 spinal nerve. These fibres give following branches:

1. *Meningeal branches*: They enter the cranial cavity through the hypoglossal canal and supply the dura mater of the posterior cranial fossa.
2. Descends hypoglossi or the upper root of ansa cervicalis: It arises from the hypoglossal nerve in front of the internal carotid artery. It descends in the anterior wall of carotid sheath and joins to the inferior root of ansa cervicalis at the level of cricoid cartilage.
3. *Nerve to thyrohyoid*: It crosses the greater cornua of the hyoid bone and supplied thyrohyoid muscle.
4. *Nerve of geniohyoid*: It arises above the hyoid bone and supply the geniohyoid muscle.

CLINICAL NEUROANATOMY

- ***Clinical testing of hypoglossal nerve***: Ask the patient to protrude the tongue. Normally, the tongue is protruded forwards in the midline. If the hypoglossal nerve of one side is paralysed, the tongue deviates to the side of paralysis due to action of contralateral genioglossus muscle.
- If both the hypoglossal nerves are paralysed, the patient cannot protrude the tongue.

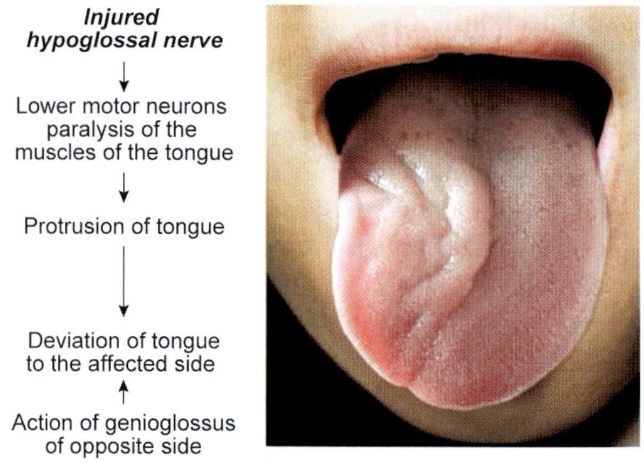

Fig. 6.52: XII nerve paralysis on right side

- ***Lesions of hypoglossal nerve***: The lesions of hypoglossal nerve are divided into intranuclear and supranuclear lesions.
  a. ***Intranuclear lesions*** or injury to the hypoglossal nerve: It results into the lower motor neuron type of paralysis of the muscles of the tongue on the side of lesion. On protrusion of tongue, it deviates to the affected side due to the action of genioglossus of opposite side (Fig. 6.52). In bilateral hypoglossal nerve injury, the patient cannot protrude the tongue. Speech and swallowing are affected.
  b. ***Supranuclear lesion*** of hypoglossal nerve: It occurs due to damage to the corticonuclear fibres connecting motor area of cerebrum to the hypoglossal nucleus. It results into upper motor neuron type of paralysis. On protrusion, the tongue deviates to the opposite side. The supranuclear lesion affects the muscles of opposite side of the tongue.

Facts to Remember

- III nerve carries parasympathetic fibres from Edinger-Westphal nucleus of midbrain to the ciliaris and constrictor pupillae muscles for accommodation.
- VII nerve carries parasympathetic fibres from lacrimatory nucleus to pterygopalatine ganglion for the lacrimal gland and glands in nasal cavity, palate and pharynx.
- VII nerve also carries parasympathetic fibres from superior salivatory nucleus to submandibular ganglion for the supply of submandibular, sublingual glands and glands in the oral cavity.
- IX nerve carries parasympathetic fibres from inferior salivatory nucleus to the otic ganglion for the supply of parotid gland.
- X nerve carries parasympathetic fibres from dorsal nucleus of vagus for the glands in the respiratory tract and glands in the digestive tract till right two-thirds of the transverse colon.
- Only trochlear nerve emerges on the dorsal aspect of the brainstem.
- V, VII, IX nerves are the nerves of 1st, 2nd, 3rd arches, respectively.
- X, XI, i.e. vagoaccessory complex supplies structures developed from 4th and 6th branchial arches.

BDC's Anatomy *e*-book

1. Nuclei of the cranial nerves
2. Highlights of the cranial nerves
3. Oculomotor nuclear complex
4. Sensory and motor components of V nerve
5. Foramina for cranial nerves and their branches
6. Further reading
7. Viva voce questions

Chapter

7

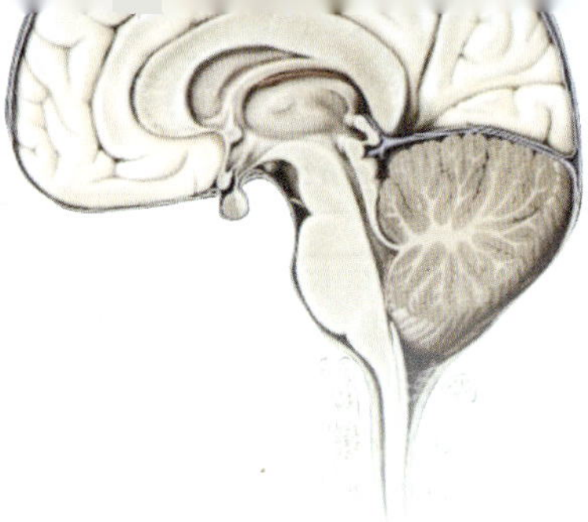

Brainstem

The brainstem is a connecting stalk between the spinal cord and cerebrum. It consists of three parts (Plates 7.1 and 7.2, Figs 7.1 to 7.3):

1. Medulla oblongata
2. Pons
3. Midbrain.

The brainstem is located in the posterior cranial fossa. It lies on the sloping clivus.

It contains:

1. Ascending and descending pathways that connect cerebrum, cerebellum, and spinal cord with each other
2. Reticular formation
3. Cranial nerve nuclei and their origin (IIIrd to XIIth)
4. Vital centres that control heart rate, blood pressure and respiration.

Note: Damage to vital centres leads to death due to respiratory and cardiac failures. A damage to ascending reticular system may lead to loss of consciousness or coma.

The gross specimens showing the transverse sections (TS) of medulla oblongata, pons, midbrain, and the spinal cord at various levels are shown in Plate 7.2 for comparison.

Plate 7.1: Brainstem (anterior view)

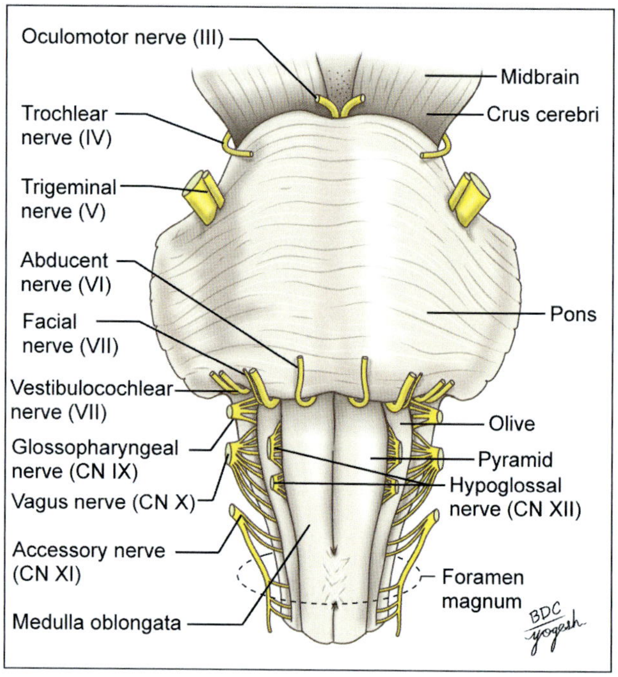

Competency:
AN58.1 Identify external features of medulla oblongata.

MEDULLA OBLONGATA

The medulla is the lowest part of brainstem (Plate 7.1, Fig. 7.1, Flowchart 7.1).

Extent

The medulla extends from the lower border of pons to a plane just above which the 1st cervical nerve arises where it is continuous with the spinal cord. It lies in the anterior part of posterior cranial fossa, extending down to the foramen magnum.

Relations

Anteriorly, it is related to the clivus and meninges and posteriorly, to the vallecula of the cerebellum. Along with other parts of the hindbrain, medulla occupies the infratentorial space.

Parts

1. *Open/superior part*—the dorsal surface of the medulla is formed by the fourth ventricle.
2. *Closed/inferior part*—fourth ventricle is narrowed at the obex and continues with the central canal.

Measurements

Length: 3 cm

Width: 2 cm at its widest part

Thickness: 1.25 cm.

EXTERNAL FEATURES

1. ***Fissures and sulci:*** The medulla is divided into right and left halves by the ***anterior and posterior median fissures***. The anterior median fissure ends in ***foramen caecum*** at its junction with pons. Each half is further divided into anterior, lateral and posterior regions by the ***anterolateral and posterolateral sulci*** (Plate 7.1, Fig. 7.1, Flowchart 7.1).

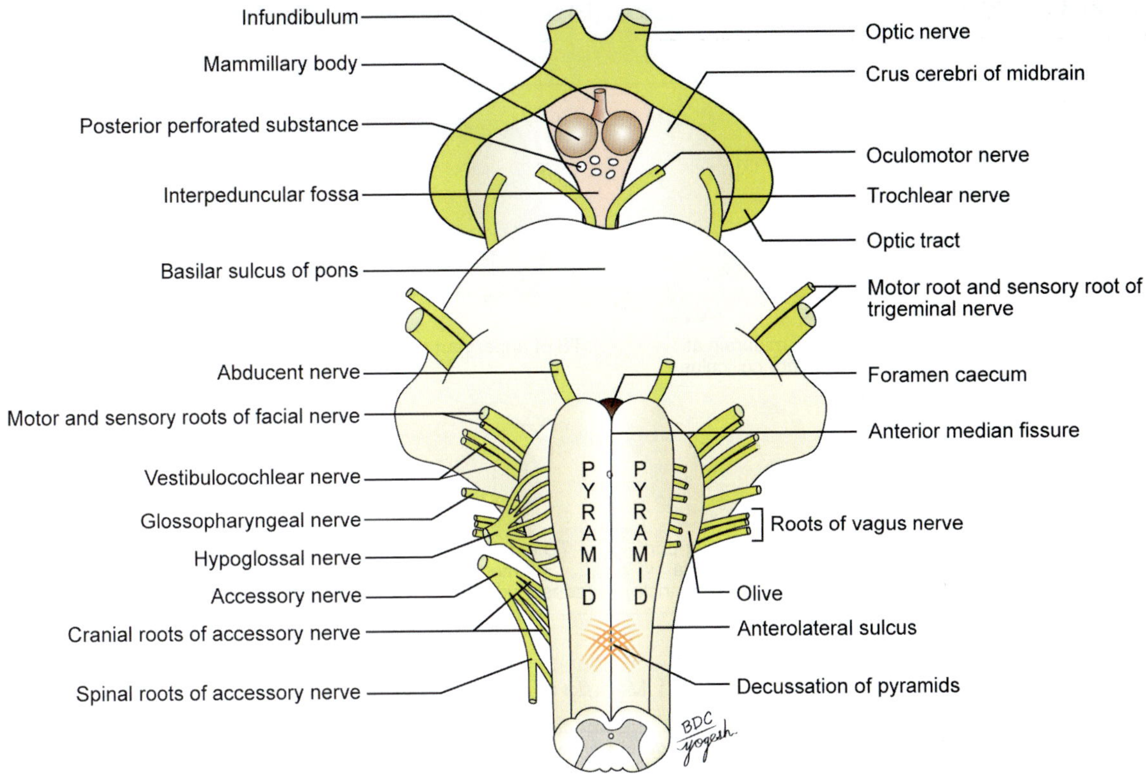

Fig. 7.1: Attachment of cranial nerves to the ventral surface of brainstem

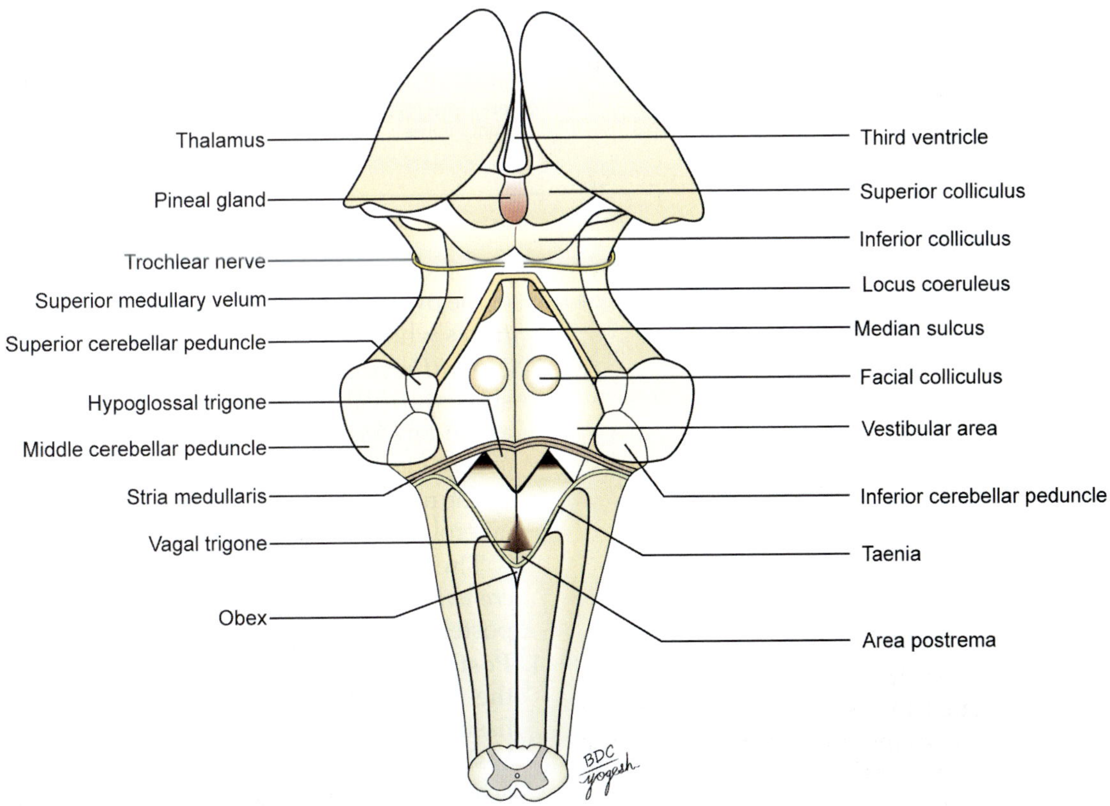

Fig. 7.2: Dorsal aspect of brainstem

2. ***Anterior region:*** The *anterior region* on either side of the fissure is formed of a longitudinal elevation called the ***pyramid***. The pyramid is made up of corticospinal and corticobulbar fibres. In the lower part of the medulla, many fibres of the right and left pyramids cross in the midline forming the ***pyramidal decussation***.

Plate: 7.2: Gross specimens showing the transverse sections (TS) of medulla oblongata, pons, midbrain, and the spinal cord at various levels

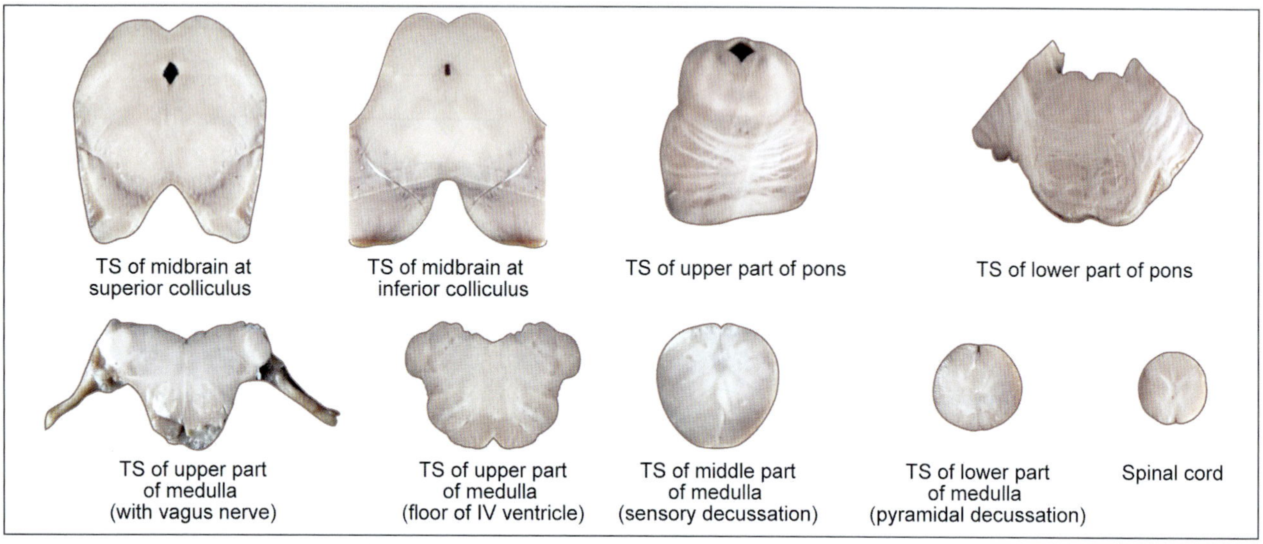

Flowchart 7.1: Medulla oblongata: Features

Medulla oblongata: Features

- ***Extent***
  - From lower border of pons to 1st pair of cervical nerves
  - L: 3 cm
  - W: 2 cm
  - Thickness: 1.25 cm
- ***Cavity***
  - Lower closed part
  - Upper open part
  - Forms 4th ventricle
- ***Sulci and fissures***
  - Anterior median fissure
  - Posterior median sulcus
  - Anterolateral and posterolateral sulci
- ***Regions***
  - ***Anterior***
    - Pyramids
    - Pyramidal decussation
    - Abducent nerve
  - ***Lateral***
    - Olives
    - Rootlets of XII nerve
    - Rootlets of IX, X, XI nerves
    - VII and VIII nerve
    - Anterior external arcuate fibres
  - ***Posterior***
    - Lower closed part:
      - Gracile, cuneate tubercles
      - Tuber cinereum
    - Upper open part:
      - Floor of 4th ventricle: Median sulcus
      - Hypoglossal, vagal triangles
      - Vestibular area, area postrema
      - Stria medullaris

BDC yogesh

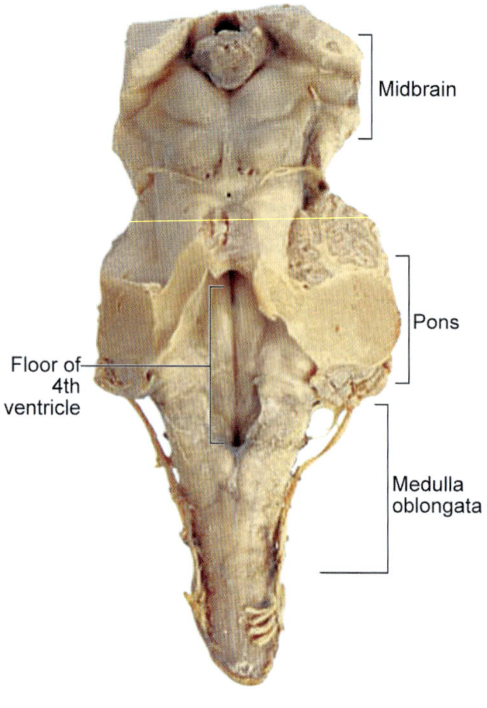

Fig. 7.3: Gross anatomy of brainstem – Dorsal view

Some fibres run transversely across the upper part of the pyramid. These are the ***anterior external arcuate fibres*** which end in the cerebellum.

3. ***Lateral region:*** The upper part of the lateral region shows an oval elevation—the ***olive***. It is produced by an underlying mass of grey matter called the *inferior olivary nucleus*.

   The rootlets of the ***hypoglossal nerve*** emerge from the anterolateral sulcus between the pyramid and the olive.

   The rootlets of the cranial nerves *IX, X and cranial part of the accessory nerve* emerge through the posterolateral fissure, behind the olive.

4. ***Posterior region:*** The posterior region lies between the posterolateral sulcus and the posterior median fissure. The upper part of this region is marked by a V-shaped depression which is the lower part of the *floor of the fourth ventricle*.

   Below the floor, there are three longitudinal elevations. From medial to lateral side, these are the fasciculus gracilis, the fasciculus cuneatus and the inferior cerebellar peduncle.

   The upper ends of fasciculus gracilis and cuneatus expand to form the ***gracile and cuneate tubercles***. These tubercles are formed by underlying masses of grey matter called the *nucleus gracilis* and *nucleus cuneatus*.

Lateral to cuneate nucleus is an accessory cuneate nucleus. Here the unconscious proprioceptive fibres of upper limb relay to terminate in the cerebellum via inferior cerebellar peduncle. This nucleus is equivalent to Clarke's column of spinal cord. These convey discriminative touch, pressure and senses of vibration, position and movements from ipsilateral part of the body. The fasciculus gracilis contains fibres from lower limb and lower part of the trunk, the fasciculus cuneatus from the upper limb and upper part of the trunk.

In the lower part of the medulla, there is another elevation the ***tuber cinerium*** lateral to the fasciculus cuneatus. It is produced by a mass of grey matter called the *spinal nucleus of the trigeminal nerve*.

Competencies:

AN58.2 Describe transverse section of medulla oblongata at the level of: (1) pyramidal decussation, (2) sensory decussation, (3) inferior olivary nucleus.

AN58.3 Enumerate cranial nerve nuclei in medulla oblongata with their functional group.

INTERNAL STRUCTURE

The internal structure (transverse section) of the medulla oblongata is studied at three levels (Plate 7.2):

1. At the lower closed part, that is, at the level of pyramidal decussation.
2. At the upper closed part – at the level of sensory decussation.
3. At the level of olives – open part of medulla.

Transverse Section through the Lower Part of the Medulla Passing through the Pyramidal Decussation

It resembles a transverse section of the spinal cord in having the same three funiculi and the same tracts (Flowchart 7.2 and Fig. 7.4).

Flowchart 7.2: Transverse sections (TS) of the medulla

TS of medulla at the level of pyramidal decussation

Grey matter
- Central grey matter with central canal
- Spinal nucleus of accessory nerve
- Nucleus gracilis and nucleus cuneatus
- Nucleus of spinal tract of trigeminal nerve
- Supraspinal nucleus (C1)

White matter
- Pyramid
- Decussation of pyramidal fibres
- Fasciculus gracilis and fasciculus cuneatus
- Spinal tract of trigeminal nerve
- Anterior and posterior spinocerebellar tract

TS of medulla at the level of sensory decussation

Grey matter
- Nucleus gracilis and nucleus cuneatus
- Nucleus of spinal tract of trigeminal nerve
- Accessory cuneate nu.
- Central grey matter:
  - Hypoglossal nucleus
  - Dorsal nucleus of vagus
  - Nucleus tractus solitarius
  - Inferior olivary nucleus

White matter
- Sensory decussation
- Pyramid
- Medial lemniscus
- Medial longitudinal bundle
- Spinal tract of trigeminal nerve
- Reticular formation
- Anterior and posterior spinocerebellar tracts
- Lateral and anterior spinothalamic tracts

TS of medulla at the level of olives (open part)

Grey matter
- Hypoglossal nucleus
- Dorsal nucleus of vagus
- Nucleus tracts solitarius
- Inferior and medial vestibular nuclei
- Nucleus ambiguus
- Dorsal and ventral cochlear nucleus
- Nucleus of spinal tract trigeminal nucleus
- Arcuate nuclei
- Inferior olivary nucleus

White matter
- Inferior cerebellar peduncle
- Olivocerebellar fibre
- Stria medullaris or external arcuate fibres
- Fibers of IXth, Xth, and XIth cranial nerves
- Pyramidal fibres

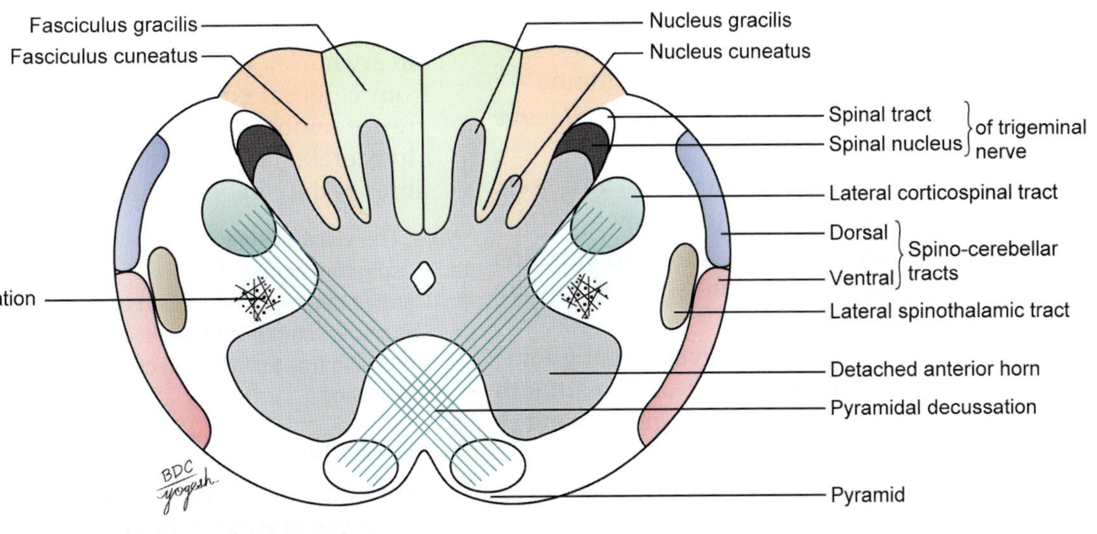

Fig. 7.4: Transverse section (TS) of medulla oblongata at the level of pyramidal decussation

Grey Matter

1. The decussating pyramidal fibres separate the anterior horn from the central grey matter. The *separated anterior horn* forms the *spinal nucleus of the accessory nerve* laterally and the ***supraspinal nucleus*** for motor fibres of the first cervical nerve medially.
2. The central grey matter (with the central canal) is pushed backwards.
3. The *nucleus gracilis* and the *nucleus cuneatus* are continuous with the central grey matter.
4. Laterally, the central grey matter is continuous with the nucleus of the *spinal tract of the trigeminal nerve*. A bundle of fibres overlying this nucleus forms the spinal tract of the trigeminal nerve.
5. *Reticular formation* made up of neurons and nerve fibres also present.

White Matter

1. The *pyramids*, anteriorly.
2. The *decussation* of the pyramidal tracts forms the most important features of the medulla at this level. The fibres of each pyramid run backwards and laterally to reach the lateral white column of the spinal cord where they form the *lateral corticospinal tract*.
3. The fasciculus gracilis and the fasciculus cuneatus occupy the broad posterior white column.
4. The other features of the white matter are similar to those of the spinal cord.

Transverse Section through the Middle of Medulla Passing through the Sensory Decussation (Fig. 7.5 and Flowchart 7.2)

Grey Matter

1. The *nucleus gracilis* and *nucleus cuneatus* increase in size. They get separated from the central grey matter. The fibers of fasciculus gracilis and fasciculus cuneatus (which carries sensation of conscious proprioception, discrimination touch, and vibration) relay in nucleus gracilis and nucleus cuneatus.
2. Lateral to the cuneate nucleus, the ***accessory cuneate nucleus*** is present which relays unconscious proprioceptive fibres from the upper limbs. It is equivalent to nucleus dorsalis/Clarke's column.
3. The ***nucleus of the spinal tract of the trigeminal nerve*** is also separate from the central grey matter.
4. The lower part of the ***inferior olivary nucleus*** is seen.
5. The ***central grey matter*** contains the following:
   - Hypoglossal nucleus—an elongated nucleus about 2 cm long, supplies muscles of tongue except palatoglossus.
   - Dorsal nucleus of the vagus—gives preganglionic parasympathetic fibres to heart and to smooth muscles and glands of respiratory and alimentary system.
   - Nucleus of tractus solitarius—receives taste fibres.
6. Reticular formation made up of neurons and nerve fibres also present.

White Matter

1. The nucleus gracilis and cuneatus give rise to the ***internal arcuate fibres***. These fibres cross to the opposite side where they form a paramedian band of fibres, called the ***medial lemniscus***. In the lemniscus, the body is represented with the head posteriorly and the feet anteriorly.
2. The ***pyramid*** lie anteriorly.
3. The ***medial longitudinal bundle*** lies posterior to the medial lemniscus.
4. The *spinocerebellar, lateral spinothalamic* and other tracts lie in the anterolateral area.
5. Emerging fibres of XII nerve.

Transverse Section through the Upper Part of Medulla Passing through the Floor of Fourth Ventricle/Open Part (Fig. 7.6 and Flowchart 7.2)

Grey Matter

1. The nuclei of several cranial nerves are seen in the floor of the fourth ventricle:
   a. *Hypoglossal nucleus,* in a paramedian position.
   b. *Dorsal nucleus of the vagus,* lateral to the XII nerve nucleus.
   c. *Nucleus of the tractus solitarius,* ventrolateral to the dorsal nucleus of vagus.
   d. *Inferior and medial vestibular nuclei,* medial to the inferior cerebellar peduncle.
2. The *nucleus ambiguus* lies deep in the reticular formation of the medulla. It gives origin to motor fibres of the cranial nerves IX, X and XI.
3. The *dorsal and ventral cochlear nuclei* lie on the surface of the inferior cerebellar peduncle. These nuclei receive fibres of the cochlear nerve.
4. The *nucleus of the spinal tract* of the trigeminal nerve lies in the dorsolateral part.
5. The *arcuate nucleus* lies anteromedial to the pyramidal tract.
6. The *inferior olivary nucleus* is the largest mass of grey matter seen at this level. It is responsible for producing the elevation of the olive. Its grey matter appears like a crumpled purse. Close to the inferior olivary nucleus, there are the medial and dorsal accessory olivary nuclei. The nucleus receives the afferent fibres from cerebral cortex, red nucleus, periaqueductal grey of midbrain and spinal cord. The efferents form olivocerebellar fibres which terminate as climbing fibres at the cerebellar cortex.

Note: The visceral centres are placed deeply. These are:
a. Respiratory centre
b. Cardiac centre for regulation of heart rate
c. Vasomotor centre for regulation of blood pressure.
d. Reflex centres for vomiting coughing, sneezing, hiccuping and swallowing.

White Matter

It shows the following important features:

1. The *inferior cerebellar peduncle* occupies the posterolateral part, lateral to the fourth ventricle.

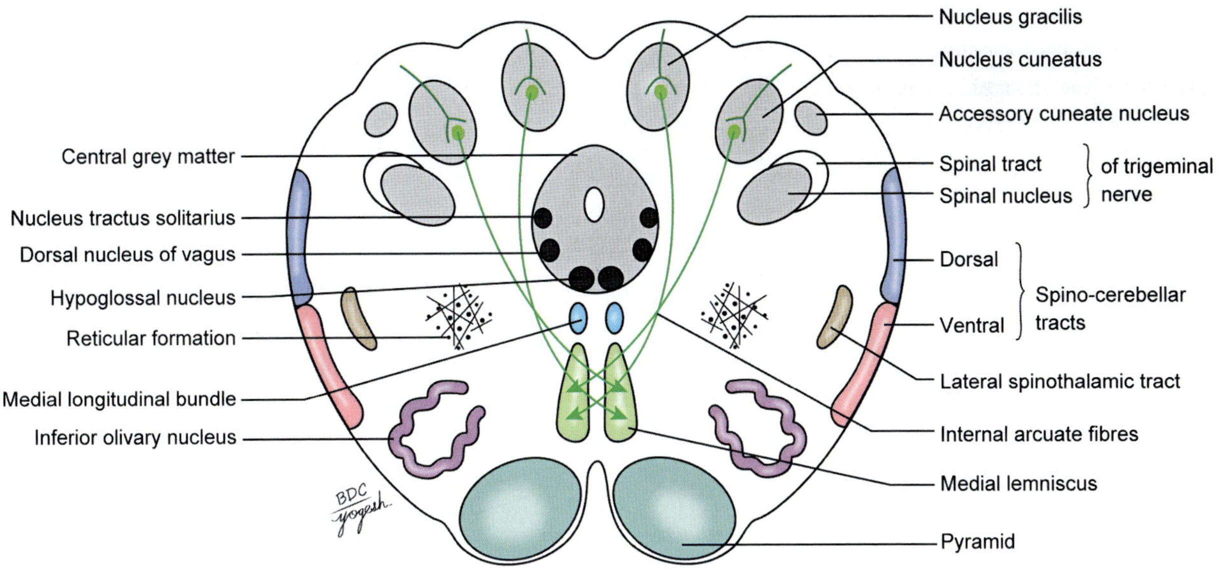

Fig. 7.5: Transverse section (TS) of medulla oblongata at the level of sensory decussation

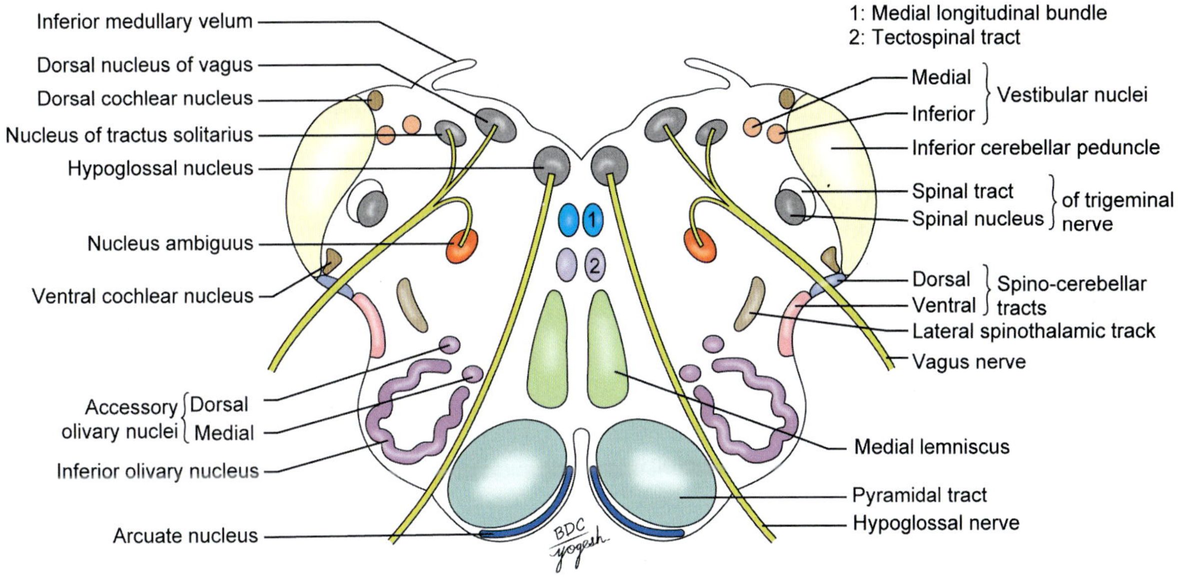

Fig. 7.6: TS of medulla oblongata at the level of olivary nucleus passing through floor of fourth ventricle

2. The *olivocerebellar fibres* are seen prominently in actual sections. The fibres emerge at the hilum of the inferior olivary nucleus and pass to the opposite inferior cerebellar peduncle, on their way to the opposite half of the cerebellum.
3. *Striae medullaris (external arcuate fibres)* are seen in the floor of the fourth ventricle.
4. Emerging fibres of IX, X, XI nerves.
5. Various ascending and descending tracts.

BLOOD SUPPLY

- *Anterior spinal artery*: This supplies the whole medial part of the medulla oblongata.
- *Posterior inferior cerebellar artery*: This supplies the posterolateral part of the medulla.

Competency:

AN58.4 Describe the anatomical basis of clinical conditions affecting the medulla oblongata (medial and lateral medullary syndromes, crossed diplegia).

CLINICAL NEUROANATOMY

Medial medullary/Dejerine syndrome/Crossed diplegia: It occurs due to blockage of anterior spinal artery. Features are:

a. Contralateral hemiplegia (Fig. 7.3, Flowchart 7.3) due to damage to pyramid of medulla.
b. Loss of sense of vibration and position due to damage to medial lemniscus.
c. Paralysis of muscles of tongue on the same side due to injury to XII cranial nerve.

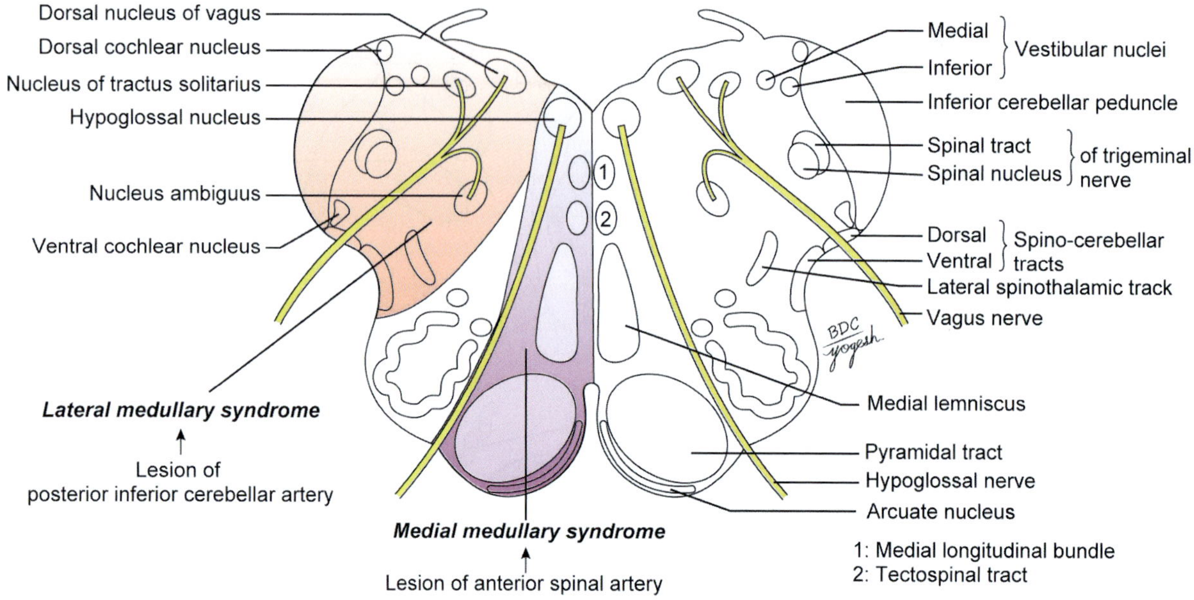

Fig. 7.7: Lesions of medulla oblongata: Light red coloured zone indicates the territory involved in lateral medullary syndrome and purple coloured zone indicates the territory involved in medial medullary syndrome (TS of medulla at the level of olives)

Lateral medullary/Wallenberg syndrome: Occurs due to blockage of posterior inferior cerebellar artery. It supplies areas behind the inferior olivary nucleus. Features are:

a. Ipsilateral paralysis of most of muscles of soft palate, pharynx and larynx due to injury to nucleus ambiguus which gives fibres to IX, X and XI cranial nerves (Fig. 7.7 and Flowchart 7.3).
b. Loss of pain and temperature on same side of face due to involvement of spinal nucleus and spinal tract of trigeminal nerve.
c. Loss of pain and temperature on opposite side of the body due to involvement of lateral spinothalamic tract.
d. Giddiness due to involvement of vestibular nuclei.
e. Damage to inferior cerebellar peduncle, spinocerebellar tracts and part of cerebellum results in loss of equilibrium, i.e. ataxia of limbs on the same side.
f. The sympathetic fibres descend from hypothalamus to cells in lateral horn of spinal cord. As these fibres descend in the lateral part of medulla (which is damaged), there is Horner's syndrome, comprising ptosis, enophthalmos, miosis and anhidrosis.

Injury to lower part of medulla oblongata: Injury in this part may be fatal due to injury to the vital centres, like respiratory centre and vasomotor centre.

Bulbar palsy: In this condition, there is weakness of muscles supplied by VII–XII cranial nerves. These nerves supply muscles of facial expression, muscles of pharynx, tongue, palate and larynx. The lesion is of lower motor neuron type. The patient has difficulty in speaking, swallowing and in usage of muscles of facial expression.

Pseudobulbar palsy: It occurs due to bilateral lesion of corticonuclear fibres. There is paralysis of muscles of tongue, lips, pharynx and palate. The causes of pseudobulbar palsy may be vascular infarction, syringomyelia and increased intracranial pressure.

Flowchart 7.3: Lateral and medial medullary syndromes

Lateral medullary syndrome
Wallenberg syndrome

Cause	*Lesion*	*Effects*
Thrombosis of posterior inferior cerebellar artery (PICA) ↓ Lesion of dorsolateral part of medulla	Spinothalamic tract	→ Contralateral loss of pain and temperature sensation in trunk and limbs
	Spinal nucleus and tract of V nerve	→ Ipsilateral loss of pain and temperature sensations over face
	Nucleus ambiguus	→ Ipsilateral paralysis of muscles of palate, pharynx, and larynx
	Inferior cerebellar peduncle	→ Ipsilateral ataxia (loss of equilibrium)
	Vestibular nuclei	→ Giddiness
	Reticular formation and descending sympathetic fibres from hypothalamus	→ Horner syndrome (miosis, ptosis, enophthalmos, anhidrosis)

Medial medullary syndrome
Dejerine syndrome

Cause	*Lesion*	*Effects*
Lesion of anterior spinal artery ↓ Lesion of paramedian region of medulla	Pyramid	→ Contralateral hemiplegia
	Medial lemniscus	→ Contralateral loss of vibration, position sense, discriminatory touch sensation
	Hypoglossal nucleus	→ Ipsilateral paralysis of muscles of tongue

PONS

The pons (Latin *bridge*) is also called metencephalon, 2.5 cm long and extends from cranial end of medulla oblongata to the cerebral peduncles of midbrain. Cranial nerves V, VI, VII, and VIII are attached here. Anteriorly, it is related to clivus separated by basilar artery, laterally to middle cerebellar peduncle and posteriorly to the fourth ventricle.

Competency:
AN59.1 Identify external features of pons.

EXTERNAL FEATURES

Surfaces

The pons has *two surfaces*—ventral and dorsal (Figs 7.1 and 7.2, Flowchart 7.4).

Ventral or Anterior Surface

1. The *ventral or anterior surface* is convex in both directions and is transversely striated. In the median plane, it shows a vertical ***basilar sulcus*** which lodges the basilar artery.
2. Laterally, the surface is continuous with the middle cerebellar peduncle.
3. The ***trigeminal nerve*** is attached to this surface at the junction of the pons with the middle cerebellar peduncle. The nerve has two roots—a small motor root which lies medial to the much larger sensory root.
4. The attached abducent, facial and vestibulocochlear nerves are at the lower border of the ventral surface at the junction of pons and medulla oblongata.

Dorsal or Posterior Surface

The *dorsal or posterior surface* is hidden by the cerebellum, and forms the upper half of the floor of the fourth ventricle.

Borders

Pons has two borders—superior and inferior.
1. ***Superior border***: Crus cerebri are attached here. III and IV nerves are also seen.
2. ***Inferior border***: Lies at the junction of pons and medulla. VI, VII and VIII nerves lie at this border.

Note: Pontomedullary junction: It is represented by a shallow groove. The following cranial nerve emerges at the pontomedullary junction from medial to lateral: Abducent (VI), facial (VII) with nervus intermedius and vestibulocochlear nerves (VIII).

Flowchart 7.4: Pons: Features

Pons: Features

- ***Location***
  - Between midbrain and medulla oblongata
  - L: 2.5 cm
  - Connected with cerebellum by middle cerebellar peduncles
- ***Anterior surface***
  - Convex
  - Basilar groove
  - Laterally continuous with middle cerebellar peduncle
  - Trigeminal nerve
    - Small medial motor root
    - Large lateral sensory root
- ***Posterior surface***
  - Forms floor of 4th ventricle
  - Median sulcus
  - Median eminence
  - Facial colliculus
  - Sulcus limitans
  - Superior fovea
  - Vestibular area

Pontomedullary junction: VIth, VIIth, VIIIth cranial nerves
Anterior inferior cerebellar arteries

BDC yogesh

Competencies:
AN59.2 Draw and label transverse section of pons at the upper and lower level.
AN59.3 Enumerate cranial nerve nuclei in pons with their functional group.

INTERNAL STRUCTURE

In transverse sections, the pons is seen to be divisible into two parts (Fig. 7.8 and Flowchart 7.5):
1. Ventral or ***basilar part*** is continuous inferiorly with the pyramids of the medulla, and on each side with the cerebellum through the middle cerebellar peduncle.
2. Dorsal or ***tegmental part*** is a direct upward continuation of the medulla (excluding the pyramids).

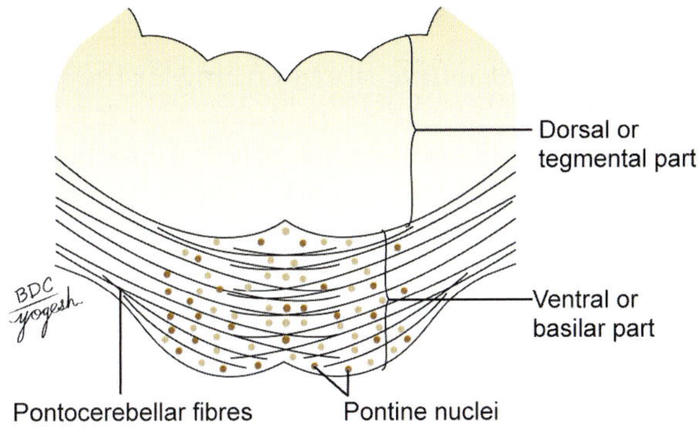

Fig. 7.8: Parts of pons (TS of pons)

Flowchart 7.5: TS of pons

TS of upper part of pons

- ***Basilar part***
  - Nuclei pontis
  - Nerve fibres
    - Corticospinal
    - Corticopontine
    - Corticonuclear
    - Pontocerebellar
- ***Tegmentum***
  - ***Grey matter***
    - Motor nucleus of V nerve
    - Main sensory nucleus of V nerve
  - ***White matter***
    - Lemnisci: MTSL
    - MLB
    - Superior cerebellar peduncles
    - Reticular formation

TS of lower part of pons

- ***Basilar part***
  - Nuclei pontis
  - Nerve fibres
    - Corticospinal
    - Corticopontine
    - Corticonuclear
    - Pontocerebellar
- ***Tegmentum***
  - ***Grey matter***
    - VIth, VIIth nerve nuclei
    - Vestibular nuclei (ventral and dorsal), cochlear nerve nuclei
    - Superior salivatory, Inferior salivatory and lacrimatory nuclei
    - Nucleus tracts solitarius
    - Spinal nucleus of Vth nerve
    - Nuclei of trapezoid body
  - ***White matter***
    - Trapezoid body
    - Medial lemniscus
    - Spinal lemniscus
    - MLB
    - Tectospinal tract
    - Spinal tract of Vth nerve
    - Intraneuronal course of VIth, VIIth nerves
    - Anterior spinocerebellar tract

BDC yogesh

(MTSL: Medial, trigeminal, spinal, and lateral; MLB: Medial longitudinal bundle)

Basilar Part/Ventral Part

The basilar part of the pons has a uniform structure throughout its length.

Grey Matter

It is represented by the ***nuclei pontis*** which are scattered among longitudinal and transverse fibres. The pontine nuclei form an important part of the cortico-pontocerebellar pathway. Some of these nuclei get displaced during development, and form the arcuate nucleus (*see* medulla) and the pontobulbar body. Fibres from all these nuclei go to the opposite half of the cerebellum.

White Matter

It consists of longitudinal and transverse fibres.

1. The longitudinal fibres include:
   a. The *corticospinal* and *corticonuclear* (pyramidal) tracts.
   b. The *corticopontine* fibres ending in the pontine nuclei.
2. The transverse fibres are *pontocerebellar* fibres beginning from the pontine nuclei and going to the opposite half of the cerebellum, through the middle cerebellar peduncle.

Tegmental Part/Dorsal Part

However, the structure of the tegmental part differs in the upper and lower parts of the pons.

1. *Tegmentum in the Lower Part of Pons*

(Fig. 7.9, Flowchart 7.5)

Grey matter

1. The 6*th nerve nucleus* lies beneath the facial colliculus.
2. The 7*th nerve nucleus* lies in the reticular formation of the pons.
3. The vestibular and cochlear nuclei lie in relation to the inferior cerebellar peduncle. The *vestibular nuclei* lie deep to the vestibular area in the floor of the fourth ventricle, partly in the medulla and partly in the pons. They are divisible into four parts—superior, inferior, medial and lateral. They receive the fibres of the vestibular nerve, and give efferents to the cerebellum (vestibulocerebellar), the medial longitudinal bundle and the spinal cord (vestibulospinal tract arising in the lateral vestibular nucleus) and the lateral lemniscus.

   The dorsal and ventral *cochlear nuclei* are situated dorsal and ventral to the inferior cerebellar peduncle. They receive the fibres of the cochlear nerve, and give efferents mostly to the superior olivary nucleus and partly to nuclei of the corpus trapezoideum, and to nuclei of the lateral lemniscus. These fibres form the trapezoid body.
4. The spinal nucleus of the trigeminal nerve lies in the lateral part.
5. Other nuclei present include the superior salivatory and lacrimatory nuclei.
6. Reticular formation also present.

White matter

1. The *trapezoid body* or corpus trapezoideum is a transverse band of fibres lying just behind the ventral part of the pons. It consists of fibres that arise in the cochlear nuclei of both sides. It is a part of the auditory pathway.
2. The medial lemniscus forms a transverse band on either side of the midline, just behind the trapezoid body. It is joined by anterior spinothalamic tract.
3. The lateral spinothalamic tract (spinal lemniscus) lies lateral to the medial lemniscus.
4. The trigeminal lemniscus conveys fibres of second sensory neurons from the opposite spinal and sensory nuclei of trigeminal nerve.

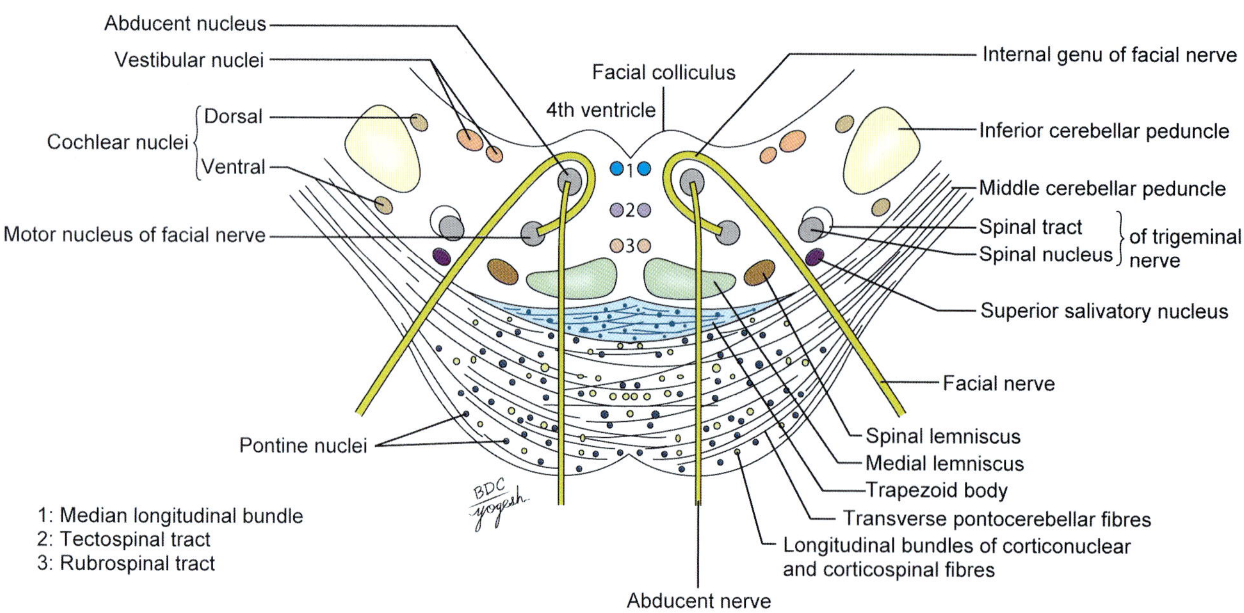

Fig. 7.9: TS of lower part of pons or TS at the level of facial colliculus

5. The inferior cerebellar peduncle lies lateral to the floor of the fourth ventricle.
6. The fibres of the facial nerve follow a peculiar course. They first pass backwards and medially to reach the medial side of the abducent nucleus. They then form a loop dorsal to the abducent nucleus. This loop is responsible for producing an elevation, the *facial colliculus*, in the floor of the fourth ventricle.

2. *Tegmentum in the Upper Part of Pons*

(Fig. 7.10, Flowchart 7.5)

Grey matter

1. The special features are the *motor, and superior sensory nuclei of the trigeminal nerve.* The motor nucleus is medial to the superior sensory nucleus.
2. Reticular formation contains pneumotaxic centre and apneustic centres in pons. These control respiration.

White matter

1. Immediately behind the ventral part of the pons, the bands of fibres made up (from medial to lateral side) of the medial lemniscus, the trigeminal lemniscus, the spinal lemniscus and the lateral lemniscus (MTSL) are present. The trigeminal lemniscus contains fibres arising in the spinal nucleus of the trigeminal nerve and travelling to the thalamus. The lateral lemniscus is a part of the auditory pathway. It is formed by fibres arising in nuclei lying in close relation to the trapezoid body (superior olivary nucleus and nucleus of trapezoid body).
2. The superior cerebellar peduncles lie dorsolateral to the fourth ventricle (replacing the inferior peduncle seen in the lower part of the pons).
3. The medial longitudinal bundle is made up of fibres that interconnect the nuclei of the cranial nerves III, IV, VI, VIII and the spinal root of the XI. It coordinates movements of the head and neck in response to stimulation of the cranial nerve VIII. However, the majority of fibres in the medial longitudinal bundle arise in the vestibular nuclei.

BLOOD SUPPLY

The pontine arteries are a number of small vessels which come off at right angles from either side of the basilar artery and supply the pons and adjacent parts of the brain.

Competency:

AN59.4 Describe the anatomical basis of clinical conditions affecting the pons (Locked-in syndrome, pontine haemorrhage, Foville syndrome, Raymond syndrome, Millard-Gubler syndrome).

CLINICAL NEUROANATOMY

Pontine haemorrhage: Occurs due to rupture of pontine branches of basilar artery. This entity has following features:

a. Bilateral paralysis of face and limbs due to involvement of VII nerve nucleus and all corticospinal fibres.
b. Deep coma due to damage to the reticular formation.
c. Hyperpyrexia due to cutting off of the temperature regulating fibres from the hypothalamus.
d. Pinpoint pupil due to damage to sympathetic ocular fibres and unopposed action of sphincter pupillae muscle which is innervated by parasympathetic fibres. Pontine haemorrhage is usually fatal.

Cerebellopontine angle (Fig. 7.11)**:** The anatomical structures located in the cerebellopontine angle include choroid plexuses of IV ventricle, flocculus, VII and VIII cranial nerves. A tumour, acoustic neuroma, in this angle arises usually in relation to VIII nerve. Features are:

a. Ipsilateral facial paralysis and loss of taste in anterior two-thirds of tongue and hyperacusis due to damage to fibres of facial nerve.
b. Deafness and vertigo due to damage to both the parts of VIII nerve.

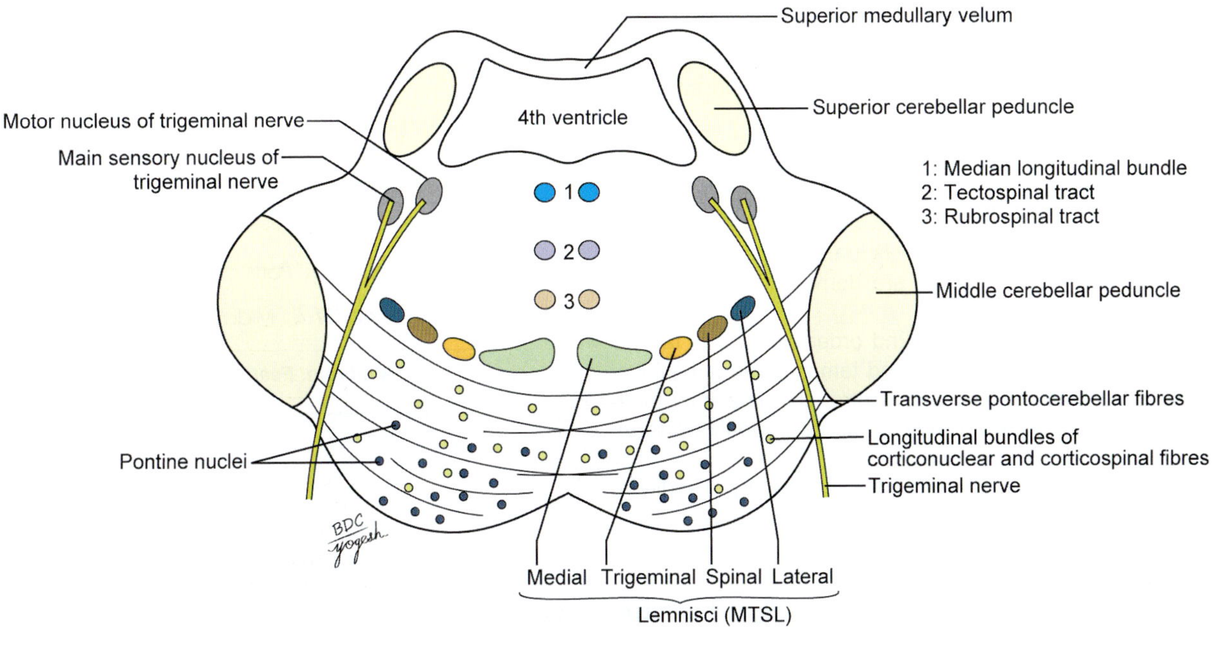

Fig. 7.10: TS of upper pons

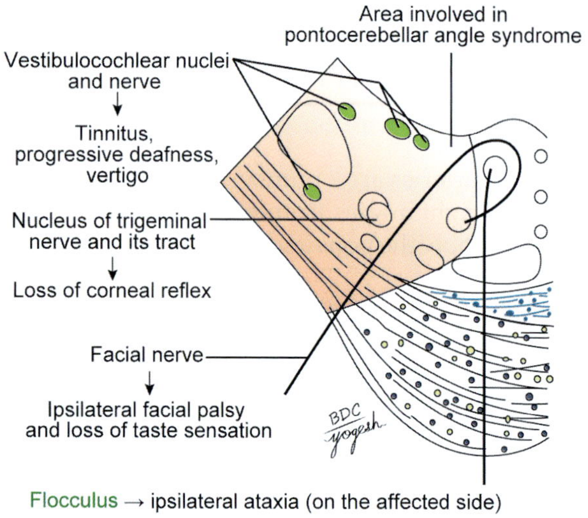

Fig. 7.11: Cerebellopontine angle tumour

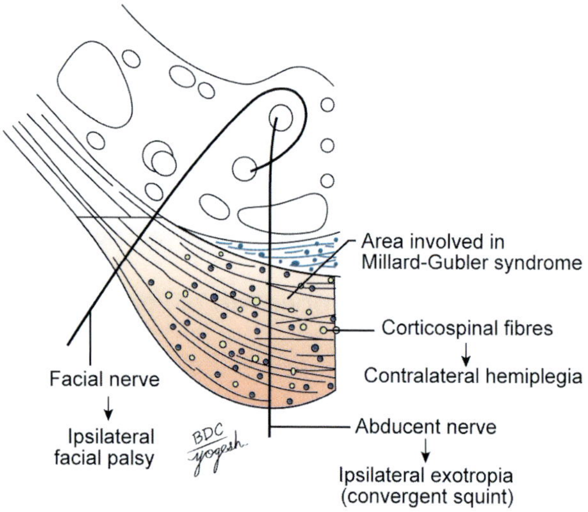

Fig. 7.12: Millard-Gubler syndrome

c. Ataxia on the affected side due to involvement of the flocculus.

d. Absence of corneal reflex on the side of lesion due to damage to nucleus of V nerve including its spinal tract.

Millard-Gubler syndrome (Fig. 7.12)**:** In this condition, there is damage to fibres of VI and VII nerves along with pyramidal fibres. Features are:

a. Ipsilateral facial paralysis due to damage to VII nerve; there is paralysis of facial muscles on the same side.

b. Ipsilateral loss of abduction of the eye due to damage to VI nerve. Due to unopposed action of adductors of eye, there is ipsilateral medial squint and diplopia on looking towards paralysed side.

c. Contralateral hemiplegia due to lesion of the pyramidal fibres.

Tumours of pons: Astrocytoma is the most common tumour of brainstem, usually in childhood. Signs and symptoms vary according to area of origin of tumour.

Foville's syndrome: It occurs due to blockage of perforating branch of a basilar artery supplying the dorsal part of pons. In this syndrome, damage to abducent nerve nucleus produces ipsilateral exotropia, and damage to facial nerve nucleus produces ipsilateral facial paralysis.

Note: ***Lemnisci:***

1. *Medial lemniscus* (*Reil's band*): It has second order neurons of tract of Goll and Burdach. It carries conscious proprioception, discriminative touch sensation and vibration sensation.
2. *Trigeminal lemniscus*: It conveys pain and temperature sensations from face. Its fibres are derived from the spinal nucleus of trigeminal nerve.
3. *Spinal lemniscus*: It consists of 2nd order neurons of lateral spinothalamic tract (carries pain and temperature sensations from opposite half of body) and ventral spinothalamic tract (carries crude touch and crude pressure sensations from opposite half of body).
4. *Lateral lemniscus*: It consists of third order neurons of auditory pathway. They are derived from superior olivary nucleus (cochlear nuclei → superior olivary nucleus → trapezoid body and its nuclei → lateral lemniscus).

[*Mnemonics:* ***Mahanagar Telephone Sitam (Nigam) Limited (MTSL)*** (from medial to lateral): **M** – Medial lemniscus; **T** – Trigeminal lemniscus; **S** – Spinal lemniscus; **L** – Lateral lemniscus]

MIDBRAIN

The midbrain is also called the *mesencephalon.* It is 2 cm long and connects the hindbrain with the forebrain. Its cavity is known as the cerebral aqueduct of Sylvius (French anatomist 1478–1555). It connects the third ventricle with the fourth ventricle (Fig. 7.13).

Location: The midbrain passes through the tentorial notch, and is related on each side to the parahippocampal gyri, the optic tracts, the posterior cerebral artery, the basal vein, the trochlear nerve, and the geniculate bodies (Flowchart 7.6). Anteriorly, it is related to the

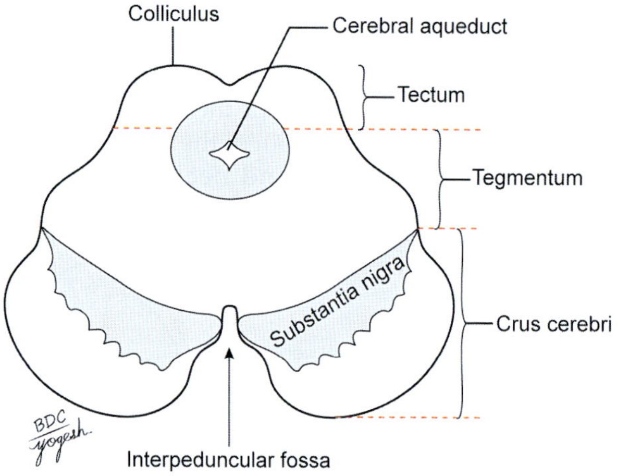

Fig. 7.13: Parts of midbrain

Flowchart 7.6: Midbrain: Features

Midbrain: Features

- ***Location***
  - Extend upward from pons
  - L: 2.5 cm
  - W: 2.5 cm
  - Cavity: cerebral aqueduct
- ***Surfaces***
  - ***Ventral surface***
    - Crus cerebri
    - Interpeduncular fossa
    - Oculomotor nerve
  - ***Dorsal surface***
    - 4 colliculi
      - 2 superior
      - 2 inferior
    - Cruciform sulcus
    - Trochlear nerve

interpeduncular structures, and posteriorly to the splenium of the corpus callosum, the great cerebral vein, the pineal body, and the posterior ends of the right and left thalami.

Dimensions

- *Length*: 2.5 cm
- *Width:* 2.5 cm.

Competency:
AN61.1 Identify external and internal features of midbrain.

EXTERNAL FEATURES

Ventral Surface

Ventral surface presents ***crus cerebri***. It is crossed by optic tract, basal vein, posterior cerebral and superior cerebellar arteries. From the medial side, of crus cerebri ***oculomotor nerve*** emerges (Figs 7.1 and 7.2).

Dorsal Surface

On the dorsal aspects, ***superior and inferior colliculi*** are present. They are called together as corpora quadrigemina (quadruplet bodies). The superior colliculus is connected to the lateral geniculate body by the *superior brachium*.

Likewise, the inferior colliculus is connected to the medial geniculate body by the *inferior brachium*.

Cruciform sulcus separates the four colliculi from each other.

The ***trochlear nerve*** emerges one on each side of frenulum veli. These nerves decussate in each superior medullary velum. Further, it curls around the lateral aspect of cerebral peduncles and runs forwards.

Competency:
AN61.2 Describe internal features of midbrain at the level of superior and inferior colliculus.

INTERNAL STRUCTURE

In the transverse section, the midbrain shows the following parts:

1. The ***tectum*** is the part posterior to aqueduct. It is made up of the right and left superior and inferior colliculi (Flowchart 7.7).
2. Each half of the midbrain anterior to the aqueduct is called the ***cerebral peduncle***. Each cerebral peduncle is subdivided into:
   a. Crus cerebri, anteriorly
   b. Substantia nigra, in the middle
   c. Tegmentum, posteriorly (Flowchart 7.7).
3. The *periaqueductal grey matter*.

It is studied conveniently by examining sections, at the level of the inferior colliculi and at the level of the superior colliculi.

Flowchart 7.7: TS of midbrain

TS of midbrain at the level of inferior colliculus

- ***Cerebral peduncle***
  - Crus cerebri
    - Fibres: Corticospinal, corticonuclear, frontopontine, temporopontine, parietopontine, occipitopontine
    - Substantia nigra
  - ***Tegmentum***
    - ***Grey matter***
      - Periaqueductal grey matter
        - Trochlear nucleus
        - Mesencephalic nucleus of Vth nerve
      - Reticular formation
    - ***White matter***
      - 4 Lemnisci: Medial, trigeminal, spinal, lateral
      - Trochlear nerve
      - Decussation of superior cerebellar peduncles
      - MLB
      - Tectospinal tract
      - Rubrospinal tract
- ***Tectum***
  - Inferior colliculus
    - Auditory pathway
    - Audio–visual reflexes

TS of midbrain at the level of superior colliculus

- ***Cerebral peduncle***
  - 1. Crus cerebri
  - 2. Substantia nigra
  - ***Grey matter***
    - Periaqueductal grey matter
    - Oculomotor nucleus
    - Edinger-Westphal nucleus
    - Mesencephalic nucleus of Vth nerve
    - Pretectal nucleus
    - Red nucleus
    - Nuclei of reticular formation
  - ***White matter***
    - Dorsal tegmental decussation
    - Ventral tegmental decussation
    - MLB
    - 3 Lemnisci: Medial, trigeminal, spinal
    - Fibers of oculomotor nerve
- ***Tectum***
  - Superior colliculus
    - Visual pathway
    - Reflex movements of eye, head, and neck in response to visual stimuli

Transverse Section of Midbrain at the Level of Inferior Colliculi

Grey Matter

1. The ***central (periaqueductal) grey matter*** contains:
   a. The ***nucleus of the trochlear nerve*** in the ventromedial part.
   b. The ***mesencephalic nucleus*** of the trigeminal nerve in the lateral part. The mesencephalic nucleus is made up of unipolar cells (first neuron) and receives proprioceptive impulses from the muscles of mastication, the facial and ocular muscles, the teeth (Fig. 7.14) and temporomandibular joint.
2. The ***inferior colliculus*** receives afferents from the lateral lemniscus, and gives efferents to the medial geniculate body. In the past, it has been considered as the centre for auditory reflexes, but the available evidence indicates that it helps in localizing the source of sounds.
3. The ***substantia nigra*** is a lamina of grey matter made up of deeply pigmented nerve cells. It is concerned with muscle tone (Fig. 7.14).
4. Reticular formation also present.

White Matter

1. The ***crus cerebri*** contains:
   a. The corticospinal tract in the middle.
   b. Frontopontine fibres in the medial one-sixth.

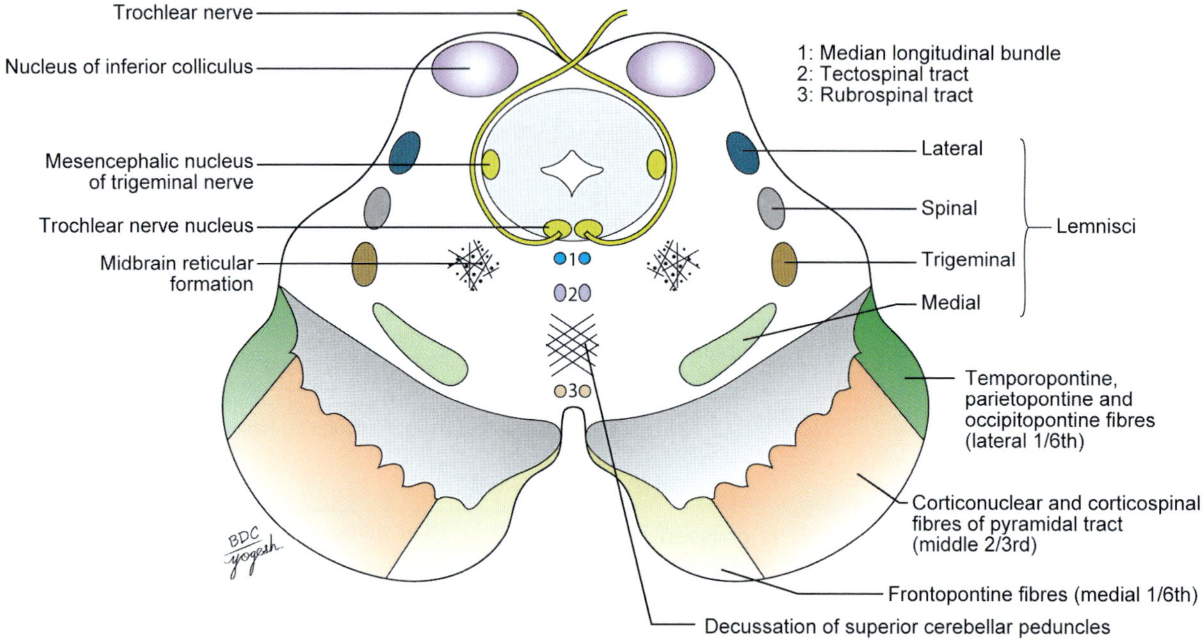

Fig. 7.14: TS of midbrain at the level of inferior colliculus

   c. Temporopontine, parietopontine and occipitopontine fibres in the lateral one-sixth.
2. The ***tegmentum*** contains ascending tracts as follows:
   a. The ***lemnisci*** (medial, trigeminal, spinal and lateral) are arranged in the form of a band in which they lie in the order mentioned (from medial to lateral side) like a necklace.
   b. The *decussation of the superior cerebellar peduncles* is seen in the median plane.
   c. The *medial longitudinal bundle* lies in close relation to the trochlear nucleus (somatic efferent column).
   d. The tectospinal tract and the rubrospinal tract are present.
3. The trochlear nerve passes laterally and dorsally round the central grey matter. It decussates in the superior medullary velum, and emerges lateral to the frenulum veli.

Transverse Section of Midbrain at the Level of Superior Colliculi

Grey Matter

1. The ***central grey matter*** contains:
   a. Nucleus of ***oculomotor nerve*** with Edinger-Westphal nucleus in the ventromedial part.
   b. ***Mesencephalic nucleus*** of the trigeminal nerve in the lateral part. The oculomotor nuclei of the two sides are very close to each other (Fig. 7.15).
2. ***Superior colliculus*** receives afferents from the retina (visual), and various other centres. It gives efferents to the spinal cord (tectospinal tract). It controls reflex movements of the eyes, and of the head and neck in response to visual stimuli (Fig. 7.15).
3. ***Pretectal nucleus*** lies deep to the superolateral part of the superior colliculus. It receives afferents from the lateral roots of the optic tract. It gives efferents to the Edinger-Westphal nuclei of both sides. The pretectal nucleus is an important part of the pathway for light reflex and the consensual reflex. Its lesion causes Argyll Robertson pupil in which the light reflex is lost but accommodation reflex remains intact.
4. ***Red nucleus*** is about 0.5 cm in diameter. It receives afferents from the superior cerebellar peduncle, globus pallidus, subthalamic nucleus and cerebral cortex. It gives efferents to the spinal cord (*rubrospinal tract*), reticular formation, thalamus, olivary nucleus, subthalamic nucleus, etc. It has an inhibitory influence on muscle tone (Fig. 7.16).
5. ***Substantia nigra*** is concerned with muscle tone. Reticular formation also present.

White Matter

1. The ***crus cerebri*** has the same tracts as described above.
2. The ***tegmentum*** contains the following:
   a. The same lemnisci as seen in the lower part except for the lateral lemniscus which has terminated in the inferior colliculus.
   b. The decussation of the tectospinal and tectobulbar tracts forms the *dorsal tegmental decussation*.
   c. The decussation of the rubrospinal tracts forms the *ventral tegmental decussation*.
   d. Medial longitudinal bundle.
   e. Emerging fibres of oculomotor nerve.
3. The ***tectum*** shows the posterior commissure connecting the two superior colliculi.

BLOOD SUPPLY

Most of the blood supply is derived from branches of the basilar artery. Besides this, it also receives from following arteries.

1. Posterior cerebral
2. Superior cerebellar
3. Posterior communicating
4. Anterior choroidal

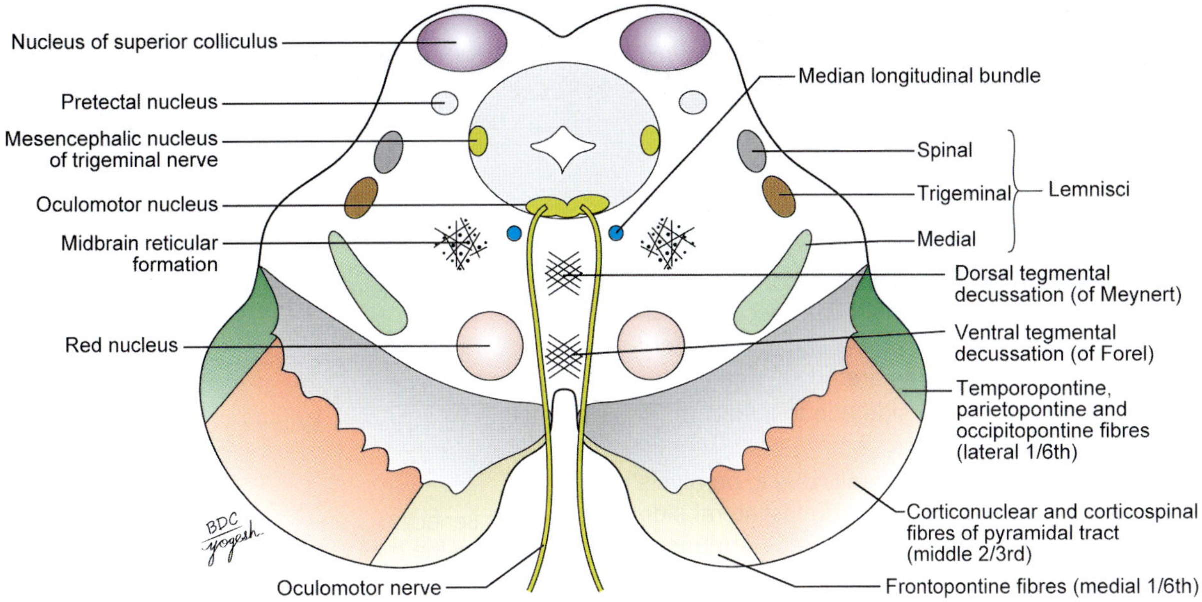

Fig. 7.15: TS of midbrain at the level of superior colliculus

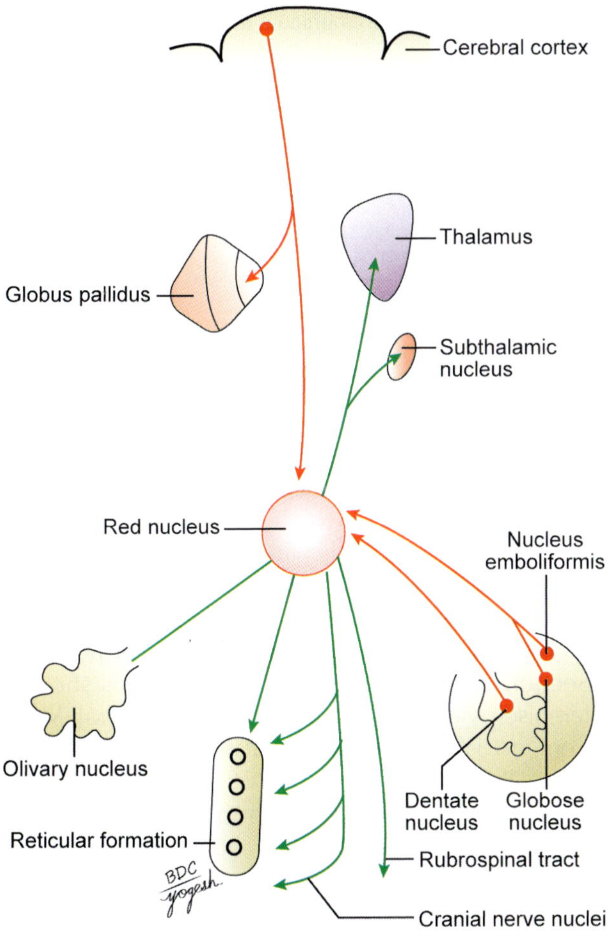

Fig. 7.16: Connections of red nucleus

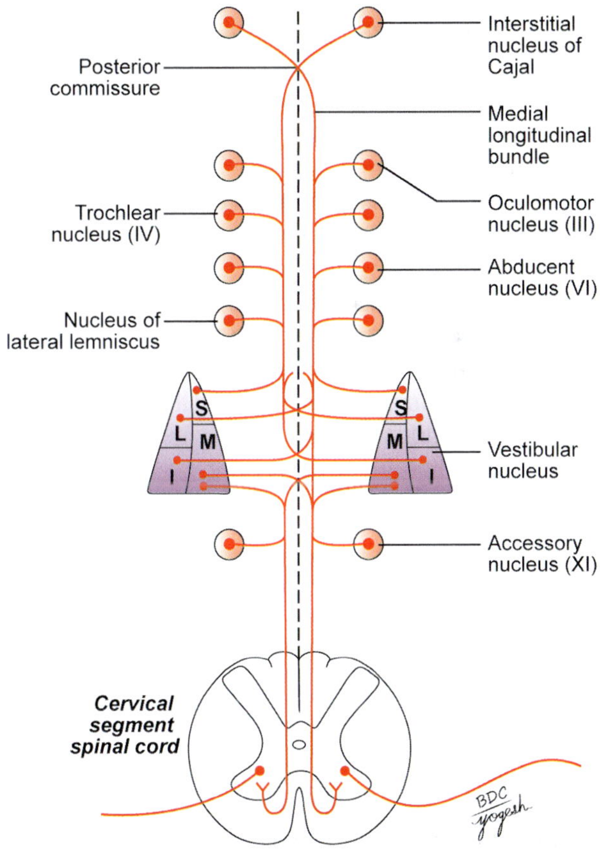

Fig. 7.17: Connections of medial longitudinal bundle

MEDIAL LONGITUDINAL BUNDLE

Main constituent fibres of medial longitudinal bundle (Fig. 7.17) are the fibres from left and right medial vestibular nuclei. These fibres reach up to interstitial nucleus of Cajal at the upper end of aqueduct. The lower end of the fibres reach up to cervical segments of spinal cord.

The bundle connects the cranial nerve nuclei of III, IV, VI, VIII and spinal root of XI nerves. It is also connected to the anterior horn cells which supply muscles of the neck.

This bundle integrates movements of eyes, and neck. It also maintains equilibrium.

Competency:

AN61.3 Describe the anatomical basis of clinical conditions affecting the midbrain (Weber's syndrome, Benedikt's syndrome, Parinaud's syndrome).

CLINICAL NEUROANATOMY

Weber's syndrome (Fig. 7.18): This syndrome involves III nerve nucleus and corticospinal fibres occur due to blockage or rupture of branch of posterior cerebral artery supplying the midbrain. Features are:

a. Hemiplegia on the opposite side due to involvement of corticospinal fibres.
b. Pupil points downwards and laterally due to paralysis of III nerve. There is lateral squint on ipsilateral side due to unopposed action of lateral rectus muscle. There is also contralateral paralysis of lower quarter of face (supranuclear facial palsy).

Benedikt's syndrome (Fig. 7.19): In this condition, most of the tegmentum of midbrain is damaged. Lesion includes loss of medial lemniscus, red nucleus, superior cerebellar peduncle and fibres of III nerve. Features are:

a. Loss of proprioception due to lesion of medial lemniscus.
b. Pupil points downwards and laterally due to injury to III nerve.
c. Tremors and twitching of opposite side due to damage to red nucleus and superior cerebellar peduncle.

Parinaud's syndrome: Lesion of superior colliculi leads to this syndrome. Features include weakness of upward gaze and vertical nystagmus due to lesion of superior colliculus.

Argyll Robertson pupil: In this condition, light reflex is lost but accommodation reflex is retained due to lesion in the vicinity of pretectal nucleus.

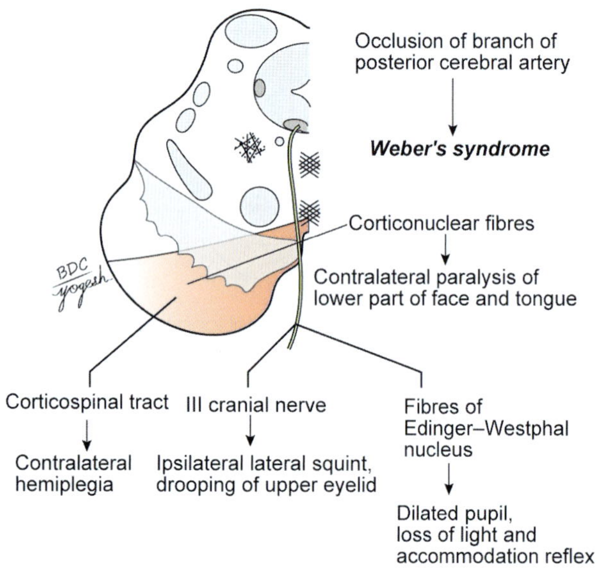

Fig. 7.18: Weber syndrome (Transverse section through the upper part of the midbrain, affected zone is shown by light red colour)

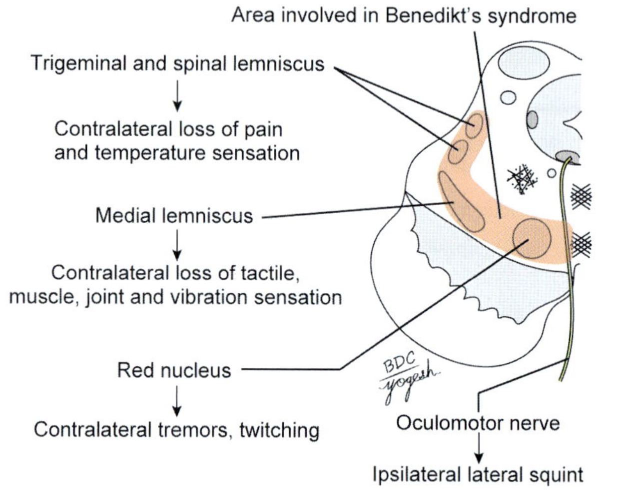

Fig. 7.19: Benedikt's syndrome (Transverse section through the upper part of the midbrain, affected zone is shown by light red colour)

Note: Locked-in syndrome is a rare disorder that shows all voluntary muscles paralysis except for the extraocular muscles. It usually results from brainstem damage, such as a stroke. Patients cannot speak or move but can communicate through eye movements.

VIDEO

Video 4.5 Brainstem

Facts to Remember

- Pyramidal decussation cuts off the anterior horn which forms nucleus of 1st cervical nerve and nucleus of spinal accessory nerve.
- Nucleus gracilis and nucleus cuneatus are equivalent of the nuclei in the posterior horn of spinal cord.
- At the lower section of pons, fibres of cochlear nuclei form trapezoid body which forms lateral lemniscus. Nuclei of VI, VII and VIII cranial nerves are present here.
- At the upper section of pons, some of the nuclei forming trigeminal nerve are situated. The nerve lies at the junction of pons with the middle cerebellar peduncle.
- Section at the level of inferior colliculus shows 4 lemnisci: Medial, trigeminal, spinal and lateral (MTSL) from medial to lateral side. It also shows nucleus of IV nerve, the delicate cranial nerve.
- Section at the level of superior colliculus shows prominent red nucleus. It also shows III nerve nucleus with Edinger-Westphal nucleus.

BDC's Anatomy *e*-book

1. Development of medulla oblongata
2. Development of pons
3. Development of midbrain
4. Further reading
5. Viva voce questions

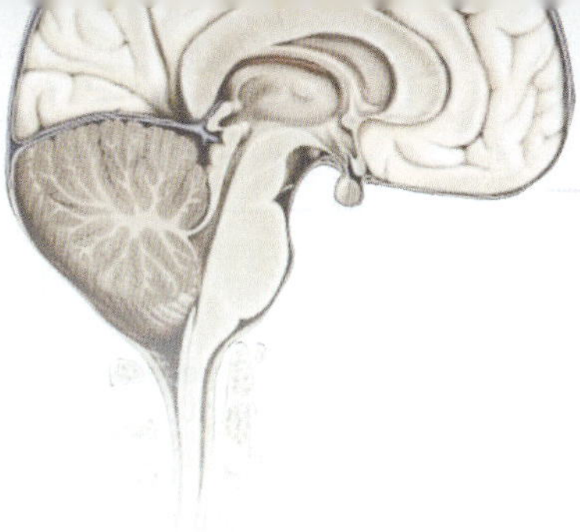

Chapter

8

Cerebellum

Cerebellum (Latin *small brain*), though small in size (weighs about 150 g), subserves important functions for maintaining tone, posture, and equilibrium of the body. It is the largest part of the hindbrain and second largest part of the brain (Plate 8.1 and Figs 8.1a and b).

The grey matter is highly folded to accommodate millions of neurons in a small area and the arrangement is called ***'arbor vitae'*** (tree of life). The structure of cerebellum is uniform throughout, i.e. homotypical.

Note:
1. Cerebellum controls the same side of the body directly or indirectly.
2. The cerebellum does not initiate movement, but it contributes to coordination, precision and accurate timing.

Location

The cerebellum is situated in the posterior cranial fossa behind the pons and medulla. The 4th ventricle separates the cerebellum from pons and upper part of medulla oblongata. It is separated from the cerebrum by tentorium cerebelli (Flowchart 8.1).

Relations

Anteriorly: Fourth ventricle, pons and medulla.
Posteroinferiorly: Squamous occipital bone.
Superiorly: Tentorium cerebelli.

Cavity

The 4th ventricle separates the cerebellum from the pons and the upper part of medulla oblongata.

Flowchart 8.1: Cerebellum: Introduction

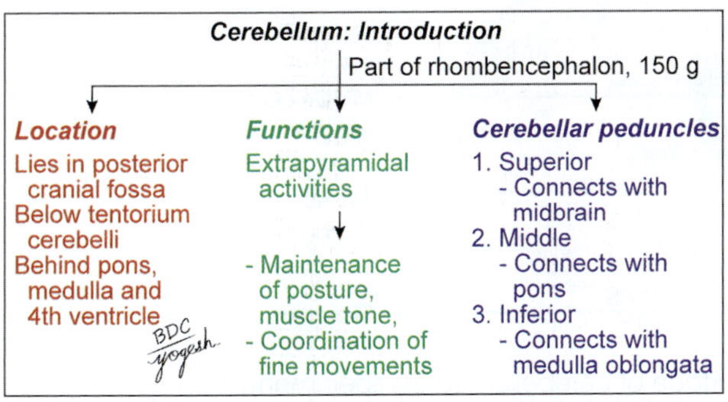

Cerebellar Peduncles

The cerebellum is connected with the brainstem by three pairs of large white fibres called cerebellar peduncles. They are as follows:
1. Superior cerebellar peduncle connects with midbrain.
2. Middle cerebellar peduncle connects with pons.
3. Inferior cerebellar peduncle connects with medulla oblongata.

Competency:
AN60.1 Describe and demonstrate external and internal features of cerebellum.

EXTERNAL FEATURES

The cerebellum is oval and flattened from above downward. Its transverse diameter is larger than the anteroposterior diameter (Flowchart 8.2). The surface of cerebellum shows numerous fissures. The cerebellum has (Fig. 8.2):
1. *Three parts*: Two cerebellar hemispheres, one vermis
2. *Two surfaces*: Superior and inferior
3. *Two notches*: Anterior and posterior
4. *Three prominent fissures*: Horizontal, posterolateral, fissura prima.

Parts of Cerebellum

It consists of:
1. Two *cerebellar hemispheres* – two lateral portions
2. *Vermis* – narrow median portion that connects two cerebellar hemispheres.

Surfaces

Superior surface: It is convex. *Superior vermis* (superior part of vermis) is continuous with superior surface of cerebellar hemispheres (Fig. 8.2).

Inferior surface: It has deep groove or notch in the median plane which is called *vallecula* (Fig. 8.2).

Vallecula (*vallecula cerebelli*) (= groove, in Latin) is a deep notch on the inferior surface of that separates cerebellar hemispheres.

Plate 8.1: Cerebellum

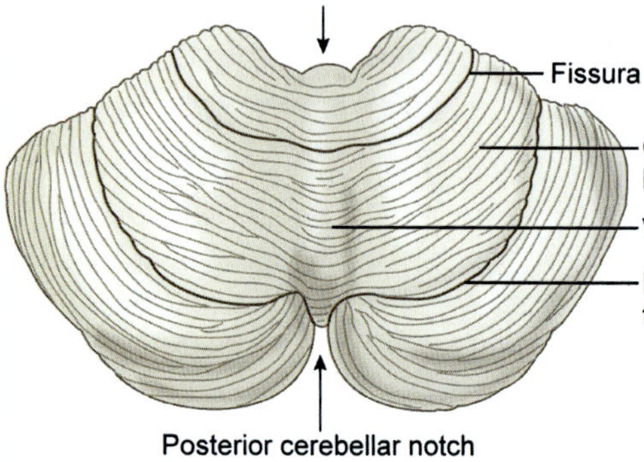

Superior view of the cerebellum

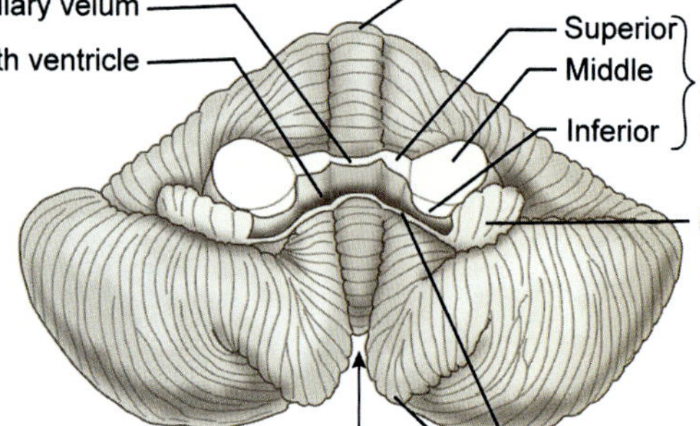

Inferior view of cerebellum

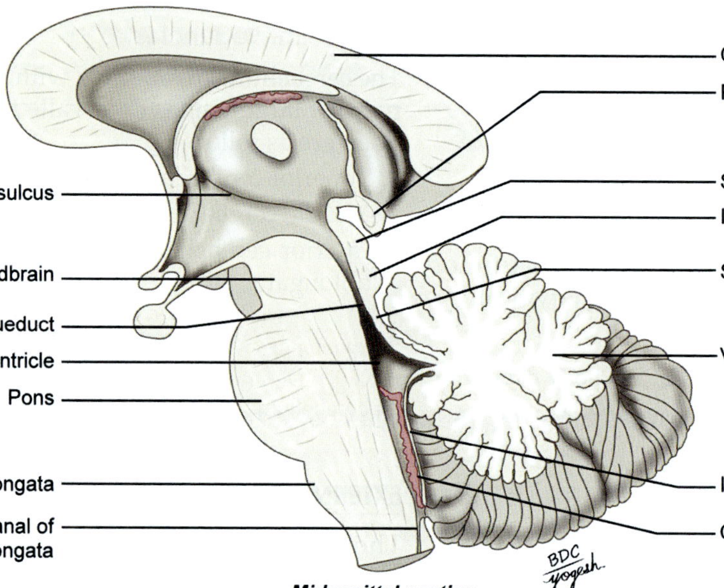

Midsagittal section

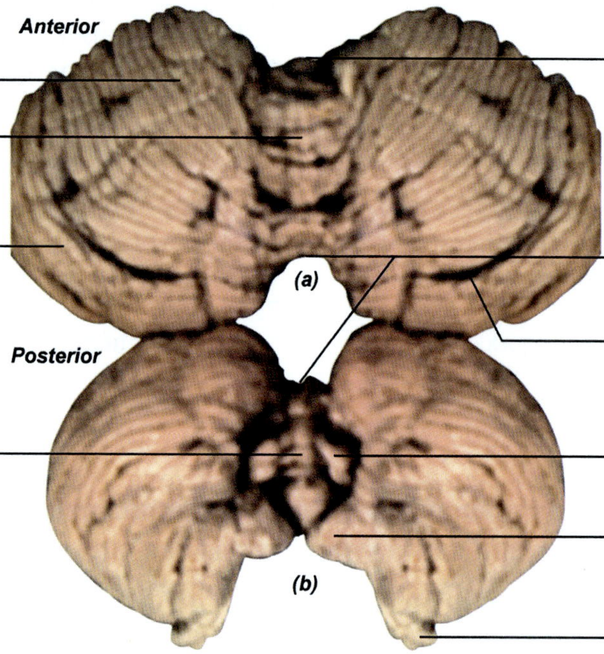

Figs 8.1a and b: (a) Superior and (b) inferior surface of cerebellum (gross specimen)

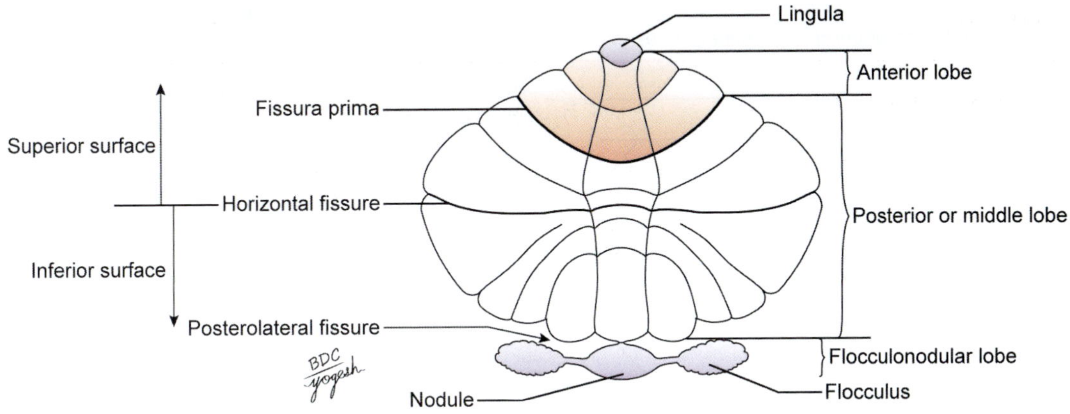

Fig. 8.2: Lobes, main fissures and surfaces of cerebellum (schematic representation)

Flowchart 8.2: Cerebellum: External features

Cerebellum: External features

- ***Parts***
  - Two cerebellar hemispheres
  - Median vermis
- ***Surfaces***
  - Superior surface
    - Convex
  - Inferior surface
    - Vallecula: Deep notch
    - Sulcus vallecula separates vermis from cerebellar hemispheres
- ***Notches***
  - Anterior
    - V-shaped
    - Lodges pons and medulla
  - Posterior
    - Deep
    - Lodges falx cerebelli
- ***Fissure***
  - Horizontal
  - Posterolateral
  - Fissura prima
  - Folia: Leaf-like lamellae separated by fissures
- ***Lobes***
  - Anterior
  - Posterior
  - Flocculonodular lobes

Sulcus vallecula: It is a sulcus that separates inferior vermis from inferior surface of cerebellar hemispheres. It is the lateral limit of vallecula.

Notches

Anterior cerebellar notch is wide, shallow, V-shaped notch on the anterior part of cerebellum. It lodges the pons and medulla.

Posterior cerebellar notch is deep and narrow. It lodges falx cerebelli (fold of dura mater).

Fissures

There are numerous transversely running furrows of varying depth on the cerebellar surface.

Folia: These are narrow leaf-like lamellae separated by fissures. Each folium consists of core of white matter covered by grey matter.

Three fissures are prominent and consistent, and they are as follows:

1. ***Horizontal fissure*:** It separates superior and inferior surface of cerebellum.
2. ***Posterolateral fissure*:** It lies on the inferior surface of cerebellum and separates the flocculonodular lobe from the rest of the cerebellum (corpus cerebelli).
3. ***Primary fissure*** (*fissura prima*): It is V-shaped fissure on the superior surface with its apex directed posterior.

The cerebellum is divided into two parts by posterolateral fissure:

1. Flocculonodular lobe
2. Corpus cerebelli.

Corpus cerebelli is divided into anterior and posterior lobes by fissura prima.

Tonsil is a part of cerebellum on its inferior surface. In raised intracranial pressure, tonsils may protrude into the foramen magnum.

PARTS AND LOBES OF CEREBELLUM

The cerebellum is subdivided into numerous small parts by fissures. Each fissure cuts the vermis and both hemispheres. Table 8.1 shows part of vermis with its respective part of cerebellar hemisphere. The *horizontal fissure* separates the superior surface from the inferior surface (Fig. 8.3).

The *primary fissure (fissura prima)* separates the anterior lobe from the middle lobe on the superior surface of the

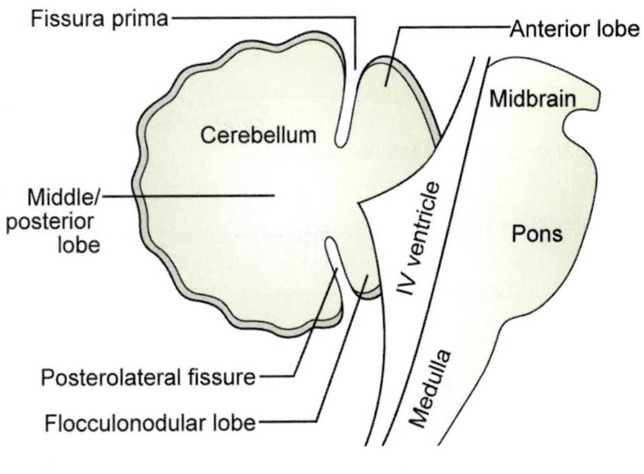

Fig. 8.3: Anatomical lobes of the cerebellum

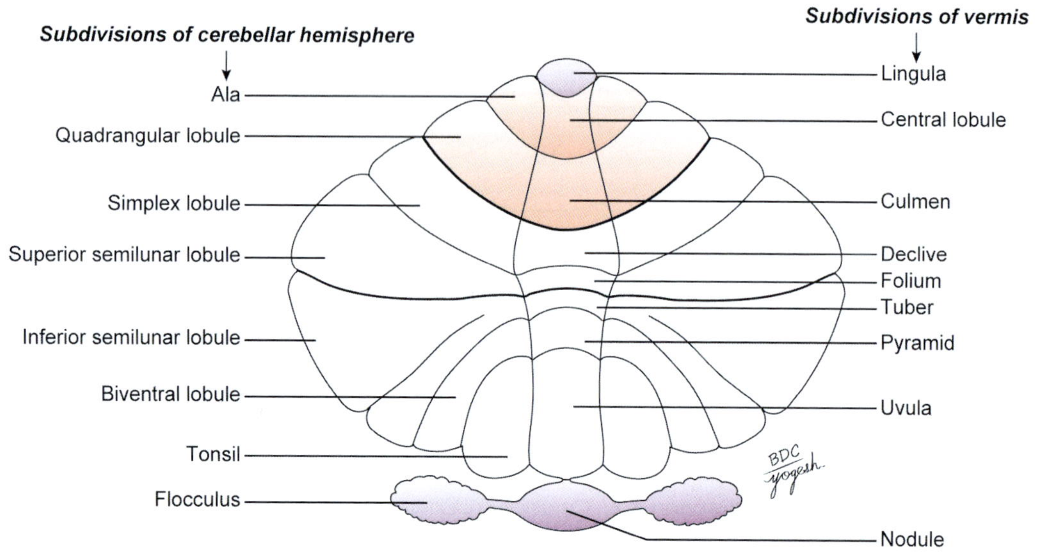

Fig. 8.4: Subdivisions of cerebellar hemispheres and vermis (schematic representation)

TABLE 8.1: Subdivisions or lobules of cerebellum

Lobes	*Subdivisions of vermis*	*Subdivisions of each cerebellar hemisphere*
Anterior lobe	Lingula	—
	Central lobule	Ala
	Culmen	Quadrangular lobule
Posterior lobe	Declive	Simplex lobule
	Folium	Superior semilunar lobule
	Tuber	Inferior semilunar lobule
	Pyramid	Biventral lobule
	Uvula	Tonsil
Flocculonodular lobe	Nodule	Flocculus

[*Mnemonics* for subdivisions of cerebellar vermis: **L**azy **C**at **D**ie **F**or **T**aka **P**izza **U**n**N**ecessarily]

cerebellum. The *posterolateral fissure* separates the middle lobe from the flocculonodular lobe on the inferior surface.

The various parts of cerebellum are shown in Fig. 8.4. Where both the superior and inferior surfaces of the cerebellum are drawn in one plane. The upper part of the diagram, above the horizontal fissure, represents the superior surface; and the lower part, below the horizontal fissure represents the inferior surface. However, the *lingula* does not have any lateral extension.

The subdivisions or lobules of cerebellum are given in Table 8.1.

MORPHOLOGICAL DIVISIONS OF CEREBELLUM

Based on function and phylogenetic (evolutionary) aspect, the cerebellum is divided into three parts:

1. ***Archicerebellum:*** The archicerebellum phylogenetically is the oldest part of the cerebellum to appear in evolution in aquatic vertebrates. It includes the flocculonodular lobe and the lingula. It is chiefly vestibular in its connections. It controls the axial musculature and the bilateral movements used for locomotion and maintenance of equilibrium (Fig. 8.5).

2. ***Paleocerebellum:*** The paleocerebellum is the next part of the cerebellum to appear in terrestrial vertebrates with the appearance of limbs. It is made up of the anterior lobe (except lingula), and the pyramid and uvula of the

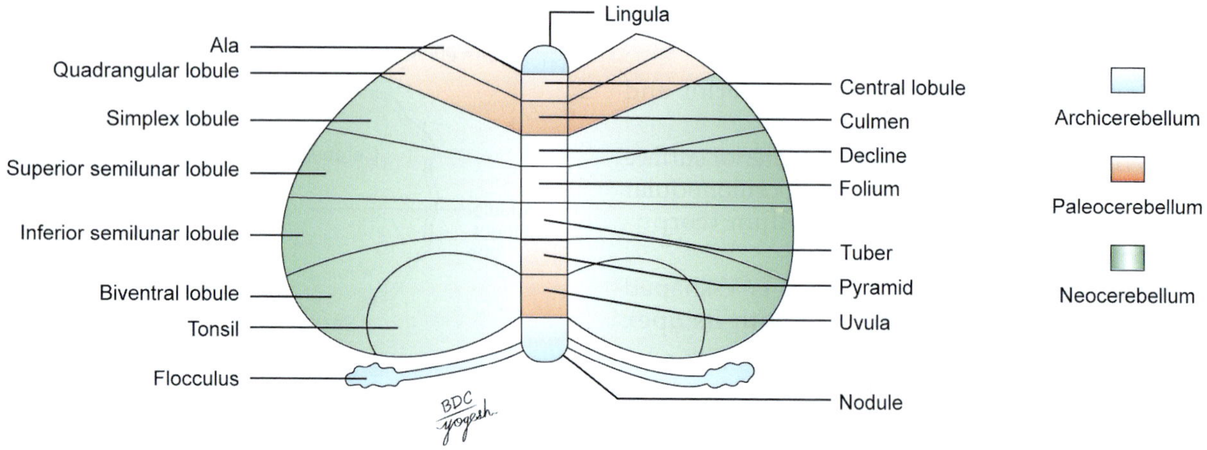

Fig. 8.5: Functional subdivisions of cerebellum

inferior vermis. Its connections are chiefly spinocerebellar. It controls tone, posture and crude movements of the limbs.

3. ***Neocerebellum:*** The neocerebellum is the newest part of the cerebellum to develop. It is made up of the posterior/middle lobe (the largest part of the cerebellum) except the pyramid and uvula of the inferior vermis. It is primarily concerned with the regulation of fine movements of the body. Table 8.1 depicts the morphological and functional divisions of cerebellum.

Competencies:

AN60.2 Describe connections of cerebellar cortex and intracerebellar nuclei.

AN64.1 Describe and identify the microanatomical features of spinal cord, cerebellum and cerebrum.

INTERNAL FEATURES AND HISTOLOGY OF CEREBELLUM

The cerebellum is highly folded to accommodate millions of neurons in a small area. These foldings are called *arbor vitae*. The cerebellum has:

1. Outer grey matter – cerebellar cortex
2. Inner white matter – cerebellar medulla
3. Cerebellar nuclei – grey matter embedded deep in the medulla.

The cerebellar cortex is uniform throughout (***homotypical***). Cerebellar cortex shows three layers: Outer molecular layer, middle Purkinje cell layer, and inner granular layer (Plate 8.2 and Fig. 8.6).

1. ***Molecular layer***: It lies just deep to the pia mater. It consists of few cells and more fibres. It has stellate cells in superficial part and few basket cells in deeper part. The molecular layer shows numerous branching processes of Purkinje cells, axons of granule cells, and climbing fibres.
2. ***Purkinje cell layer***: This layer consists of a single row of Purkinje cell bodies that are arranged between molecular and granular layer. The Purkinje cells are large, flask-shaped neurons. Dendrites of Purkinje cells arise from apex of flask and enter into the molecular layer. A single axon arises from their base that passes through the granular layer and white matter to the cerebellar nuclei.
3. ***Granular layer:*** It lies between Purkinje cell layer and white matter. It stains dark with haematoxylin because of closely packed, numerous, small granule cells. The granular layer has granule cells and Golgi cells. Granule cells are small neurons with round nucleus. Golgi cell are large, stellate cells.

The granule cells has mossy fibres that bring information from pons to granule cells (pontocerebellar fibres). Climbing fibres and axons of Purkinje cells pass through the granular layer.

Table 8.2 shows the neurons of cerebellum.

The white matter is composed of fibres and neuroglial cells.

Note: ***Cerebellar glomeruli***: Mossy fibres end as dilated terminals. This dilated terminal is surrounded by dendrites of granule cells and axons of Golgi cells. Mossy fibre terminal with surrounding dendrites and axons form light-stained areas in granular layer. These areas are called *glomeruli of cerebellum*.

Plate 8.2: Histology of cerebellum

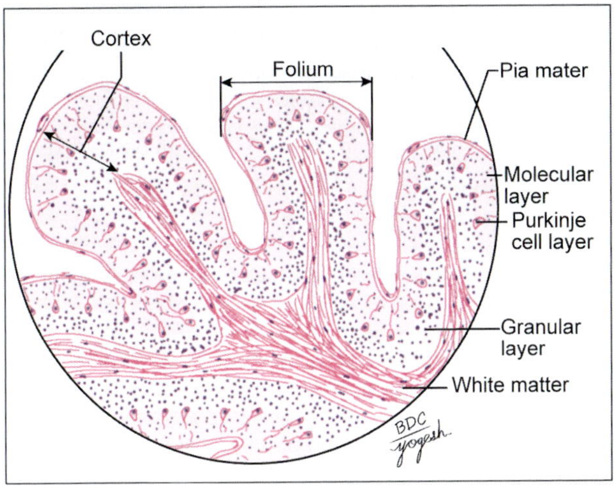

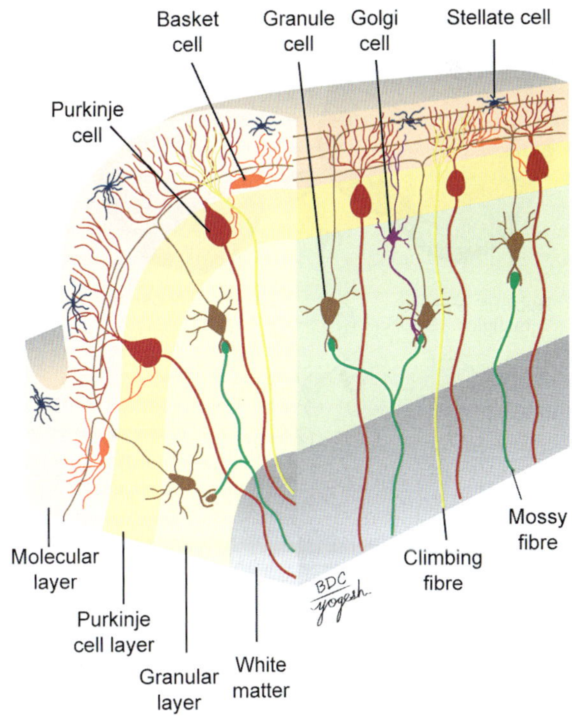

Fig. 8.6: Cerebellar neurons and layers

CEREBELLAR NUCLEI

There are four cerebellar nuclei on each side (Figs 8.7a and b). These are masses of grey matter embedded deeply in the substance of white matter of cerebellum.

1. *Dentate nucleus*: It is the largest cerebellar nucleus. It has a shape like a crumpled purse. Its hilus faces medially. It is the nucleus of neocerebellum and highly evolved in human.
2. *Emboliform nucleus*: It is oval. It lies lateral to globose nucleus and medial to dentate nucleus.
3. *Globose nucleus*: It is round. It lies between emboliform and fastigial nuclei. The emboliform and globose nuclei are the part of paleocerebellum. They are collectively called nucleus interpositus.

TABLE 8.2: Neurons of cerebellum

Neurons	*Location*	*Features*	*Dendrites*	*Axon*
Stellate cells	Just beneath the surface of cerebellum in molecular layer	Star-shaped (stellate) dendritic trees	Confined to molecular layer Synapse with parallel fibre of granule cells	Confined to molecular layer Synapse with dendrites of Purkinje cells
Basket cells	Deeper part of molecular layer	Form basket-like structure	Few dendrites Synapse with parallel fibres bodies of granule cells, Purkinje cells, climbing and mossy fibres	Synapse with Purkinje cell
Purkinje cells	Purkinje cell layer	Large flask-shaped cells	Arborize in molecular layer	Single axon to deep cerebellar nuclei
Granule cells	Granular layer	Small, spherical neurons	Dendrites form glomeruli with mossy fibres	Axon runs parallel to each other and enters into molecular layer
Golgi neurons	Superficial part of granular layer	Large stellate cells GABAergic inhibitory neurons	Dendrites enter molecular synapse with parallel fibres	Axon ends in glomeruli

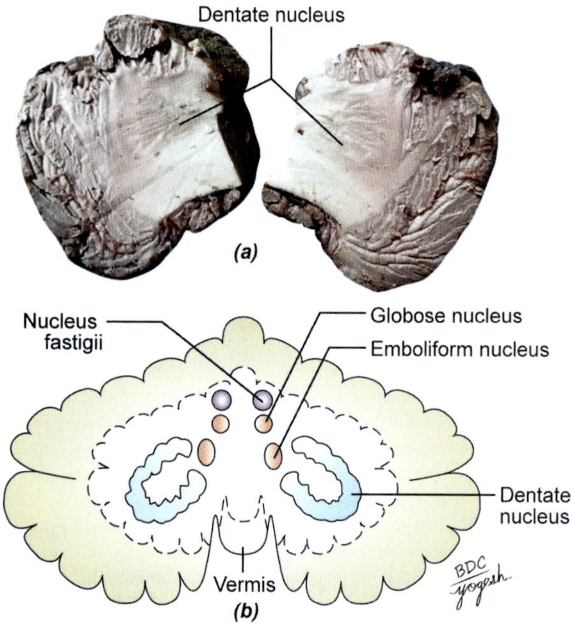

Figs 8.7a and b: Positions of intracerebellar nuclei

4. *Nucleus fastigii*: It lies close to midline in the vermis just dorsal to the 4th ventricle. It is spherical. It is the nucleus of archicerebellum.

WHITE MATTER OF CEREBELLUM

The white matter of cerebellum forms the medulla of cerebellum. It has typical tree-like branching appearance called *arbor vitae cerebelli*. The white matter consists of intrinsic, afferent and efferent fibres.

1. *Intrinsic fibres*: They do not leave the cerebellum and remain confined to cerebellum. They connect the different regions of cerebellum.
2. *Projection fibres*: They are afferent and efferent fibres. They connect the cerebellum with the other parts of brain. They are arranged into three large bundles on each side as superior, middle, and inferior cerebellar peduncles.

Sensory Fibres of Cerebellum

Cerebellum receives input from mossy fibres and climbing fibres.

1. *Climbing fibres:* These are olivocerebellar fibres (axons) arising from inferior olivary nucleus. They synapse in molecular layer with Purkinje cells (one fibre for one cell).
2. *Mossy fibres:* These are other than olivocerebellar fibres. These include vestibulocerebellar, pontocerebellar, and spinocerebellar fibres. Mossy fibres have dilated terminals in granular layer. They synapse with dendrites of granule cells and axons of Golgi cells. This synapse forms light staining cerebellar glomeruli (Fig. 8.8).

CONNECTIONS OF CEREBELLUM

The fibres entering or leaving the cerebellum are grouped to form three peduncles (Latin *small foot*) which connect the cerebellum to the midbrain, the pons and the medulla (Figs 8.9 and 8.10 and Flowchart 8.3).

Inferior cerebellar peduncle: It connects the cerebellum with medulla oblongata. It is also called *restiform body*. It consists of mainly afferent fibres that carry sensory information.

Afferent fibres

1. *Posterior spinocerebellar fibres* from ipsilateral thoracic nuclei (Clarke's column) of spinal cord.

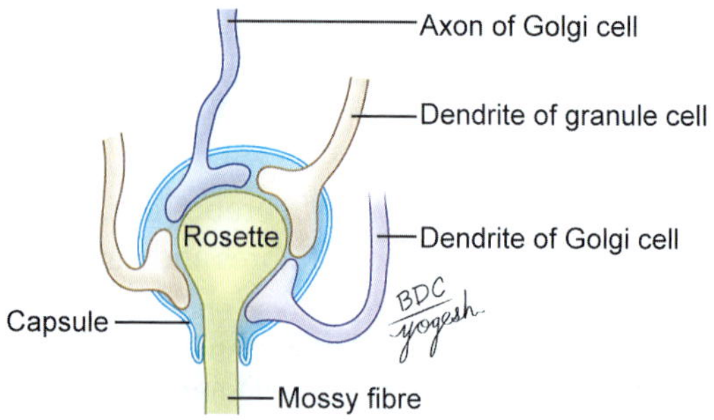

Fig. 8.8: Structure of cerebellar glomerulus

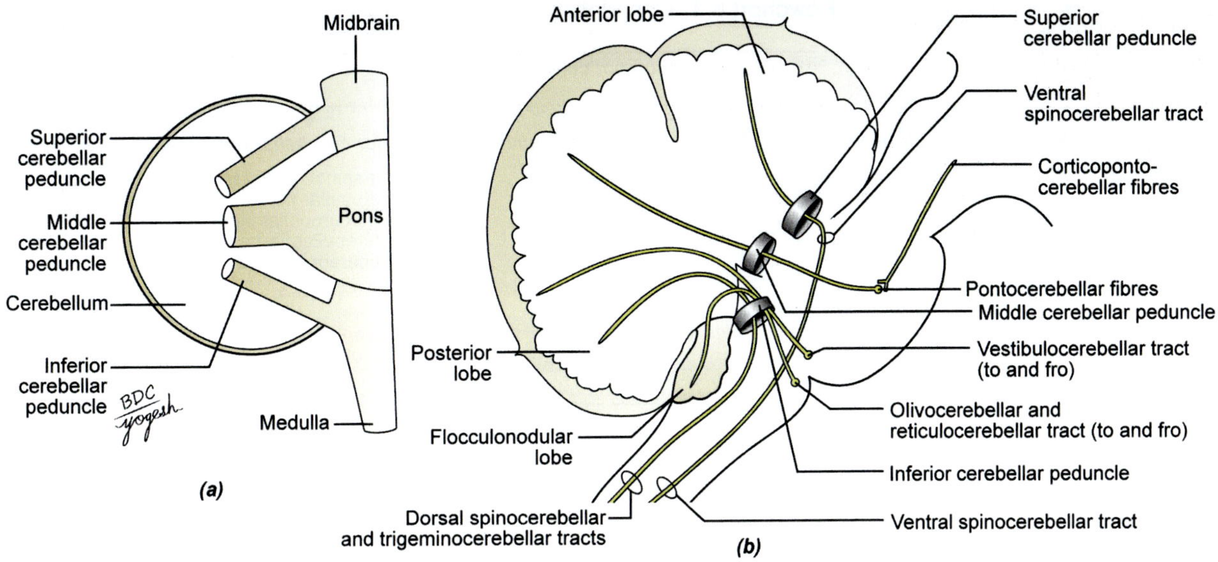

Figs 8.9a and b: (a) The three cerebellar peduncles and (b) main connections of cerebellum

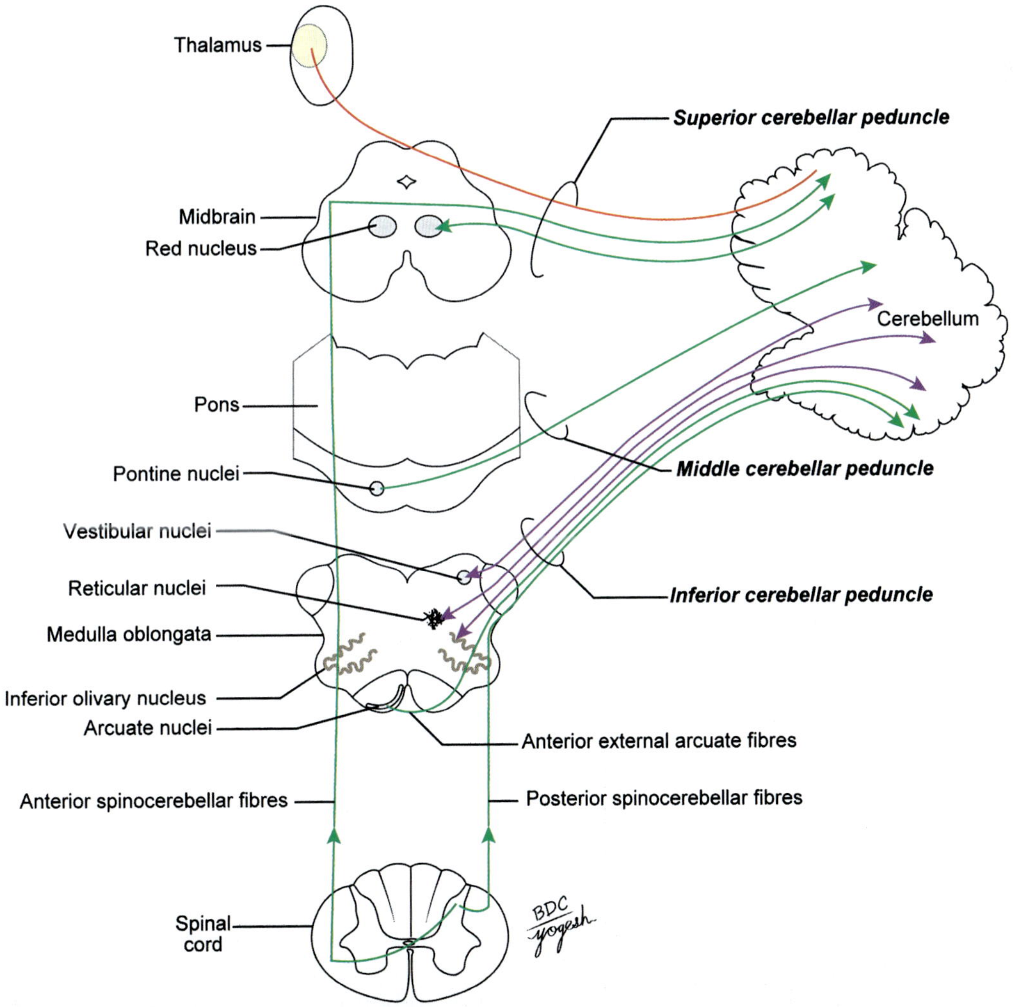

Fig. 8.10: Major connections of cerebellum

2. *Vestibulocerebellar tract* from vestibular nerve and vestibular nuclei.
3. *Olivocerebellar tract* from opposite inferior olivary nucleus (they form climbing fibres).
4. *Par-olivocerebellar tract* from opposite medial olivary nuclei.
5. *Cuneocerebellar* or *posterior external arcuate fibres* from ipsilateral accessory cuneate nuclei.
6. *Reticulocerebellar fibre* from reticular nuclei of medulla oblongata.
7. *Anterior external arcuate fibres* from both arcuate nuclei.

Flowchart 8.3: Connections of cerebellum

Connections of cerebellum

	Inferior cerebellar peduncle	Middle cerebellar peduncle	Superior cerebellar peduncle
Afferent	Posterior spinocerebellar fibres Vestibulocerebellar tract Olivocerebellar tract Par-olivocerebellar tract Cuneocerebellar fibres Reticulocerebellar fibre Anterior external arcuate fibres	Pontocerebellar fibres Reticulocerebellar fibres	Anterior spinocerebellar tract Tectocerebellar fibres Trigeminocerebellar fibres Rubrocerebellar fibres Ceruleocerebellar fibres
Efferent	Cerebelloreticular fibres Cerebellovestibular fibres Cerebello-olivary fibres	Nil	Cerebellorubral fibres Dentatorubral and dentatothalamic fibres Cerebello-olivary fibres

Efferent fibres:

1. *Cerebelloreticular fibres* from both fastigial nuclei to reticular formation.
2. *Cerebellovestibular fibres* from ipsilateral flocculonodular lobe and fastigial nuclei of both sides to vestibular nuclei.
3. *Cerebello-olivary fibres.*

Middle cerebellar peduncle

Afferent fibres:

1. *Pontocerebellar fibres* from opposite pontine nuclei
2. *Reticulocerebellar fibres* from pontine reticular nuclei.

Efferent fibres: Nil.

Superior cerebellar peduncle

Afferent fibres:

1. *Anterior spinocerebellar tract* from spinal cord.
2. *Tectocerebellar fibres* from tectum (superior and inferior colliculi) of midbrain.
3. *Trigeminocerebellar fibres* from superior sensory nucleus of V nerve.
4. *Rubrocerebellar fibres* from red nucleus.
5. *Ceruleocerebellar fibres* from locus coeruleus (located in the pons).

Efferent fibres:

1. *Cerebellorubral fibres* from globose and emboliform nucleus to contralateral red nucleus.
2. *Dentatorubral* and *dentatothalamic fibres* from dentate nucleus to opposite red nucleus and thalamus, respectively.
3. *Cerebello-olivary fibres* from dentate nucleus to contralateral olivary nucleus.

BLOOD SUPPLY

Arterial Supply

The cerebellum is supplied by three pairs of cerebellar arteries:

1. Superior cerebellar artery – branch of basilar artery.
2. Anterior inferior cerebellar artery – branch of basilar artery.
3. Posterior inferior cerebellar artery – branch of vertebral artery.

Venous Drainage

1. Superior cerebellar veins drain into straight, transverse, and superior petrosal sinuses.
2. Inferior cerebellar veins drain into the transverse and inferior petrosal sinuses.

FUNCTIONS OF CEREBELLUM

1. Cerebellum controls the same side of the body. Its influence is ipsilateral.
2. The *neocerebellum* coordinates voluntary movements so that they are smooth, balanced and accurate. Neocerebellum is responsible for fine tuning of motor performance for precise movements. It helps in planning and production of skilled movements along with cerebrum.
3. Cerebellum controls tone, posture and equilibrium. This is chiefly done by the archicerebellum and paleocerebellum.
4. Cerebellum controls movements of eyeballs. It controls and coordinates these by affecting agonists, antagonists and synergists. It also helps in learning of special motor skills. It plays a role in cognition.
5. Flocculonodular lobe is connected to vestibular nuclei. It is involved in maintenance of muscle tone and posture. Spinocerebellum, vermis and intermediate regions receive afferents from motor cortex via corticopontocerebellar fibres.
6. All sensory information from muscles, joints, cutaneous, auditory and visual parts are relayed here. Spinocerebellar tracts carry information from the same side.
7. Vermis controls axial muscles, and thus maintains posture. Paramedian areas are involved in control of distal group of muscles to bring smooth coordinated activity.
8. Cerebellum functions as '***comparator***'. It receives information from cerebrum and spinal cord. It corrects and modifies ongoing movements through thalamo-cortical projections, reticulospinal and rubrospinal tracts.

Note: It has been seen by functional magnetic resonance imaging (fMRI) that if fingers of right hand are moved repetitively, the activity is seen in precentral gyrus of left cerebral cortex and in anterior quadrangular lobule of right cerebellar hemisphere (Fig. 8.11).

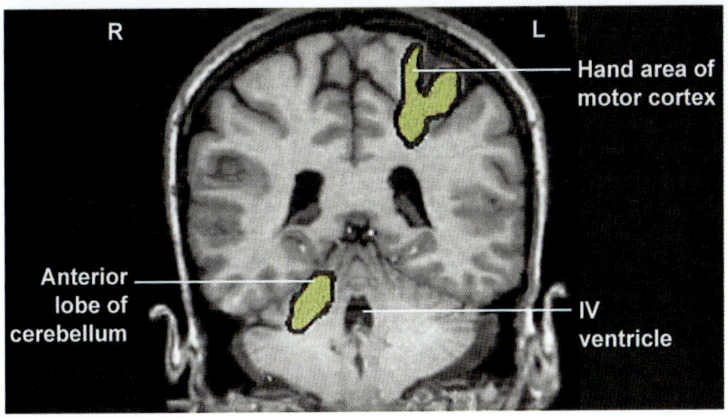

Fig. 8.11: MRI showing activity in left cerebral cortex and right cerebellum on moving the fingers of right hand

Competency:

AN60.3 Describe anatomical basis of cerebellar dysfunction.

CLINICAL NEUROANATOMY

Cerebellar syndrome

It is a group of signs and symptoms produced due to lesion of the cerebellum (Flowchart 8.4). The components of cerebellar syndrome are divided into three sets as follows:

1. Lesion of archicerebellum or flocculonodular lobe (vestibular cerebellum)
2. Lesion of paleocerebellum (spinal cerebellum)
3. Lesion of neocerebellum (cerebral cerebellum)

Lesion in flocculonodular lobe or archicerebellum: As the archicerebellum maintains equilibrium, tone, and posture of the *trunk* muscles with the help of inputs from vestibular nuclei, its lesion leads to:

1. *Disequilibrium*: It is characterized by unsteady and *staggering gait*. The patient tends to fall forward, backward, or laterally on standing – this is called *cerebellar ataxia*.
2. *Waddling gait*: The person stands and walks with the legs wide apart.
3. *Nystagmus*: The involuntary to and fro oscillatory movements of the eyeballs while looking to either side.

Lesion in paleocerebellum (spinal cerebellum): As the paleocerebellum maintains the tone, posture, and crude movements of the *limbs* by sensory inputs from the spinal cord, its lesion leads to hypotonia and asthenia of limb muscles. It causes:

1. *Flail joints* – lack of joint stability
2. *Pendular knee jerk* – tapping of patellar tendon produces oscillating movements of leg, that is, leg swings backward and forward
3. *Cerebellar ataxia* (= disorderly, Greek) – inability to maintain balance while walking

Lesion of neocerebellum (cerebral cerebellum): As the neocerebellum controls the smooth performance of skilled voluntary movements, its lesion produces the following signs:

1. *Asynergy*: Loss of smooth movements. The movements are intermittent and jerky.
2. *Dysmetria*: Errors in measurement of rates, range, force, and direction of movement.
   Pastpointing (finger–nose test): Inability to touch the nose by finger. The patient overshoots or undershoots the tip of nose.
3. *Intention tremors*: The tremors come on initiation of voluntary movement and disappear during rest.
4. *Dysdiadochokinesia* or *adiadochokinesia*: Inability to perform respect alternating movements, that is, supination and pronation of forearm, tapping of one hand with other hand.
5. *Dysarthria* or *scanning speech*: The muscular incoordination produces slurred, prolonged, explosive speech with pause in wrong place.
6. *Rebound phenomenon*: The patient is unable to stop action suddenly. For example, if patient pushes some object, on sudden removal of the object, the patient is not able to stop the pushing act.
7. *Hypotonia* (diminished muscle tone) results in excess movements of limbs (loose joints or ragdoll appearance).

Note: Lesion of vermis and paravermal zone results to truncal ataxia and nystagmus, abnormal stance, and gait. The l*esion of cerebellar hemisphere* results in ataxia and tremor on the ipsilateral side body. It also produces nystagmus, intention tremor, delayed initiation of motor activity, abnormal stance, and gait, hypotonia, dysarthria, dysmetria, dysdiadochokinesia, dysrhythmias, and rebound phenomenon.

Flowchart 8.4: Cerebellar syndrome

Cerebellar syndrome

Lesion of archicerebellum	***Lesion of paleocerebellum***	***Lesion of neocerebellum***
Affects trunk muscles	Affects limb muscles	Affects skilled movements
Disequilibrium	Flail joints	Asynergy
Staggering gait	Pendular knee jerk	Dysmetria (finger–nose test)
Cerebellar ataxia	Cerebellar ataxia	Intention tremors
Waddling gait		Dysdiadochokinesia
Nystagmus		Adiadochokinesia
		Dysarthria/scanning speech
		Rebound phenomenon
		Hypotonia

BDC yogesh

VIDEO

Video 4.6 Cerebellum

Facts to Remember

- Cerebellum or a little brain acts like younger sibling of the large cerebrum. It controls tone, posture, equilibrium and fine movements of the body. It cannot initiate the movement.
- It is connected to medulla oblongata by inferior cerebellar peduncle, to pons by middle cerebellar peduncle, and to midbrain by superior cerebellar peduncle.

- Number of neurons are about half of the cerebrum, though it is much smaller than the cerebrum.
- Its structure is uniform throughout, i.e. homotypical. It has outer molecular, middle Purkinje cell layer, and inner granular layer.
- Its control is ipsilateral side of the body.
- *Climbing fibres* are olivocerebellar fibres and *mossy fibres* are other than olivocerebellar fibres reaching to cerebellum.
- Cerebellar nuclei – dentate nucleus, emboliform nucleus, globose nucleus, and nucleus fastigius.

BDC's Anatomy *e*-book

1. Functional divisions of cerebellum
2. Morphological and functional divisions of cerebellum
3. Constituents of the cerebellar peduncles
4. Development of cerebellum
5. Further reading
6. Viva voce questions

Chapter

9

Fourth Ventricle

Competency:

AN63.1 Describe and demonstrate parts, boundaries and features of IIIrd, IVth and lateral ventricle.

The cavity of hindbrain is called the fourth ventricle. It is a tent-shaped space situated between the pons and upper part of medulla oblongata in front and cerebellum behind. So it lies dorsal to pons and upper part of medulla oblongata and ventral to cerebellum.

It has lateral boundaries, floor, roof and a cavity (Fig. 9.1, Plate 9.1 and Flowchart 9.1) with recesses and angles.

Communication

The cavity of the fourth ventricle communicates inferiorly with the central canal and superiorly with cerebral aqueduct.

Lateral Boundaries of Fourth Ventricle

On each side, fourth ventricle is bounded:

1. Inferolaterally by gracile, cuneate tubercles and inferior cerebellar peduncles.
2. Superolaterally by the superior cerebellar peduncles.

Floor of Fourth Ventricle

It is also called ***'rhomboid fossa'*** because of its rhomboidal shape. The floor is formed by:

1. Posterior (dorsal) surface of lower part of pons (Plate 9.2).
2. Posterior (dorsal) surface of open or upper part of medulla oblongata.

Structural Layers

The floor is lined by:

1. Ependyma
2. A thin layer of the neuroglia beneath the ependyma
3. A layer of grey matter, forming the various nuclei deep to neuroglia.

Parts

It is divisible into:

1. An upper triangular part formed by dorsal surface of pons.

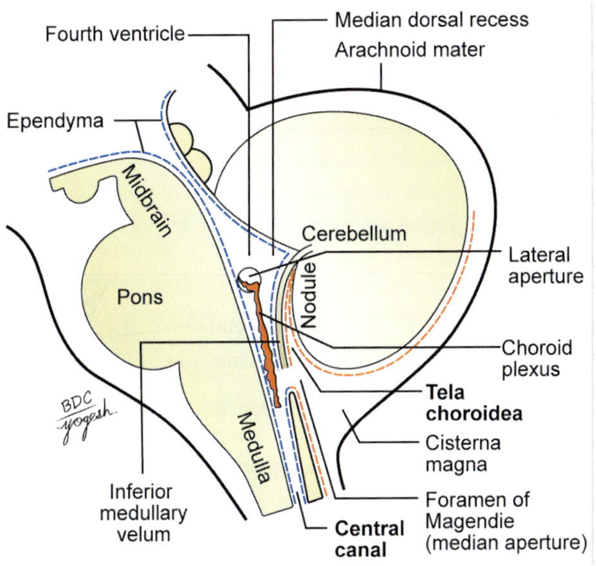

Fig 9.1: Fourth ventricle

2. A lower triangular part formed by dorsal surface of medulla.
3. The intermediate part is at the junction of pons and medulla. The intermediate part is prolonged laterally over the inferior cerebellar peduncle as the floor of lateral recess. This part is marked by transversely running fibres which are fibres of *stria medullaris*. These fibres represent fibres from arcuate nucleus to the opposite cerebellum.

Features of the Floor

1. ***Dorsal median sulcus*** divides the floor into two symmetrical halves.
2. ***Sulcus limitans*** divides each half into median eminence and lateral vestibular area. The sulcus limitans presents depression at the cranial end called superior fovea and towards caudal part called inferior fovea (Fig. 9.2).
3. ***Median eminence***: The eminence is wider above and narrow below. It presents facial colliculus just opposite and medial to superior fovea. Deep to the colliculus is the genu of the facial nerve formed by this nerve looping around the abducent nucleus.

Plate 9.1: Fourth ventricle (midsagittal section, right medial view)

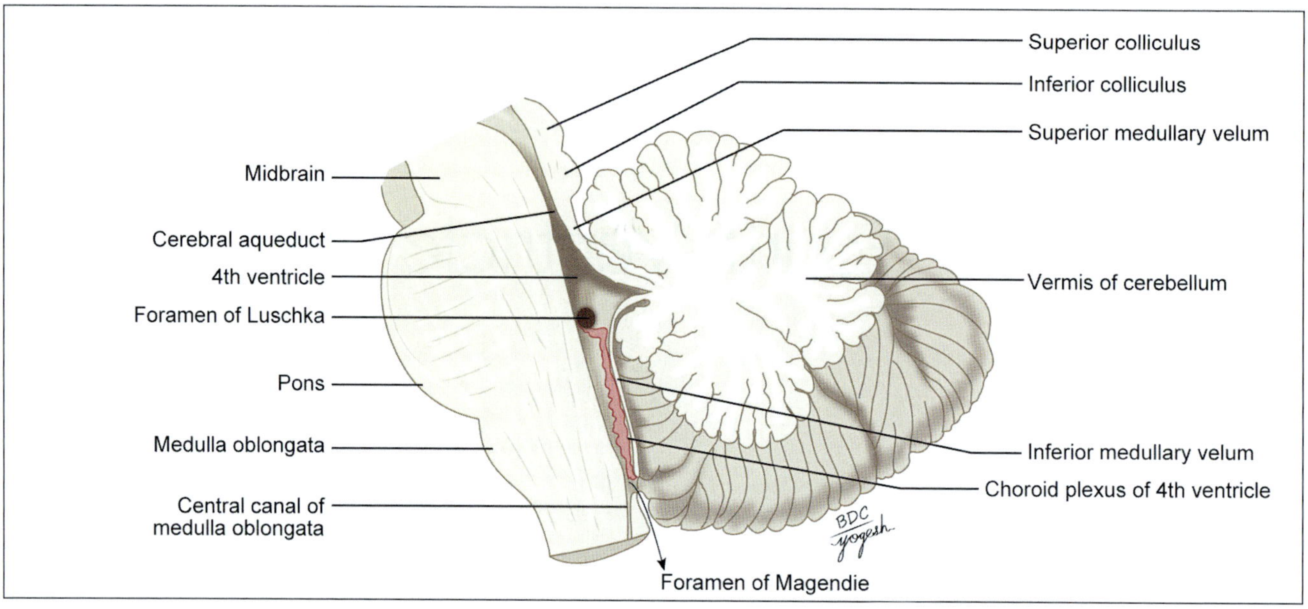

Plate 9.2: Floor of fourth ventricle

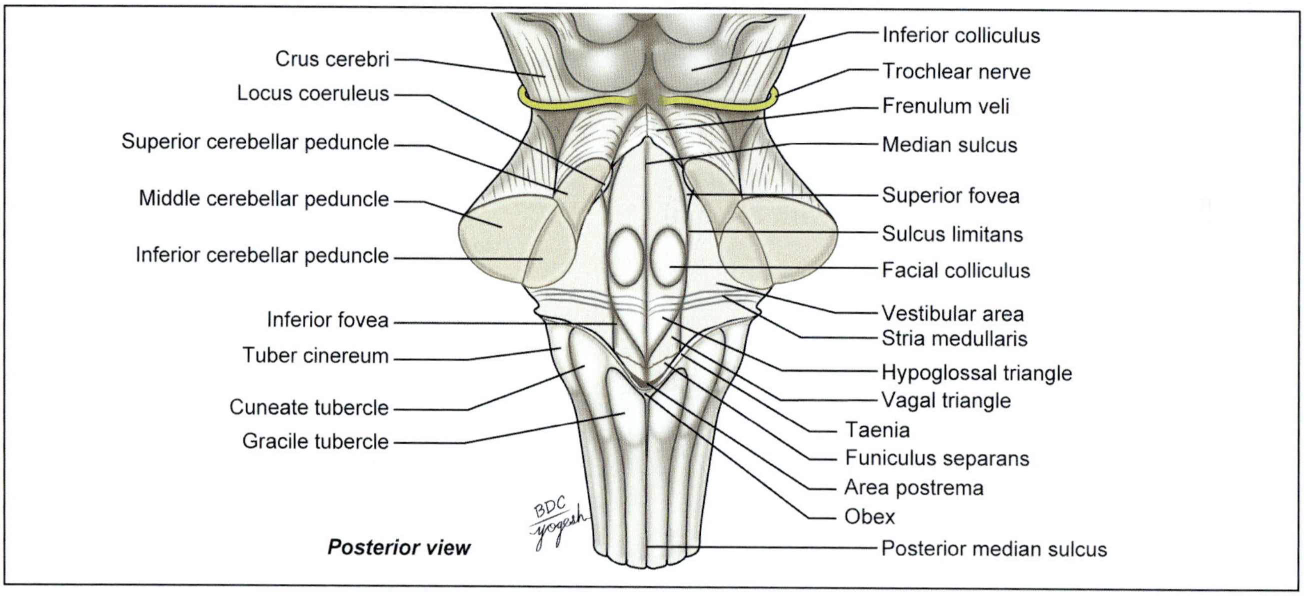

Posterior view

Flowchart 9.1: Fourth ventricle

Fourth ventricle

Tent-like cavity of rhombencephalon

Location
- Cavity of hindbrain
- Lies between cerebellum behind and pons and medulla anteriorly

Continuity
- Superiorly
  - Cerebral aqueduct
- Inferiorly
  - Central canal of medulla

Lateral boundaries
- Inferolateral:
  - Gracile and cuneate tubercles, inferior cerebellar peduncles
- Superolateral:
  - Superior cerebellar peduncles

Roof
- Tent-shaped
- Upper part
  - superior medullary velum
- Inferior part
  - Inferior medullary velum
  - Ependyma and fold of pia mater

Communications
- With 3rd ventricle
  – cerebral aqueduct
- With central canal of medulla
- Foramen of Magendie
- Two foramina of Luschka

Recesses
- Two lateral
- Two dorsolateral
- One median dorsal

Floor

Rhomboid fossa

Sulci and depressions
- Median sulcus
- Median eminence
- Sulcus limitans
- Superior fovea
- Inferior fovea

Areas/ structures
- Facial colliculus
- Locus coeruleus
- Hypoglossal triangle
- Vagal triangle
- Funiculus separans
- Area postrema
- Taenia
- Obex

Clinical integration: Blockage of 4th ventricle → hydrocephalus, medulloblastoma, vital centers

BDC yogesh

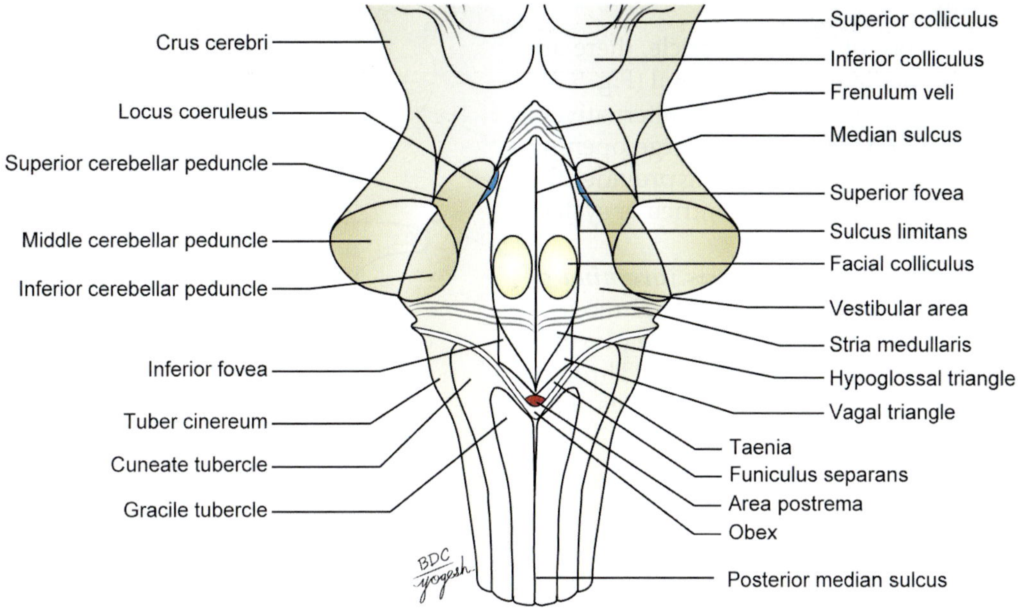

Fig. 9.2: Floor of fourth ventricle

4. In the uppermost part (pontine part), the sulcus limitans overlies an area that is bluish in colour and is called ***locus coeruleus***. The colour is due to presence of pigmented neurons which constitute ***substantia ferruginea***. These neurons belong to the reticular formation. They are rich in noradrenaline and help in paradoxical sleep.
5. Descending from the inferior fovea, there is a sulcus that runs obliquely towards midline. This sulcus divides median eminence into two triangles. These are ***hypoglossal triangle*** medially and ***vagal triangle*** laterally. These overlie the hypoglossal nerve nucleus and of vagus nerve, respectively.
6. Between the vagal triangle above and gracile tubercle below, there is small area called the ***area postrema*** which may function as chemoreceptor. An ependymal thickening called ***funiculus separans*** separates both. This area is devoid of blood–brain barrier.
7. ***Vestibular area*:** This lies lateral to the inferior fovea (sulcus limitans) which overlies the vestibular nuclei. This area is partly in the pons and partly in the medulla.

Note: The lowest part of the floor resembles the pointed nib of writing pen so it is described as calamus scriptorius.

Roof of Fourth Ventricle

The roof of the ventricle is diamond-shaped and can be divided into superior and inferior parts (Fig. 9.3).

1. The superior or cranial part of roof is formed by superior cerebellar peduncles and superior medullary velum. The superior cerebellar peduncles on emerging from central white matter of cerebellum pass first cranially and ventrally forming at first lateral boundaries of ventricles. On approaching the inferior colliculi, they converge and then intermingle over the ventricles and form part of the roof.

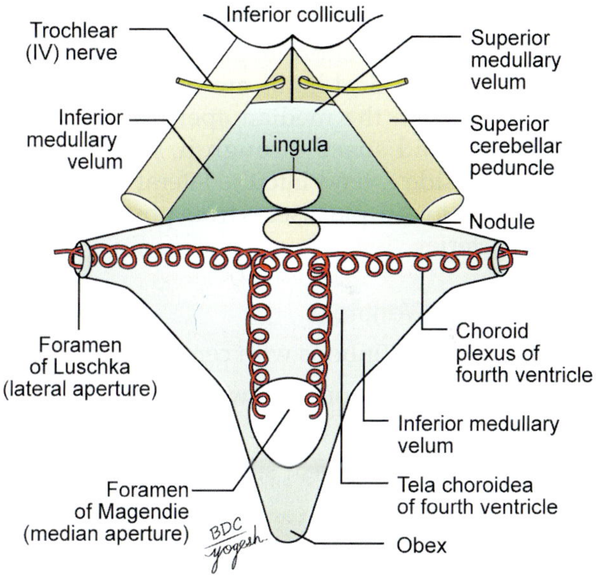

Fig. 9.3: Roof of fourth ventricle

Superior medullary velum (white matter) lies in between the two superior cerebellar peduncles. It is triangular in shape. Frenulum veli is a vertical ridge on the posterior surface of superior medullary velum. Trochlear, the 4th cranial nerve, emerges on each side of this ridge.

2. The lower part of roof is also sloping like the upper part. It is formed by fold of pia mater and ependyma of the ventricle. Laterally, it is formed by semilunar inferior medullary velum. Its outer surface is covered by fold of pia mater, while inner surface is covered by ependyma. It gets continuous with white matter of cerebellum. Two narrow bands of white matter extend down from inferior medullary velum to form lower part of roof of ventricle called the obex.

Openings in the Roof

In the caudal part of roof of fourth ventricle, there are three openings—one median and two lateral (Fig. 9.3).

1. The median aperture of fourth ventricle, alternatively known as *foramen of Magendie,* is a large opening situated caudal to nodule. This opening provides the principal communication between ventricular system and subarachnoid space.
2. The lateral apertures, also known as *foramina of Luschka,* are situated at the ends of lateral recesses and are partly occupied by parts of choroid plexuses which protrude into subarachnoid space. Through these also fourth ventricle communicates with subarachnoid space.

Tela Choroidea of Fourth Ventricle

Tela choroidea of 4th ventricle is a fold (double layer) of pia mater with capillaries. This fold enters 4th ventricle in the interval between lower part of roof of the ventricle and the cerebellum.

Choroid Plexuses of Fourth Ventricle

The fold of pia mater with capillaries lined by secretory ependyma forms the choroid plexus. This plexus is "T-shaped", the vertical limbs are two in number, lie side by side, reach the median aperture and project into subarachnoid space through it. The horizontal limbs on each side extend into the lateral recesses. The arterial supply for the plexuses is from posterior inferior cerebellar arteries.

Angles of Fourth Ventricle

Superior angle: Continuous with cerebral aqueduct.

Inferior angle: Continuous below with central canal of spinal cord.

Lateral angles: One on each side towards the inferior cerebellar peduncles.

Cavity and Recesses of Fourth Ventricle

The cavity lies between roof and floor of the ventricle. It reveals some recesses. These are extensions of the main cavity of ventricle. Five recesses have been identified (Fig. 9.4).

1. Two lateral recesses—one on each side. Each lateral recess passes laterally in the interval between the inferior cerebellar peduncle (ventrally) and the peduncle of flocculus dorsally reaching as far as the medial part of flocculus.
2. One recess present in the median plane, is known as median dorsal recess. It extends dorsally into white core of cerebellum and lies above the cerebellar nodule (Fig. 9.5).
3. Two lateral dorsal recesses—one on each side. Each lateral dorsal recess extends dorsally lateral to the nodule and cranial to the inferior medullary velum. These lie on either side of median dorsal recess.

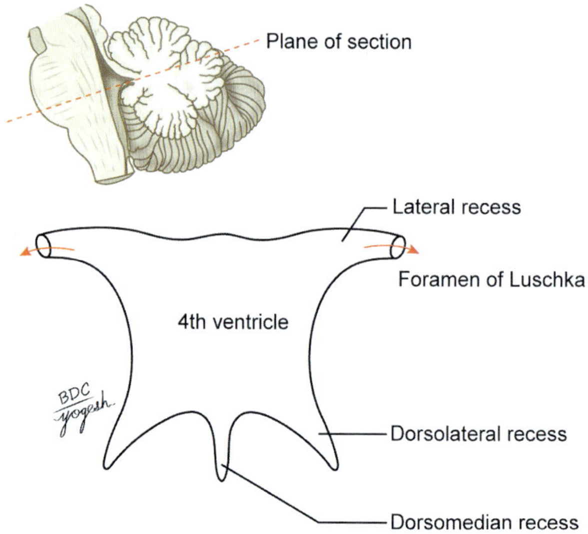

Fig. 9.4: Recesses and apertures of the fourth ventricle

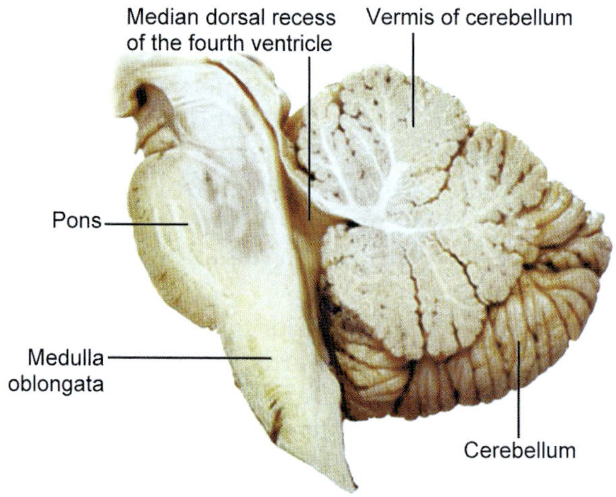

Fig. 9.5: Median dorsal recess of the fourth ventricle

CLINICAL NEUROANATOMY

- ***Vital centres*** are situated in the vicinity of vagal triangle. An injury to this area, therefore, would prove fatal.
- ***Hydrocephalus*** is a condition that occurs due to abnormal increase in CSF within the ventricle system. It may occur due to occlusion of outflowing channels of CSF (ventricle → subarachnoid space → dural venous sinuses). Sometimes, the foramen of Magendie or foramen of Luschka may get occluded due to growing tumours or fibrous adhesions after meningitis. It may produce hydrocephalus, headache, vomiting, papilloedema, etc.
- ***Medulloblastoma***: It is the most common tumour in the region of 4th ventricle. It arises from poorly differentiated primitive neuroectodermal cells of cerebellar vermis.
- The 4th ventricle can be visualised in MRI (Fig. 9.6).

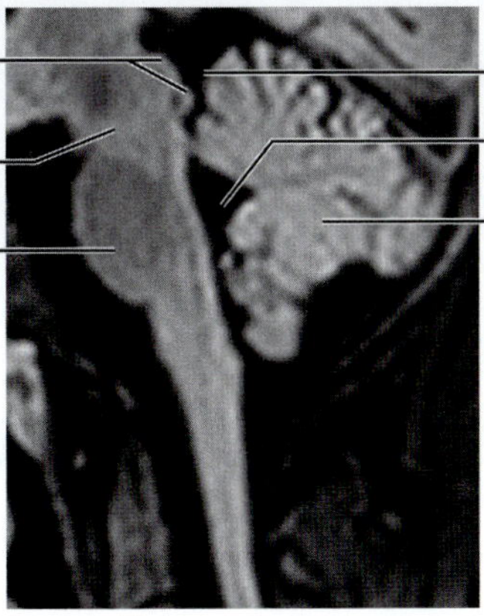

Fig. 9.6: MRI showing fourth ventricle

Facts to Remember

- Vital centres like respiratory and cardiovascular are situated in the floor of fourth ventricle.
- Fourth ventricle has 3 openings, one foramen of Magendie and two foramina of Luschka for the exit of used CSF into the subarachnoid space for absorption in the superior sagittal venous sinus.
- It also has 5 recesses to accommodate the CSF.
- In its floor are nuclei of VI, VII, VIII, X and XII cranial nerves.

BDC's Anatomy *e*-book

1. Further reading
2. Viva voce questions

Chapter

10

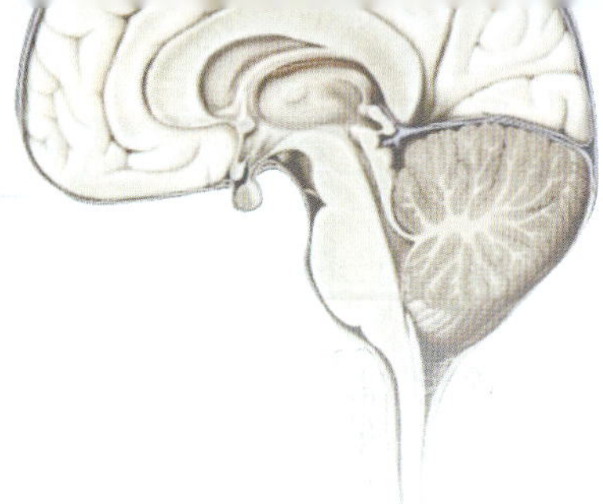

Diencephalon and Third Ventricle

DIENCEPHALON

The diencephalon is a middle structure which is largely embedded in the cerebrum, and, therefore, hidden from surface view. Its cavity forms the greater part of the third ventricle. The hypothalamic sulcus, extending from the interventricular foramen to the cerebral aqueduct, divides each half of the diencephalon into dorsal and ventral parts (Plate 10.1).

The diencephalon consists of pairs of:

1. Thalamus
2. Hypothalamus
3. Metathalamus: Medial geniculate body (MGB), lateral geniculate body (LGB)
4. Subthalamus
5. Epithalamus: Pineal body, habenular nuclei and commissure, posterior commissure, and stria medullaris thalami.

Competency:

AN62.5 Describe boundaries, parts, gross relations, major nuclei and connections of dorsal thalamus, hypothalamus, epithalamus, metathalamus and subthalamus.

THALAMUS

The thalamus (Greek *inner chamber*) is a large mass of grey matter 4 cm each in transverse, vertical and anteroposterior diameters situated in the lateral wall of the third ventricle and the floor of the central part of the lateral ventricle (Figs 10.1 to 10.5 and Flowchart 10.1).

Major Functions of Thalamus

1. *Sensory relay station*: Thalamus is a sensory station for all impulses except olfactory sensation.
2. *Pain and temperature perception*: Thalamus is capable of poor recognition of pain and temperature sensations.
3. *Extrapyramidal function*: It conveys sensory inputs of cerebellum and basal ganglia to motor cortex and influences motor activity.
4. *Maintenance of wakefulness and alertness* through influencing ascending reticular activating system.
5. *Emotional behavior and recent memory*: These play a role as a part of limbic system in emotional behaviour and recent memory mechanism.
6. *Autonomic control of viscera*: It takes part in autonomic control through the hypothalamus.
7. Mood and emotional balance.
8. Personality and intellect of an individual.

External Features of Thalamus

Measurements

- Length (anteroposterior): 4 cm
- Vertical: 1.5 cm
- Width (transverse): 1.5 cm.

Flowchart 10.1: Thalamus

Thalamus
Ovoid mass of grey matter; L: 4 cm; W: 1.5 cm

- ***Features of thalamus***
  - ***External features***
    - Two ends
      - Anterior
      - Posterior
    - 4 surfaces
      - Superior
      - Medial
      - Inferior
      - Lateral
  - ***Body***
    - ***White matter***
      - Stratum zonulae
      - External medullary lamina
      - Internal medullary lamina (Y-shaped)
    - ***Grey matter***
      - Anterior part
      - Medial part
      - Lateral part
- ***Thalamic nuclei***
  - ***Anterior part***
    - Anterior N
  - ***Lateral part***
    - ***Dorsal group***
      - Lateral dorsal N
      - Lateral posterior N
      - Pulvinar
    - ***Ventral group***
      - Ventral anterior N
      - Ventral lateral N
      - Ventral posterior N: VPL, VPM
  - ***Medial part***
    - Medial dorsal N
  - ***Other nuclei***
    - MGB, LGB
    - Intralaminar N
    - Centromedian N
    - Midline N
    - Reticular N
- ***Functions***
  - Sensory relay station
  - Pain and temperature perception
  - Extrapyramidal function
  - Maintenance of wakefulness
  - Emotional behaviour
  - Recent memory
  - Autonomic control

BDC yogesh

Plate 10.1: Location of diencephalon (sagittal section of the brain)

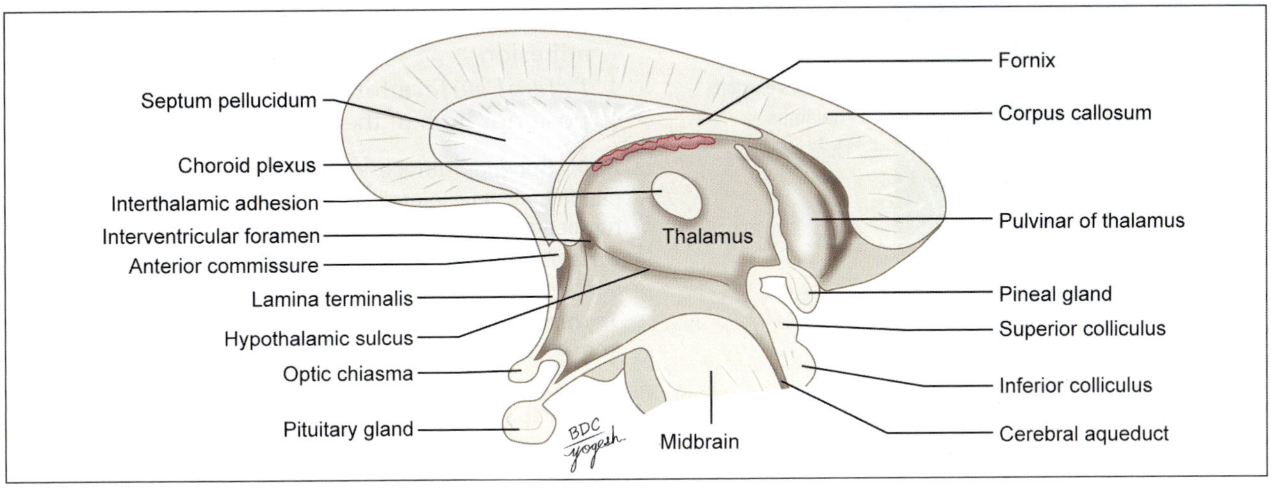

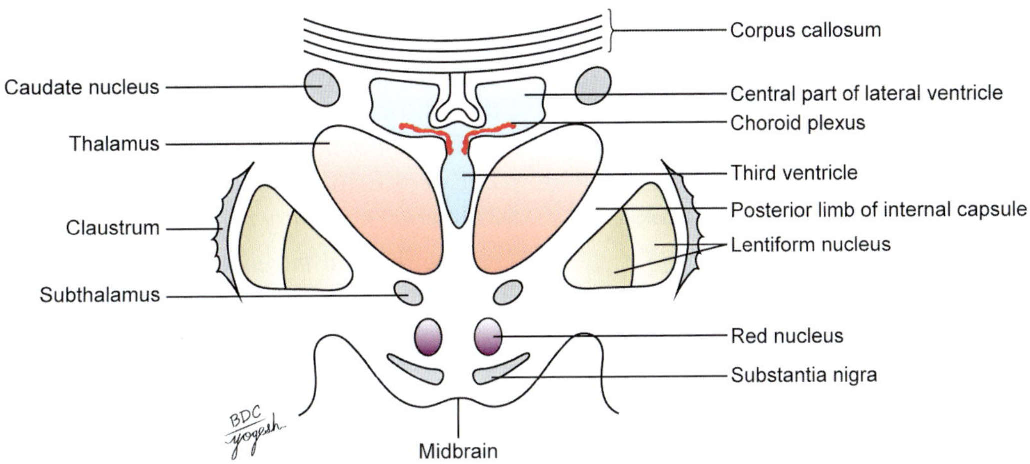

Fig. 10.1: Relations of thalamus (posterior view, coronal section of the brain)

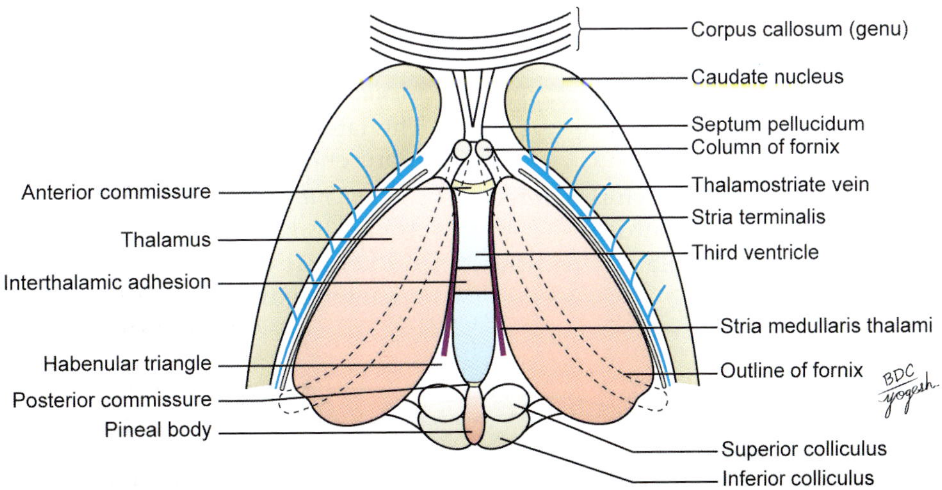

Fig. 10.2: Relation of thalamus with third ventricle (superior view, *Note*: overlying tela choroidea of third ventricle is removed)

Each thalamus has
- Two ends: Anterior and posterior
- Four surfaces: Superior, inferior, medial, and lateral.

Ends

1. ***Anterior end*** with anterior nucleus is narrow and forms the posterior boundary of the interventricular foramen.
2. ***Posterior end*** is expanded and is known as the ***pulvinar***. It overhangs the lateral and medial geniculate bodies, and the superior colliculus with its brachium.

Surfaces

1. ***Superior surface*** is divided into:
   a. A lateral ventricular part which forms the floor of the central part of the lateral ventricle

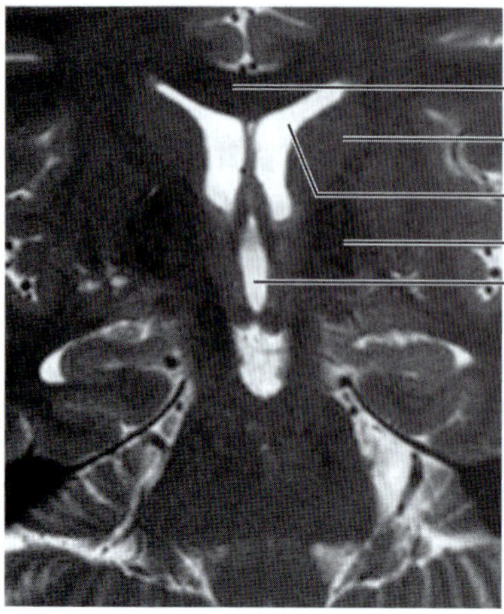

Fig. 10.3: MRI of thalamus

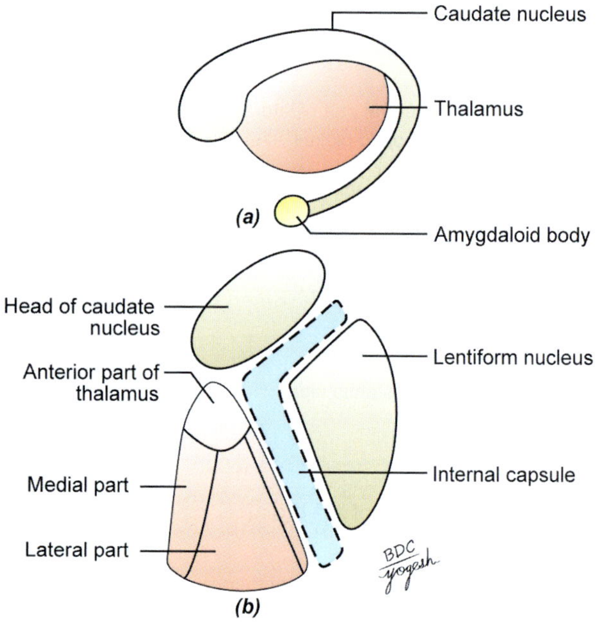

Figs 10.4a and b: (a) Lateral view of thalamus and caudate nucleus and (b) thalamus as seen in horizontal section

b. A medial extraventricular part which is covered by the tela choroidea of the 3rd ventricle.

2. ***Inferior surface*** rests on the subthalamus and the hypothalamus.
3. ***Medial surface*** forms the posterosuperior part of the lateral wall of the third ventricle. The medial surfaces of two thalami are interconnected by an interthalamic adhesion.
4. ***Lateral surface*** forms the medial boundary of the posterior limb of the internal capsule.

Note: Superior surface thalamus is related to the body of the caudate nucleus laterally. *Stria terminalis* and *thalamostriate vein* run between the thalamus and caudate nucleus.

Stria medullaris thalami separates superior surface from medial surface of thalamus.

Taenia thalami is a line of reflection of ependyma of 3rd ventricle from its lateral wall to its roof.

Internal Structure of Thalamus

The thalamus is mainly consisting of grey matter and a thin layer of white matter.

White Matter

The thalamus contains small quantity of white matter as the following thin laminae:

1. *Stratum zonulae* on the superior surface
2. *External medullary lamina* on the lateral surface
3. *Internal medullary lamina* lies within the thalamus.

The *internal medullary lamina* is a vertical sheet of Y-shaped white matter that bifurcates anterosuperiorly.

Grey Matter

The Y-shaped internal medullary lamina divides the thalamus into anterior, medial, and lateral parts. The anterior part lies between the limbs of the 'Y' and medial and lateral parts on either side of the stem of 'Y'. The grey matter of the thalamus consists of number of nuclei as follows:

1. *Anterior nucleus* in the anterior part (Fig. 10.5).
2. *Medial nucleus* in the medial part.
3. The lateral part of the thalamus is the largest and represents the *neothalamus*. It is divided into:
   a. *Lateral nucleus* in the dorsolateral part
   b. *Ventral nucleus* in the ventromedial part. The ventral nucleus is subdivided into anterior, intermediate and posterior groups. The posterior

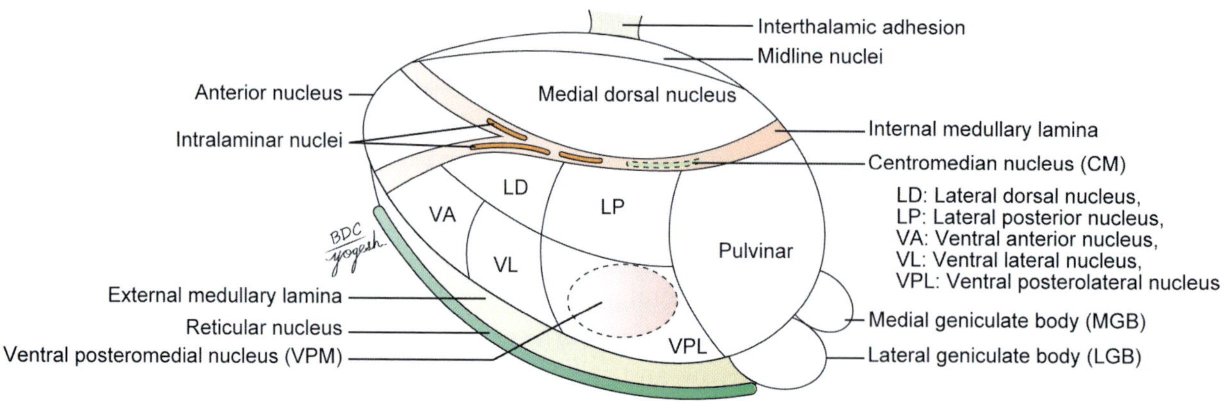

Fig. 10.5: Thalamic nuclei (schematic representation, note: Centromedian nucleus and VPM nucleus lies deep)

group is further subdivided into the posterolateral and posteromedial groups.

4. *Intralaminar nuclei* including *centromedian nucleus* (located in the internal medullary lamina), midline nuclei (periventricular grey on the medial surface) and reticular nuclei (on the lateral surface) are also present. The *medial geniculate body* (*MGB*) and *lateral geniculate body* (*LGB*) are also considered as a part of thalamus which forms metathalamus.

The thalamic nuclei are listed in Table 10.1 (Fig. 10.6) and their major connections and functions are given in Table 10.2. Medial and lateral geniculate bodies are described below separately.

CLINICAL NEUROANATOMY

- ***Thalamic syndrome:*** A vascular lesions of thalamogeniculate branch of posterior cerebral artery results in thalamic syndrome. It is characterized by the following features:
  1. Hyperesthesia – exaggerated sensations.
  2. Severe spontaneous pain on the opposite side of body.
  3. Emotional instability, that is, patient may laugh or cry without any reason.
  4. *Thalamic phantom limb*, that is, patient is unable to locate the limb with the eyes closed and develops the illusion that the limb is lost.
  5. *Thalamic hand*: It may occur in thalamic lesions. The opposite hand is involved. The forearm is pronated, wrist flexed, metacarpophalangeal joint flexed, and interphalangeal joint extended.
- ***Thalamic pain syndrome (Dejerine-Roussy syndrome):*** It involves loss of sensation followed by progressive agonizing pain in the parts of body where loss of sensation has occurred. It shows:
  a. *Allodynia* – a painful sensation elicited from an innocuous stimulus on normal skin
  b. *Hyperpathia* – an unusual and intense response to nociceptive stimuli
  c. *Dysesthesia* – an abnormal sensation triggered by sense of touch.

TABLE 10.1: Thalamic nuclei

Part	*Nuclei*
Anterior part	Anterior nucleus
Medial part	Medial dorsal nucleus (only one in humans)
Lateral part 1. Dorsal tier nuclei	 Lateral dorsal nucleus Lateral posterior nucleus Pulvinar
2. Ventral tier nuclei	Ventral anterior nucleus Ventral lateral nucleus Ventral posterior nucleus: Ventral posterolateral (VPL) and ventral posteromedial (VPM)
Other nuclei	Medial geniculate body (MGB) Lateral geniculate body (LGB) Intralaminar nuclei Centromedian nucleus (CM) Midline nuclei Reticular nucleus

METATHALAMUS

The metathalamus consists of the medial and lateral geniculate bodies, which are situated on each side of the midbrain, below the thalamus (Plate 10.2 and Flowchart 10.2).

Medial Geniculate Body (MGB)

It is an oval elevation situated just below the pulvinar of the thalamus and lateral to the superior colliculus. The

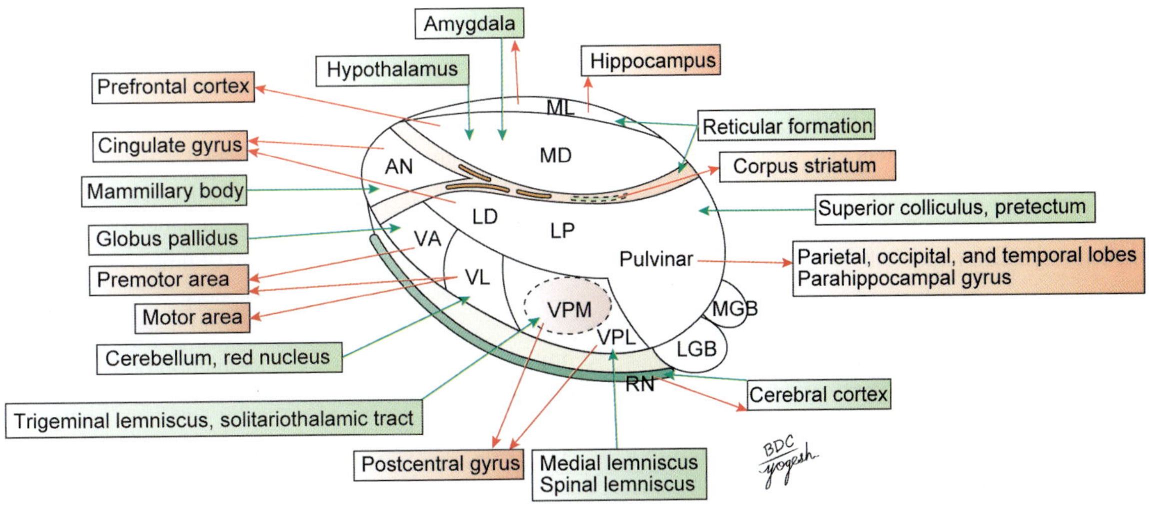

Fig. 10.6: Major afferent connections of the thalamus (schematic representation, green arrows – afferent fibres and red arrows – efferent fibres)

Plate 10.2: Geniculate bodies (posterior view of brainstem)

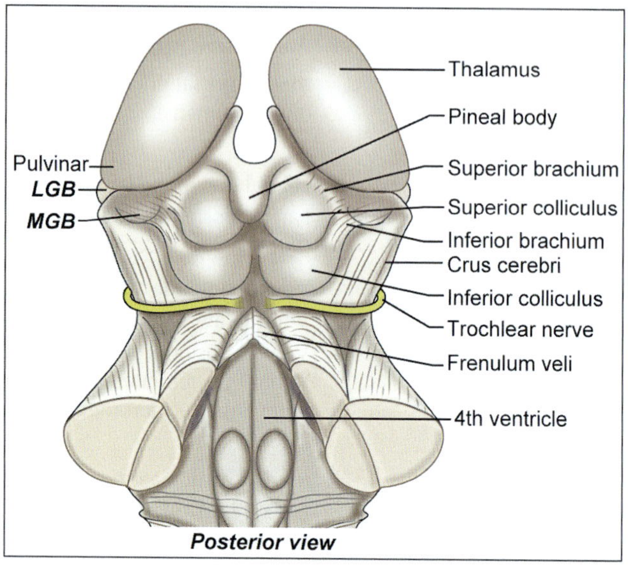

inferior brachium connects the medial geniculate body to the inferior colliculus. The connections of the medial geniculate body are as follows:

Afferents

1. Lateral lemniscus
2. Fibres from both inferior colliculi
3. Ascending reticular pathway and perception of painful and nociceptive stimuli.

Efferents

1. It gives rise to the acoustic (auditory) radiation going to the auditory area of the cortex (in the temporal lobe) through the sublentiform part of the internal capsule.
2. To secondary somatosensory area.

Function: Medial geniculate body is the last relay station on the pathway of auditory impulses to the cerebral cortex and for perception of painful and nociceptive stimuli.

TABLE 10.2: Connections and functions of thalamic nuclei

Nucleus	*Afferent*	*Efferent*	*Functions*
Anterior nucleus	From mammillary body (mammillothalamic tract)	To cingulate gyrus	Associate with limbic system Emotional behaviour, recent memory
Medial dorsal nucleus	From hypothalamus, amygdala, other thalamic nuclei	Prefrontal cortex	Association or integration of visceral and somatic activities Personality of individual mood and feelings
Lateral dorsal group (LD, LP, pulvinar)	Ventral thalamic nuclei, superior colliculus, pretectum	Cingulate gyrus, parahippocampal gyrus, parietal, occipital, and temporal lobes	Forms part of limbic system Helps in sensory analysis
Ventral posteromedial nucleus (VPM)	Trigeminal lemniscus Solitariothalamic tract	Postcentral gyrus	Relay station for pain, temperature, touch, proprioceptive sensations from head and face
Ventral posterolateral nucleus (VPL)	Medial lemniscus Spinal lemniscus	Postcentral gyrus	Relay station for pain, temperature, touch, proprioceptive sensations from whole body except face and head
Ventral anterior (VA) nucleus	Globus pallidus through subthalamic fasciculus	Premotor area	Relay station for striatal impulses Modifies motor activity
Ventral lateral (VL) nucleus	Cerebellum (dentatothalamic) Red nucleus (dentato-rubrothalamic)	Motor and premotor areas Influences motor activity	Relay station for cerebellar impulses
Intralaminar nuclei (centromedian and parafascicular nuclei)	Reticular formation	Other thalamic nuclei and corpus striatum	General awareness of painful stimuli Sensory motor integration Maintenance of arousal
Midline nuclei	Reticular formation	Hippocampus, amygdala	Part of limbic system Memory Arousal responses
Thalamic reticular nucleus (lies between external medullary lamina and internal capsule)	Corticothalamic fibres	Other nuclei of thalamus Thalamocortical fibres	Regulation of interthalamic activity
Medial geniculate body	Auditory fibres from inferior colliculus	Primary auditory areas 41, 42	Relay station for auditory impulses and perception of painful and nociceptive stimuli
Lateral geniculate body	Optic tract	Primary visual cortex area 17	Relay station for visual impulses

Flowchart 10.2: Medial and lateral geniculate bodies

Medial geniculate body

- ***Definition***
  - Part of metathalamus
  - Oval elevation on inferior aspect of pulvinar
- ***Connections***
  - Afferent: From inferior colliculus through inferior brachium
  - Efferent: Auditory radiation to areas 41 and 42
- ***Functions***
  - Relay station for auditory pathway

Lateral geniculate body

- ***Definition***
  - Part of metathalamus
  - Oval elevation at the posterior end of optic tract
- ***Structure***
  - 6 layers
  - Layers 1, 4, 6: Receive fibres from nasal side of opposite retina
  - Layers 2, 3, 5: Receive fibres from temporal side of same retina
- ***Connections***
  - Afferent: Optic tract
  - Efferent: Optic radiation to areas 17, 18 and 19
- ***Functions***
  - Relay station on visual pathway

Clinical integration: Lesion of LGB → Contralateral homonymous hemianopia

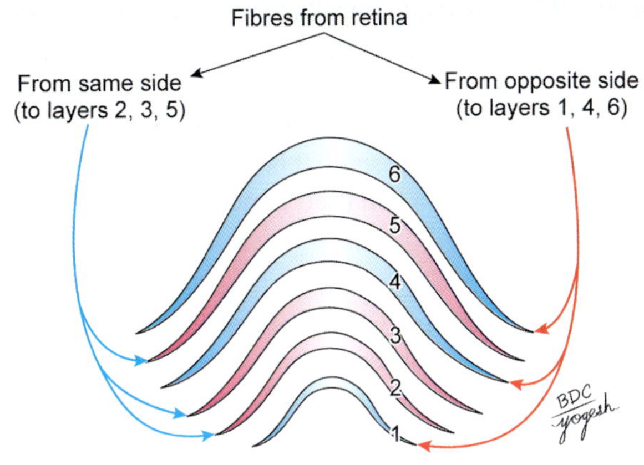

Fig. 10.7: Six layers of lateral geniculate body

Lateral Geniculate Body (LGB)

It is a small oval elevation situated anterolateral to the medial geniculate body, below the thalamus. It is overlapped by the medial part of the temporal lobe, and is connected to the superior colliculus by the superior brachium (Fig. 10.7).

Structure: It is six-layered structure. Layers 1, 4 and 6 receive contralateral optic fibres, and layers 2, 3 and 5 receive ipsilateral optic fibres.

Connections

1. *Afferents:* Optic tract (lateral root).
2. *Efferents:* It gives rise to optic radiations going to the visual area of cortex through retrolentiform part of internal capsule.

Function: Lateral geniculate body is the last relay station on the visual pathway to the occipital cortex.

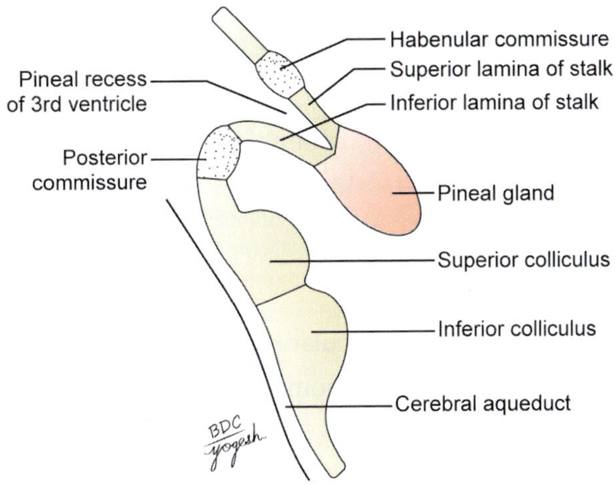

Fig. 10.8: Components of the epithalamus

Flowchart 10.3: Epithalamus

Epithalamus

- ***Pineal gland***
  - Small conical projection
  - 100–200 mg
  - Pineal stalk: Superior and inferior lamina
  - Functions:
    - Secretes melatonin
    - Maintains circadian rhythm
- ***Habenular nucleus and commissure***
  - Habenular trigone:
    - Small depressed triangular area
  - Habenular nucleus
  - Habenular commissure connects two habenular nuclei
  - Functions:
    - Part of limbic system
    - Emotional drives
- ***Posterior commissure***
  - Lies in inferior lamina of pineal stalk
  - Function not known

EPITHALAMUS

The epithalamus (Fig. 10.8 and Flowchart 10.3) occupies the caudal part of the roof of the diencephalon and consists of:

1. Pineal body or epiphysis cerebri.
2. Right and left habenular nuclei, each situated beneath the floor of the corresponding habenular trigone.
3. Habenular commissure lies superior to suprapineal recess.
4. Posterior commissure lies inferior to the suprapineal recess.

Pineal Body/Pineal Gland

The pineal (Latin *pine, cone*) body is a small, conical organ, projecting backwards and downwards between the two superior colliculi. It is placed below the splenium of the corpus callosum, but is separated from it by the tela choroidea of the third ventricle.

Weight: About 100–200 mg.

It consists of a conical *body* about 8 mm long, and a *stalk* or *peduncle* which divides anteriorly into two laminae separated by the pineal recess of the 3rd ventricle. The superior lamina of the stalk contains the habenular commissure; and the inferior lamina contains the posterior commissure.

Note: ***Morphological significance:*** In many reptiles, the epiphysis cerebri is represented by a double structure. The anterior part *(parapineal organ)* develops into the pineal or parietal eye. The posterior part is glandular in nature. The human pineal body represents the persistent posterior glandular part only. The parietal eye has disappeared.

Structure: Pineal gland consists of pinealocytes and interstitial cells. The pinealocytes are chief cells of pineal gland. They secrete ***melatonin*** hormone. The interstitial cells are a few cells that support the pinealocytes.

Corpora arenacea or brain sand: It is a characteristic feature of pineal gland. It is a calcified concretion (deposit) that increases with age.

Functions:

1. Secretion of melatonin that inhibits secretion of gonadotropins from hypothalamus.
2. Maintenance of circadian rhythm (*biological clock*).

Habenular Nucleus

The nucleus lies beneath the floor of the habenular trigone (*habenula* = little rein, in Latin). The trigone is a small, depressed triangular area, situated above the superior colliculus and medial to the pulvinar of the thalamus. Medially, it is bounded by the stria medullaris thalami and stalk of the pineal body. The habenular nucleus forms a part of the limbic system.

Afferents

- Hypothalamus
- Amygdaloid body
- Hippocampus

Efferents: To interpeduncular nucleus.

Functions: Acts as nodal point for convergence of basic emotional drives.

Habenular Commissure

These are the fibres that connect the habenular nucleus of two sides across the midline. They lie in the superior lamina of pineal stalk. They form a part of limbic system and are responsible for primitive visceral response to basic emotional drives.

Posterior Commissure

It is a bundle of fibres that cross the midline in the inferior lamina of pineal stalk. It contains fibres from medial longitudinal bundle, interstitial nuclei, and many other adjacent areas. Its exact function is not listed.

Note: ***Stria medullaris thalami*** is a bundle of fibres lying deep to taenia thalami (ependyma of 3rd ventricle). It lies along the junction of medial and superior surfaces of thalamus. It connects the septal nucleus, basal nuclei of Meynert and hypothalamus with habenular nucleus and thus forms a part of limbic system.

HYPOTHALAMUS

The hypothalamus is a part of the diencephalon (Figs 10.9a and b and Flowchart 10.4). It lies in the floor and lateral wall of the third ventricle. It has been designated as the head ganglion of the autonomic nervous system because it takes part in the control of many visceral and metabolic activities of the body.

Anatomically, it includes:

a. The floor of the third ventricle, or structures in the interpeduncular fossa.
b. The lateral wall of the third ventricle below the hypothalamic sulcus.

Weight: 4 g (forms less than 1% of total brain weight).

Boundaries

Anteriorly: Lamina terminalis
Posteriorly: Subthalamus
Superiorly: Thalamus
Inferiorly: Floor of 3rd ventricle
Medially: Cavity of 3rd ventricle
Laterally: Internal capsule.

Note: *Hypothalamic sulcus* extends from the interventricular foramen to the cerebral aqueduct. This sulcus separates hypothalamus from thalamus.

Flowchart 10.4: Hypothalamus

Hypothalamus
Part of diencephalon

Functions
Regulates
- Autonomic nervous system
- Body temperature
- Food and water intake
- Pituitary gland
- Emotion, sexual behaviour, and reproduction

Boundaries
Anteriorly: Lamina terminalis
Posteriorly: Subthalamus
Superiorly: Thalamus
Inferiorly: Floor of 3rd ventricle
Medially: Cavity of 3rd ventricle
Laterally: Internal capsule

Parts
Preoptic part
Supraoptic region
Tuberal region
Mammillary region

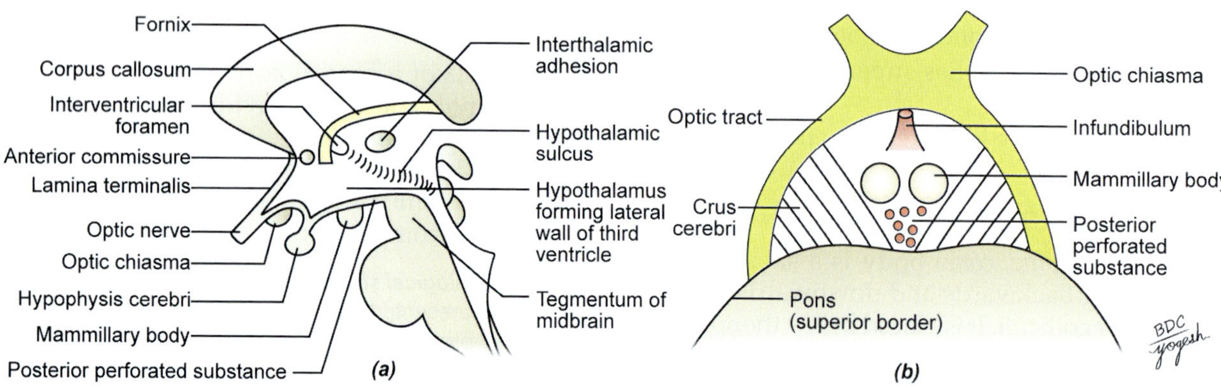

Figs 10.9a and b: (a) Hypothalamus as seen in sagittal section and (b) hypothalamus viewed at the base of brain

Parts of the Hypothalamus

The hypothalamus is divided into four regions or parts:

1. *Preoptic part*: It lies anteriorly between optic chiasma and anterior commissure. It consists of preoptic nucleus.
2. *Supraoptic region*: It lies above the optic chiasma. It consists of supraoptic, anterior, and paraventricular nuclei.
3. *Tuberal region*: It includes tuber cinereum, arcuate nucleus, ventromedial and dorsomedial nuclei.
4. *Mammillary region*: It includes mammillary body and posterior nucleus.

Note:

- Anterior column of fornix, mammillothalamic tract, and fasciculus retroflexes traverse the hypothalamus.
- *Tuber cinereum* is an elevation produced by grey matter. It lies between optic chiasma and mammillary bodies.
- *Infundibulum* is a pituitary stalk which passes inferiorly from the centre of tuber cinereum.
- *Median eminence* is an elevated part of tuber cinereum at the attachment of infundibulum.
- *Mammillary bodies* are paired, small spherical masses. They lie in between tuber cinereum and posterior perforated substance of interpeduncular fossa. They are masses of gray matter covered by white fibres. They form a part of limbic system.

Hypothalamic Nuclei and Connections

The hypothalamic nuclei are named according to their location as preoptic, supraoptic, paraventricular, anterior, arcuate, ventromedial, dorsomedial, posterior, mammillary, and lateral nuclei (Fig. 10.10, Flowchart 10.5). Their functions are listed in Table 10.3.

TABLE 10.3: Hypothalamic nucleus and their functions

Nucleus	*Function*
Preoptic	Controls the release of gonadotropic hormones from the adenohypophysis
Supraoptic	Produces ADH and oxytocin
Paraventricular	Produces hypothalamic releasing and inhibiting hormones
Anterior	Regulates parasympathetic activity Regulates body temperature
Arcuate or infundibular	Produces hypothalamic releasing and inhibiting hormones
Ventromedial	It is a satiety and hunger centre
Dorsomedial	It causes obesity
Posterior	Regulates sympathetic activity Regulates body temperature by conservation of heat and production of heat (thermostat centre)
Mammillary	Emotional expression (part of limbic system)
Lateral	It is a feeding centre
Suprachiasmatic	Regulates circadian rhythm (acts as master clock)

ADH: Antidiuretic hormone.

Afferent Fibres for Hypothalamus

1. *Medial forebrain bundle* connects medial olfactory area (that is olfactory bulb and anterior perforated substance) to the preoptic and lateral nuclei.
2. *Fornix* connects the hippocampus to mammillary body.
3. *Stria terminalis* connects the amygdaloid nucleus to preoptic and anterior thalamic nuclei.
4. *Ansa lenticularis* (pallido-hypothalamic fibres) connects the lentiform nucleus of basal ganglia to ventromedial nucleus of hypothalamus.
5. *Thalamohypothalamic fibres* from thalamus.
6. Corticohypothalamic fibres.
7. *Mammillary peduncle* connects the spinal cord and brainstem to the lateral hypothalamus nuclei.

Efferent Fibres of Hypothalamus

1. *Mammillothalamic* tract connects mammillary body to anterior nucleus of hypothalamus.
2. *Mammillotegmental* tract connects mammillary body to the reticular formation of brainstem.
3. Descending fibres to spinal cord and brainstem.
4. *Supraoptico-hypophyseal* and *tubero-infundibular fibres* are axons of supraoptic and paraventricular nuclei

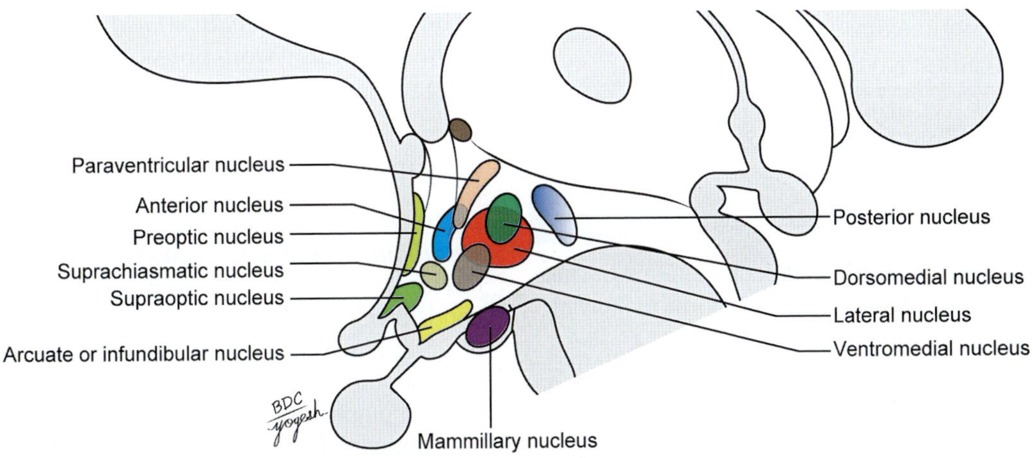

Fig. 10.10: Nuclei of hypothalamus

Flowchart 10.5: Major connections of hypothalamus

Source	Pathway	Destination
Medial olfactory area	Medial forebrain bundle	Hypothalamus
Hippocampus	Fornix	Mammillary body
Amygdaloid nucleus	Stria terminalis	Preoptic nucleus Anterior thalamic nuclei
Lentiform nucleus	Ansa lenticularis	Ventromedial nucleus
Thalamus	Thalamohypothalamic fibres	Hypothalamus
Cerebral cortex	Corticohypothalamic fibres	Hypothalamus
Spinal cord and brainstem	Mammillary peduncle	Lateral hypothalamus nuclei
Mammillary body	Mammillothalamic tract	Anterior nucleus of thalamus
Mammillary body	Mammillo-tegmental tract	Midbrain
Supraoptic and paraventricular nuclei	Supraoptico-hypophyseal and tubero-infundibular fibres	Posterior pituitary

of hypothalamus that pass through infundibulum to the posterior pituitary. The hormones stored in their axon terminals produce *Herring bodies*. They secrete vasopressin and oxytocin hormones.

Functions of Hypothalamus

The hypothalamus is a complex neuroglandular mechanism concerned with regulation of visceral and vasomotor activities of the body. Its functions are as follows:

1. Controls autonomic nervous system
2. Regulates body temperature
3. Regulates food and water intake
4. Regulates endocrine function of anterior and posterior pituitary gland
5. Regulates emotion, sexual behavior, and reproduction
6. Maintains circadian rhythm (biological clock).

For details of hypothalamo-hypophyseal portal circulation, *see* Volume 3, Chapter 12.

CLINICAL NEUROANATOMY

Hypothalamic disorders: The vascular lesions or any other disorder of hypothalamus result on the following conditions:

1. Diabetes insipidus due to lack of ADH secretion
2. Polydipsia and polyuria
3. Obesity due to overeating (polyphagia)
4. Somnolence (drowsiness or sleepiness)
5. Loss of temperature control (poikilothermia), may be hyperthermia
6. Loss of sexual desires
7. Dehydration due to lack of water intake
8. Aggressive behaviour, rage, or extreme passivity.

These symptoms may not be completely observed. There may be aphagia instead of polyphagia.

SUBTHALAMUS

The subthalamus lies between the midbrain and thalamus, medial to internal capsule and the globus pallidus (Fig. 10.11). It consists of the following:

Grey Matter

1. The cranial ends of the red nucleus and substantia nigra extend into it.
2. Subthalamic nucleus
3. Zona incerta.

White Matter

1. Cranial ends of lemnisci—lateral to the red nucleus
2. Dentatothalamic tract along with the rubrothalamic fibres
3. Ansa lenticularis (ventral)
4. Fasciculus lenticularis (dorsal)
5. Subthalamic fasciculus (intermediate fibres).

The ***subthalamic nucleus*** is a lens-shaped nucleus lying on the medial aspect of internal capsule just above the substantia nigra. It is one of the extrapyramidal nuclei that modifies motor activity.

The ***zona incerta*** is a thin lamina of grey matter situated between the thalamus and the subthalamic nucleus. Laterally, it is continuous with the reticular nucleus of the thalamus. Its activity influences drinking of water.

The ***fasciculus lenticularis*** (*lenticular fasciculus*) consists of fibres of globus pallidus that pass through the internal capsule to the subthalamus nucleus.

The ***ansa lenticularis*** is an inferior bundle of fibres from globus pallidus to thalamus and other subthalamic nuclei.

The ***thalamic fasciculus*** (*Field H1 of Forel*) is a group of fibres extending from prerubral field to the thalamus. It also has some fibres from fasciculus.

CLINICAL NEUROANATOMY

Discrete lesions of the subthalamic nucleus result in ***hemiballismus*** characterised by involuntary choreiform movements on the opposite side of the body. The condition is abolished by ablation of the globus pallidus or of its efferent tracts, the anterior ventral nucleus of the thalamus, area 4 of the cerebral cortex, or of the corticospinal tract. From these facts, it appears that the subthalamic nucleus has an inhibitory control on the globus pallidus and on the cerebral cortex.

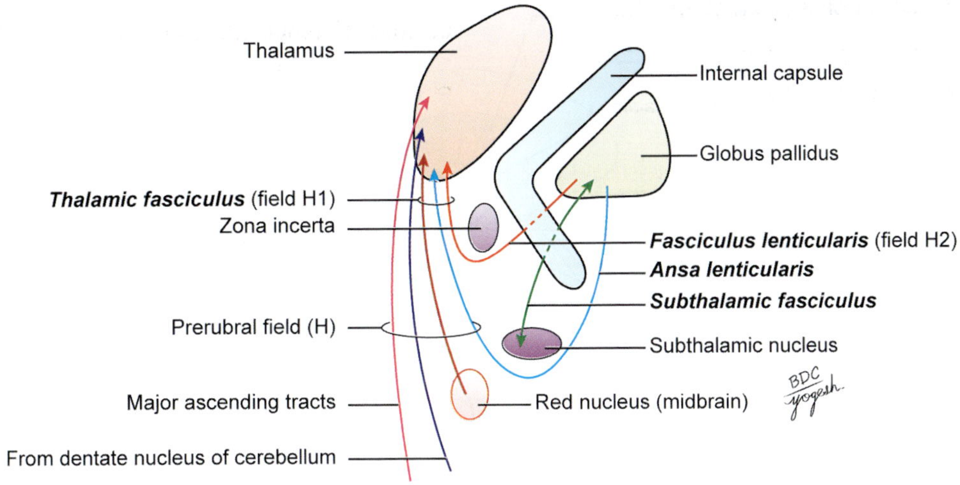

Fig. 10.11: Important fibre bundle running through subthalamic region

Competency:

AN63.1 Describe and demonstrate parts, boundaries and features of IIIrd ventricle.

THIRD VENTRICLE

The third ventricle is a median cleft between the two thalami. Developmentally, it represents the cavity of the diencephalon, except for the area in front of the interventricular foramen which is derived from the median part of the telencephalon. The cavity is lined by ependyma (Fig. 10.12 and Flowchart 10.6).

Extent

It extends from lamina terminalis anteriorly to the cerebral aqueduct posteriorly.

Contents

1. Cerebrospinal fluid
2. Interthalamic adhesion (covered by ependyma lining).

Communications

Anterosuperiorly, on each side, it communicates with the lateral ventricle through the ***interventricular foramen*** (foramen of Monro). This foramen is bounded anteriorly by the column of the fornix, and posteriorly by the tubercle of the thalamus.

Posteroinferiorly, in the median plane, it communicates with the fourth ventricle through the cerebral aqueduct.

Boundaries

Anterior Wall

1. Lamina terminalis
2. Anterior commissure
3. Anterior columns of fornix. The two columns of the fornix diverge, pass downwards and backwards, and sink into the lateral wall of the third ventricle to reach the mammillary body.

Posterior Wall

1. Pineal body
2. Posterior commissure (in the lower lamina of the pineal stalk)
3. Cerebral aqueduct.

Roof

It is formed by body of fornix and the ependyma lining the under surface of the tela choroidea of the 3rd ventricle. The choroid plexus of the third ventricle projects downwards from the roof.

At the junction of the roof with the anterior and lateral walls, there is the interventricular foramen.

Floor

It is formed by hypothalamic structures:

1. Optic chiasma
2. Infundibulum (pituitary stalk) and tuber cinereum
3. Mammillary bodies
4. Posterior perforated substance
5. Tegmentum of the midbrain.

At the junction of the floor with the anterior wall, there is the optic recess.

Lateral Wall

It is formed by the following:

1. Medial surface of thalamus (in its posterosuperior part)
2. Hypothalamus (in its anteroinferior part)
3. The hypothalamic sulcus which separates the thalamus from the hypothalamus. The sulcus extends from the interventricular foramen to the cerebral aqueduct.

Note:

a. The interthalamic adhesion connects the medial surfaces of the two thalami and crosses the ventricular cavity.
b. The habenular stria lies at the junction of the roof and the lateral wall. The two striae join posteriorly at the habenular commissure.
c. The columns of the fornix, as already indicated, run downwards and backwards to reach the mammillary bodies. The columns lie beneath the lateral wall of the ventricle.

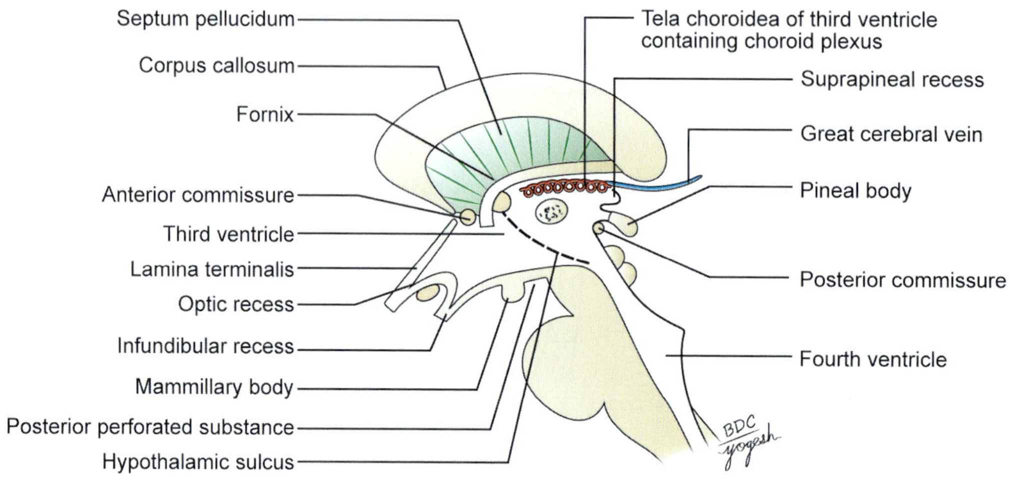

Fig. 10.12: Boundaries of third ventricle

Flowchart 10.6: Third ventricle

Third ventricle

- ***Location, extent, contents***
  - Location:
    - Midline slit-like cavity
    - Lies between two thalami and in hypothalamus
  - Extent: From lamina terminalis to cerebral aqueduct
  - Contents:
    - CSF
    - Interthalamic adhesion
- ***Communications***
  - Interventricular foramen ↕ Lateral ventricles
  - Cerebral aqueduct ↕ 4th ventricle
- ***Boundaries of 3rd ventricle***
  - ***Anterior wall***: Anterior column of fornix; Anterior commissure; Lamina terminalis
  - ***Posterior wall***: Habenular commissure; Pineal gland; Posterior commissure
  - ***Roof***: Ependymal lining
  - ***Floor***: Optic chiasma; Infundibulum and tuber cinereum; Mammillary bodies; Posterior perforated substance; Tegmentum of midbrain
  - ***Lateral walls***: Thalamus; Hypothalamus
  - ***Recesses***: Infundibular; Optic; Pineal; Suprapineal

Clinical integration: Obstruction in 3rd ventricle→Increased ICT, endoscopic third ventriculostomy

Recesses

Recesses are extensions of the cavity. They are as follows:

1. *Infundibular recess* – extends downward into the infundibulum of pituitary gland.
2. *Optic or chiasmatic recess* – extends anteriorly into the optic chiasma
3. *Pineal recess* – extends posteriorly into the stalk of the pineal gland
4. *Suprapineal recess* – extends posteriorly above the stalk of pineal gland and below the tela choroidea.

Note:

- ***Tela choroidea*** is the region where pia mater and ependyma adhere with each other without intervening neuronal tissue. (*Tela* = Woven, in Latin). It contains a thin layer of connective tissue and numerous blood vessels. It forms choroid plexuses in ventricles that produce cerebrospinal fluid (CSF).
- ***Choroid plexuses of 3rd ventricle*** hang downwards from tela choroidea of 3rd ventricle as two longitudinal finger-like projections that run anteroposteriorly. They are continuous with the choroid plexus of lateral ventricle.

CLINICAL NEUROANATOMY

- ***Obstruction in 3rd ventricle:*** The third ventricle is a narrow space which is easily obstructed by local brain tumours or by developmental defects. The obstruction leads to raised intracranial pressure in adults and hydrocephalus in infants.
- Tumours in the lower part of the third ventricle give rise to hypothalamic symptoms, like diabetes insipidus, obesity, sexual disturbance, disturbance of sleep, hyperglycaemia and glycosuria.
- ***Endoscopic third ventriculostomy:*** It is an endoscopic procedure that may be performed to release excess CSF in hydrocephalus cases. It is performed through the floor of the 3rd ventricle, in between two mammillary bodies.

DISSECTION

Identify the extent of the third ventricle from the lamina terminalis anteriorly to the upper end of the aqueduct and root of pineal body posteriorly. Examine its anterior wall, posterior wall, roof, floor and lateral walls.

Facts to Remember

- Thalamus is the inner chamber receiving and coordinating motor, sensory, visceral, visual, auditory and emotional impulses.
- Third ventricle is a slit-like ventricle in between the two thalami.
- Aqueduct is the narrow duct connecting 3rd ventricle above with the fourth ventricle below.
- All the sensory pathway relay in thalamus except olfactory pathway.
- Lateral geniculate body is a relay centre for the visual pathway, whereas the medial geniculate bosy is for the auditory pathway.
- Pineal gland is called third eye and it secretes melatonin.
- Hypothalamus is the main centre of autonomic nervous system.

BDC's Anatomy *e*-book

1. Location of thalamic nuclei
2. Stria medullaris thalami
3. Further reading
4. Viva voce questions

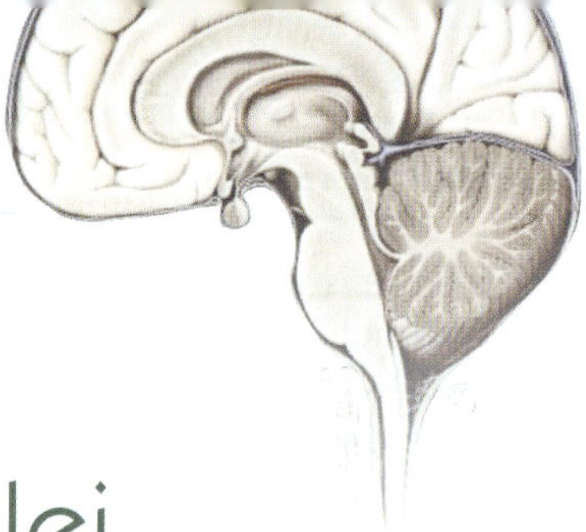

Chapter

11

Cerebrum, Basal Nuclei and White Matter

CEREBRUM

The cerebrum (Latin *brain*) is the ***largest part of the brain***. It is also known as ***pallium***. It occupies anterior, middle cranial fossae and the supratentorial part of the posterior cranial fossa (Figs 11.1a and b and 11.2).

Components of Cerebral Hemisphere

It is made up of:

1. Outer grey matter
2. Inner white matter
3. Basal ganglia or nuclei – some neuronal masses within the white matter
4. Diencephalon
5. A cavity called lateral ventricle.

The cerebrum is made of two cerebral hemispheres which are incompletely separated from each other by the median ***longitudinal fissure***.

The two hemispheres are connected to each other across the median plane by the ***corpus callosum***. Each hemisphere contains a cavity, called the ***lateral ventricle***. The surface area of cerebrum is 2000 cm^2.

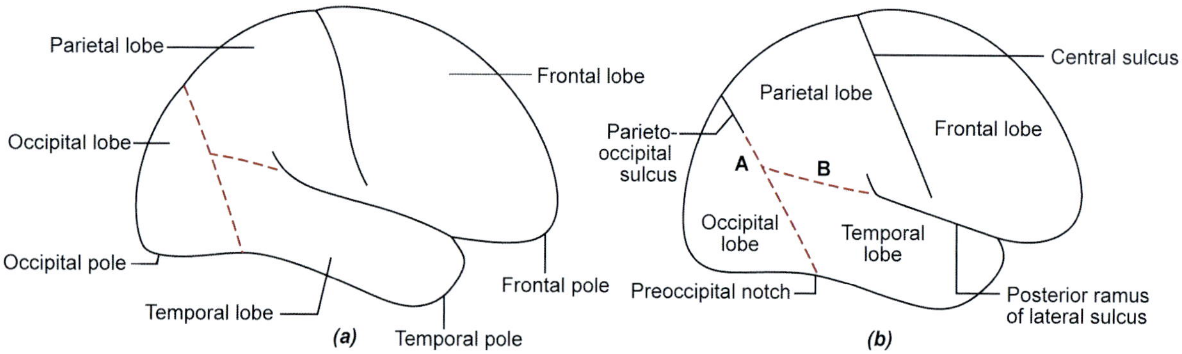

Figs 11.1a and b: Superolateral surface of cerebral hemisphere

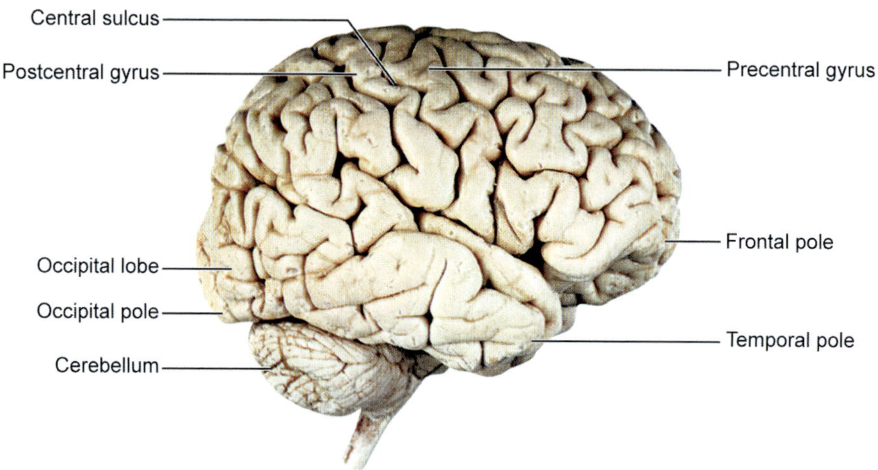

Fig. 11.2: Superolateral surface of cerebral hemisphere

Cerebral Sulci and Gyri

Cerebral cortex is folded into ***gyri*** (Greek *circle*) which are separated from each other by ***sulci*** (Figs 11.3 to 11.5).

Note: Sulci and gyri increase the surface area of the cortex. In human brain, the total area of the cortex is estimated to be more than 2000 cm^2, and approximately 2/3rd of this area is hidden from the surface within the sulci.

The pattern of folding of the cortex is not entirely haphazard. It is largely determined by the differential growth of specific functional areas of the cortex, because many of the sulci bear a definite topographical relation to these areas. The formation of sulci in the intrauterine life begins from 5th–6th month and ends almost at the end of 9th month.

DISSECTION

Keep the cerebrum in a position so that the longitudinal fissure faces superiorly. Identify the convex strong band of white matter, the corpus callosum, binding parts of the medial surfaces of the two cerebral hemispheres. Define splenium as the thick rounded part of corpus callosum.

Divide the corpus callosum in the median plane starting from the splenium towards the trunk, genu and rostrum. Inferior to the trunk of corpus callosum extend the incision into the tela choroidea of the lateral and third ventricles, and the interthalamic adhesion connecting the medial surfaces of two thalami.

Identify the thin septum pellucidum connecting the inferior surfaces of corpus callosum to a curved band of white matter—anterior column of the fornix. Look for the anterior commissure just at the anterior end of the anterior column of fornix.

Turn the brain upside down and identify optic chiasma. Divide the optic chiasma, anterior communicating artery, infundibulum and a thin groove between the adjacent mammillary bodies, posterior cerebral artery close to its origin. Carry the line of division around the midbrain to

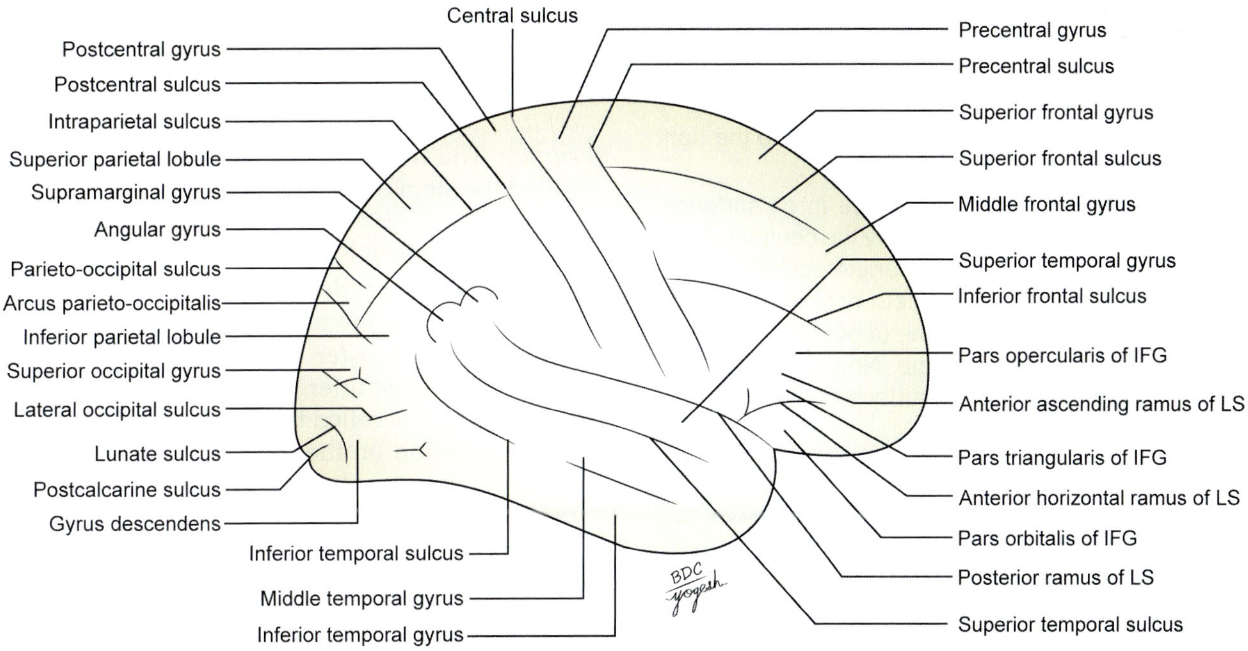

Fig. 11.3: Sulci and gyri on superolateral surface of cerebral hemisphere (IFG: Inferior frontal gyrus; LS: Lateral sulcus)

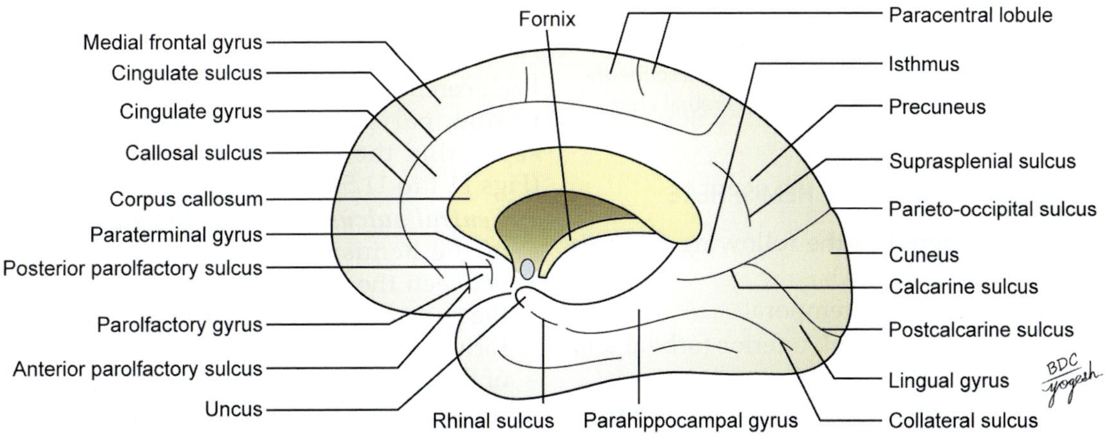

Fig. 11.4: Sulci and gyri on the medial surface of cerebral hemisphere

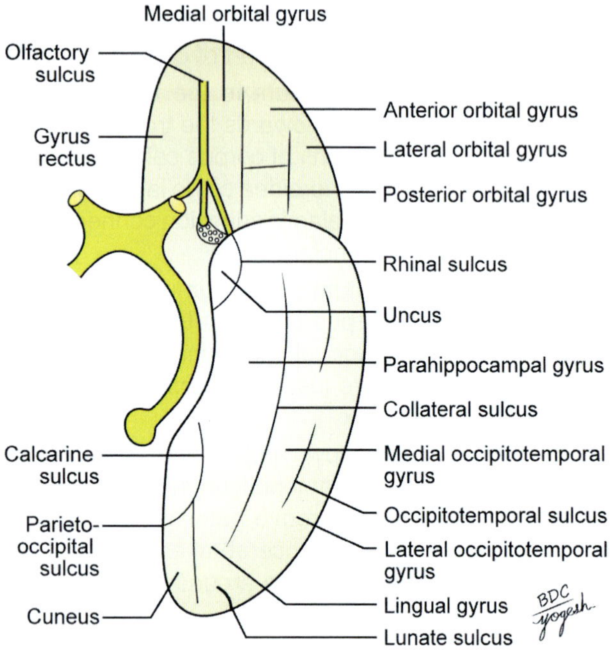

Fig. 11.5: Gyri and sulci on the inferior aspect of cerebral hemisphere

join the two ends of the median cut. Separate the right and the left cerebral hemispheres.

In the two hemispheres, identify the three surfaces, four borders, and three poles. Identify the central sulcus, posterior ramus of lateral sulcus, parieto-occipital sulcus and preoccipital notch. Join parieto-occipital sulcus to preoccipital notch. Extend the line of posterior ramus of lateral sulcus till the previous line. Now demarcate the four lobes of the superolateral surface of each cerebral hemisphere.

Strip the meninges from the surfaces. Identify the vessels on the surfaces of hemisphere. Demarcate the main sulci and gyri on the superolateral surface, medial surface and inferior surface of hemisphere.

Make thin slice through the part of the calcarine sulcus, posterior to its junction with the parieto-occipital sulcus. Identify the stria running through it. On cutting series of thin slices try to trace the extent of visual stria.

Competency:

AN62.2 Describe and demonstrate surfaces, sulci, gyri, poles, and functional areas of cerebral hemisphere. Also describe the effects of damage to various functional areas of cerebral cortex.

EXTERNAL FEATURES OF CEREBRAL HEMISPHERE

Each cerebral hemisphere has the following features (Figs 11.1 to 11.5, Flowchart 11.1):

- Poles: Frontal, occipital, and temporal
- Surfaces: Superolateral, medial, inferior (orbital and tentorial)
- Borders: Superomedial, superciliary, inferolateral, medial orbital, inferomedial, medial occipital.
- Lobes: Frontal, parietal, temporal, occipital, insula.

Flowchart 11.1: Cerebrum: External features

Cerebrum: External features

Poles	Surfaces	Borders	Lobes
Frontal	Superolateral	Superomedial	Frontal
Occipital	Medial	Superciliary	Parietal
Temporal	Inferior:	Inferolateral	Temporal
	- Orbital	Medial orbital	Occipital
	- Tentorial	Inferomedial	Insula
		Medial occipital	

Poles of Cerebral Hemisphere

1. *Frontal pole,* at the anterior end.
2. *Occipital pole,* at the posterior end.
3. *Temporal pole,* at the anterior end of the temporal lobe.

Surfaces of Cerebral Hemisphere

1. ***Superolateral surface*** is convex and is related to the cranial vault.
2. ***Medial surface*** is flat and vertical. It is separated from the corresponding surface of the opposite hemisphere by the falx cerebri and the longitudinal fissure.
3. ***Inferior surface*** is divided into an anterior part—the *orbital surface,* and a posterior part—the *tentorial surface.* The two parts are separated by a deep cleft called the stem of the lateral sulcus.

Borders of Cerebral Hemisphere

1. ***Superomedial border*** separates the superolateral surface from the medial surface.
2. ***Inferolateral border*** separates the superolateral surface from the inferior surface. The anterior part of this border is called the ***superciliary border.*** There is a depression on the inferolateral border situated about 5 cm in front of the occipital pole, it is called the ***preoccipital notch.***
3. ***Medial orbital border*** separates the medial surface from the orbital surface.
4. ***Medial occipital border*** separates the medial surface from the tentorial surface.
5. The ***inferomedial (hippocampal) border*** surrounds the cerebral peduncle. It is formed by the medial aspect of the uncus and parahippocampal gyrus.

Lobes of Cerebral Hemisphere

Each cerebral hemisphere is divided into four lobes—frontal, parietal, occipital and temporal. The sulci separating the lobes on this surface are as follows (Figs 11.1 to 11.5):

1. ***Central sulcus*** begins at the superomedial border of the hemisphere a little behind the midpoint between the frontal and occipital poles. It runs on the superolateral surface obliquely downwards and forwards and ends a little above the posterior ramus of the lateral sulcus.
2. It is seen that the ***lateral sulcus*** separates the orbital and tentorial parts of the inferior surface. Laterally, this sulcus reaches the superolateral surface where

it divides into anterior, ascending and posterior branches. The largest of these, the *posterior ramus of the lateral sulcus* passes backwards and slightly upwards over the superolateral surface.

3. ***Parieto-occipital sulcus*** is a sulcus of the medial surface. Its upper end cuts off the superomedial border about 5 cm in front of the occipital pole.
4. ***Preoccipital notch*** is an indentation on the inferolateral border, about 5 cm in front of the occipital pole.

The division is completed by drawing an imaginary vertical line joining the parieto-occipital sulcus to the preoccipital notch; and another horizontal line continuing backwards from the posterior ramus of the lateral sulcus to meet the first line as follows:

1. ***Frontal lobe*** lies anterior to central sulcus and above the posterior ramus of lateral sulcus.
2. ***Parietal lobe*** lies behind the central sulcus and in front of an imaginary vertical line joining the parieto-occipital sulcus and preoccipital notch. It lies above the horizontal line drawn from the horizontal part of posterior ramus of lateral sulcus.
3. ***Temporal lobe*** lies below the posterior ramus of lateral sulcus and horizontal line extending backward from horizontal part of this sulcus. It lies anterior to imaginary vertical line joining the parieto-occipital sulcus and preoccipital notch.
4. ***Occipital lobe*** lies behind the vertical line joining the parieto-occipital sulcus and preoccipital notch.

Insula (Island of Reil or Central Lobe)

Insula lies deep in the floor of lateral fissure surrounded by a circular sulcus and overlapped by adjacent cortical areas—the ***opercula*** (Plate 11.1 and Flowchart 11.2):

1. Insula comprises ***frontal operculum*** between anterior and ascending rami of lateral sulcus.
2. ***Parietal operculum*** lies between ascending and posterior rami of lateral sulcus.
3. ***Temporal opercula*** below posterior ramus of lateral sulcus formed by superior temporal gyri.

Insula is a pyramidal area, apex near anterior perforated substance.

The insula is divided into two regions: Anterior and posterior by a central sulcus. The anterior region presents 3 or 4 short gyri called *gyri brevia* and the posterior region presents 1 or 2 long gyri called *gyri longa*.

Functions:

1. Role of anterior insular cortex is in olfaction and taste.
2. Role of posterior insular cortex is in language function.

Flowchart 11.2: Insula

Insula — Surface projection

Location	***Insular operculae***	***Parts***	***Functions***
Central lobe	Temporal	Limen insulae	Olfaction
Lies deeply at the bottom of lateral sulcus	Frontal	Central sulcus	Taste.
Triangular	Frontoparietal	Gyri brevia	Language
	Orbital	Gyri longa	

Sulci and Gyri on Superolateral Surface

(Fig. 11.3, Table 11.1)

1. ***Central sulcus*** *(of Rolando)* (Latin *furrow*): It begins at the superomedial border of the hemisphere about 1 cm behind the midpoint between the frontal and occipital poles. It runs on the superolateral surface obliquely downwards and forwards and ends a little above the posterior ramus of the lateral sulcus. The upper end of the sulcus extends for a short distance onto the medial surface.
2. ***Lateral sulcus*** begins on the inferior surface. On reaching the lateral surface, it divides into three rami.
   - ***Anterior ramus*** (2.5 cm) passes forward into the inferior frontal gyrus.
   - ***Anterior ascending ramus*** (2.5 cm) runs upward in the inferior frontal gyrus.
   - ***Posterior ramus*** (7.5 cm) runs posteriorly and upward up to the inferior parietal lobule. Its posterior end upturns sharply.
3. ***In the frontal lobe*:** The frontal lobe is further divided by the following sulci:
   a. ***Precentral sulcus*** runs parallel to the central sulcus, a little in front of it. The ***precentral gyrus*** lies between the two sulci.
   b. The area in front of the precentral sulcus is divided into ***superior, middle and inferior frontal gyri*** by the ***superior and inferior frontal sulci.***
   c. The anterior horizontal and anterior ascending rami of the lateral sulcus subdivide the inferior frontal gyrus into three parts: *Pars orbitalis, pars triangularis,* and *pars opercularis.*
4. ***In the parietal lobe*:** The parietal lobe is further subdivided by the following sulci:
   a. ***Postcentral sulcus*** runs parallel to the central sulcus, a little behind it. The ***postcentral gyrus*** lies between the two sulci.
   b. The area behind the postcentral gyrus is divided into the ***superior* and *inferior parietal lobules*** by the ***intraparietal sulcus.***
   c. The inferior parietal lobule is invaded by the upturned ends of the posterior ramus of the lateral sulcus, and of the superior and inferior temporal sulci. They divide the inferior parietal lobule into anterior, middle and posterior parts:
      - The anterior part that surrounds the posterior ramus of lateral sulcus is called ***supramarginal gyrus.***
      - The middle part surrounding the superior temporal sulcus is the angular gyrus.
      - The posterior and lower part surrounding the inferior temporal sulcus is the arcus temporo-occipitalis.
5. ***In the temporal lobe:*** The ***superior and inferior temporal sulci*** divide the temporal lobe into ***superior, middle and inferior temporal gyri.***

Plate 11.1: Insula (island of Reil) (exposed by pulling the opercula)

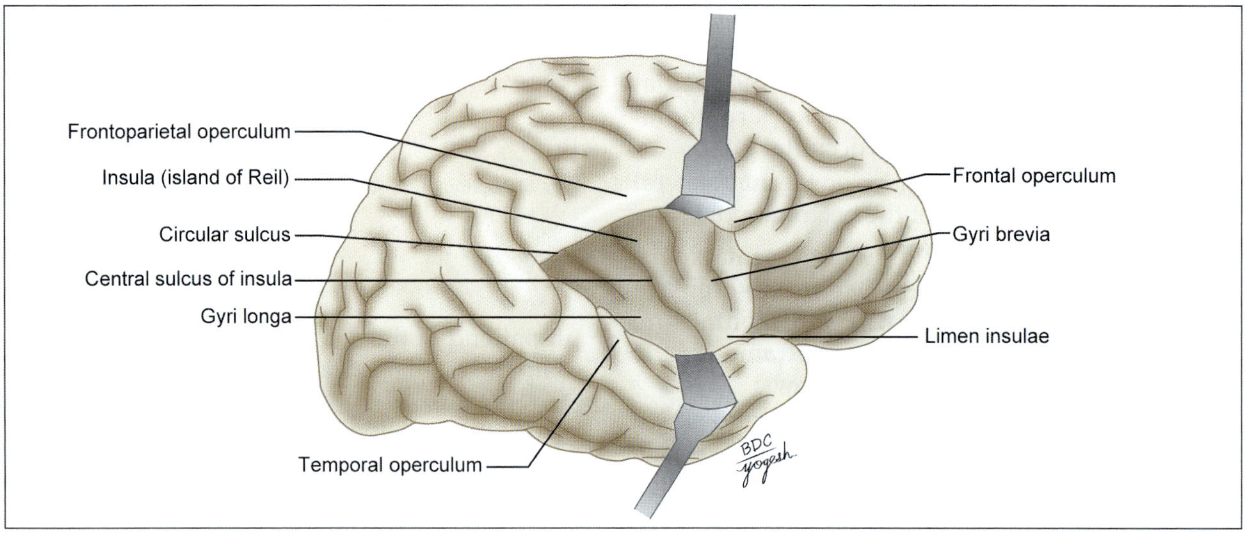

TABLE 11.1: Sulci and gyri of the cerebrum

Surface/lobe	*Sulci*	*Gyri*
I. Superolateral surface		
Frontal lobe	1. Precentral 2. Superior frontal 3. Inferior frontal	a. Precentral b. Superior frontal c. Middle frontal d. Inferior frontal which also contains anterior horizontal and anterior ascending rami of the lateral sulcus, and the pars orbitalis, pars triangularis and pars opercularis
Parietal lobe	1. Postcentral 2. Intraparietal	a. Postcentral b. Superior parietal lobule c. Inferior parietal lobule, which is divided into 3 parts: i. Anterior – supramarginal ii. Middle – angular iii. Posterior – over the upturned end of inferior temporal sulcus
Temporal lobe	1. Superior temporal 2. Inferior temporal	a. Superior temporal b. Middle temporal c. Inferior temporal
Occipital lobe	1. Lateral occipital 2. Lunate 3. Superior and inferior polar 4. Calcarine 5. Transverse occipital	a. Arcus parieto-occipitalis b. Superior occipital c. Inferior occipital d. Gyrus descendens
II. Medial surface	1. Anterior parolfactory 2. Posterior parolfactory 3. Cingulate 4. Callosal 5. Suprasplenial or subparietal 6. Parieto-occipital 7. Calcarine	a. Paraterminal b. Paraolfactory (subcallosal area) c. Medial frontal d. Paracentral lobule e. Cingulate f. Cuneus g. Precuneus
III. Inferior surface	1. Olfactory 2. H-shaped orbital sulci 3. Collateral 4. Rhinal 5. Occipitotemporal	a. Gyrus rectus b. Anterior orbital c. Posterior orbital d. Medial orbital e. Lateral orbital f. Uncus g. Parahippocampal h. Medial occipitotemporal i. Lateral occipitotemporal j. Lingual

6. ***In the occipital lobe:*** The occipital lobe is further subdivided by the following sulci:
   a. ***Lateral occipital sulcus*** divides this lobe into the ***superior and inferior occipital gyri.***
   b. ***Lunate sulcus*** separates these gyri from the occipital pole.
   c. The area around the ***parieto-occipital sulcus*** is the ***arcus parieto-occipitalis.*** It is separated from the superior occipital gyrus by the ***transverse occipital sulcus.***
   d. ***Calcarine sulcus*** begins near the occipital pole and runs forward to a point below the splenium of corpus callosum, where it is joined at an acute angle by medial part of the parieto-occipital sulcus.

Note: The **arcus parieto-occipitalis** lies in both parietal and occipital lobes.

Sulci and Gyri on Medial Surface (Fig. 11.4)

1. ***Corpus callosum*:** The central part of the medial aspect of the hemisphere is occupied by the ***corpus callosum.*** The corpus callosum is divisible into the *genu* (anterior end), the *body,* and the *splenium* (posterior end). It is made up of nerve fibres connecting the two cerebral hemispheres. Below the corpus callosum, there are the *septum pellucidum,* the *fornix* and the *thalamus.*
2. *Sulci on the medial surface*
   a. ***Cingulate sulcus*** starts in front of the genu of corpus callosum and runs backwards parallel to the upper margin of the corpus callosum.
   b. ***Callosal sulcus*** separates the cingulate gyrus from the corpus callosum.
   c. ***Suprasplenial sulcus*** lies above and behind the splenium.
   d. ***Calcarine sulcus*** begins a little below the splenium and runs towards the occipital pole. It extends for a short distance on the superolateral surface.
   e. ***Parieto-occipital sulcus*** begins at the midpoint of the calcarine sulcus. It runs upward and slightly backward to intersect the superomedial border about 5 cm in front of the occipital pole. It extends slightly on the superolateral surface.
   f. A little below the genu, there are two small anterior and posterior ***paraolfactory sulci.***
3. *Gyri on the medial surface*
   a. ***Cingulate gyrus*** lies between the corpus callosum and the cingulate sulcus. Its posterior part is bounded above by the ***suprasplenial sulcus*** and is divided into anterior and posterior parts.
   b. The U-shaped gyrus around the end of the central sulcus is the ***paracentral lobule.*** It is usually divided into anterior and posterior parts.
   c. The area between the cingulate gyrus and the superomedial border in front of the paracentral lobule is called the ***medial frontal gyrus.***
   d. The quadrangular area between the suprasplenial sulcus and the superomedial border is called the ***precuneus.***
   e. The triangular area between the parieto-occipital sulcus (above) and the calcarine sulcus (below) is called the ***cuneus.***
   f. A narrow strip between the splenium and the stem of the calcarine sulcus is the ***isthmus.***
   g. ***Paraterminal gyrus*** lies just in front of the lamina terminalis.
   h. ***Paraolfactory gyrus*** lies between the anterior and posterior paraolfactory sulci.

Sulci and Gyri on the Orbital Surface (Fig. 11.5)

1. Parallel to the medial orbital border, there is the ***olfactory sulcus;*** between these two, there is the ***gyrus rectus.*** The rest of the orbital surface is subdivided by an H-shaped sulcus into *anterior, posterior, medial and lateral* ***orbital gyri.***
2. The stem of the lateral sulcus lies deep between the temporal pole and orbital surface.

Sulci and Gyri on the Tentorial Surface (Fig.11.5)

This area presents two sulci running anteroposteriorly. The medial one is the ***collateral sulcus,*** and the lateral is the ***occipitotemporal sulcus.*** On the medial side of the temporal pole, there is the ***rhinal sulcus.***

The gyri are as follows:

1. The part medial to the rhinal sulcus is the ***uncus.***
2. The part medial to the collateral sulcus is the ***parahippocampal gyrus.*** Its posterior part is limited medially by the calcarine sulcus. It is joined to the cingulate gyrus through the isthmus.
3. The part lateral to the collateral sulcus is divided into ***medial and lateral occipitotemporal gyri*** by the ***occipitotemporal sulcus.***
4. ***Lingual gyrus*** lies between parahippocampal gyrus and occipital pole.

Types of the Cerebral Cortex

Allocortex (archipallium): It is the original olfactory cortex, and is represented by rhinencephalon (piriform area and hippocampal formation). Structurally, it is simple and is made up of only three layers.

Paleocortex or paleopallium: It is intermediate in development. It includes cingulate gyrus.

Isocortex (neopallium): It is the lately acquired cortex, containing various centres other than those for smell. Structurally, it is thick and six layered. It is subdivided into the following:

a. Granular cortex (koniocortex or dust cortex). It is basically a sensory cortex.
b. Agranular cortex. This is the motor cortex.

FUNCTIONAL OR CORTICAL AREAS OF CEREBRAL CORTEX

Functionally, the cortex is divided into number of areas by many neurobiologists. **Brodmann's areas** are taken normally according to whom there are 200 areas.

Types of Cortical Areas

There are three basic functional divisions of cerebral cortex (Table 11.2):

1. ***Motor areas:*** They control motor activity and give rise to corticospinal and corticonuclear fibres.
2. ***Sensory areas:*** In these areas receive afferent sensory fibres from thalamus and subthalamic nuclei.
3. ***Association areas:*** They are responsible for modification of motor activities, interpretation of sensory inputs, intellect, emotions and so on.

Note: The motor and sensory functions also overlap in the same region of cortex. If the motor function is predominant, it is known as motor-sensory (Ms) and where sensory function is predominant, it is called sensorimotor (Sm).

Motor Areas (Figs 11.6 to 11.8)

Primary Motor Area (Area 4)

It is located in the precentral gyrus, including the anterior wall of central sulcus, and in the anterior part of paracentral lobule on the medial surface of cerebral hemispheres. This corresponds to area 4 of Brodmann.

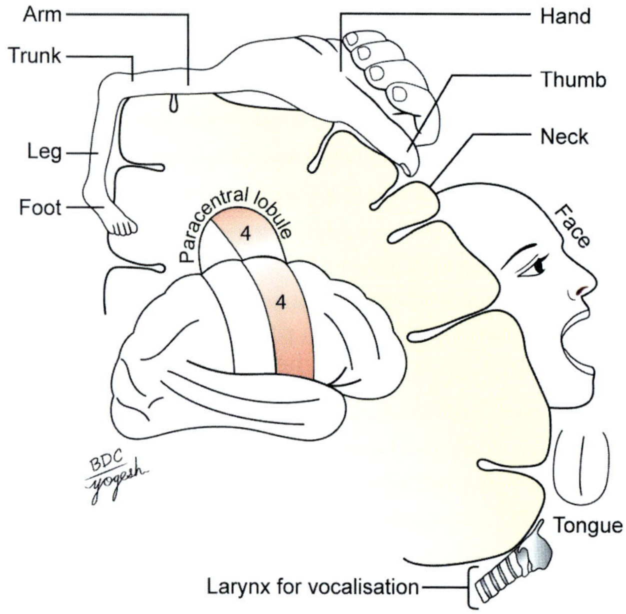

Fig. 11.6: Motor homunculus on the precentral gyrus

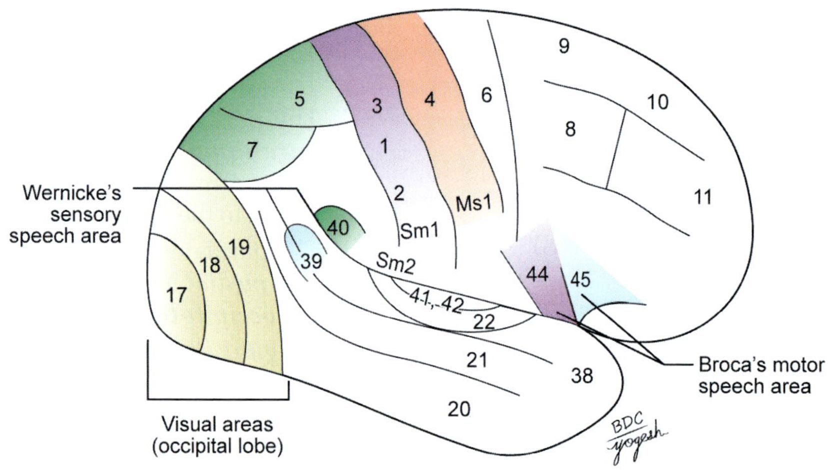

Fig. 11.7: Functional areas of the superolateral surface of cerebral hemisphere

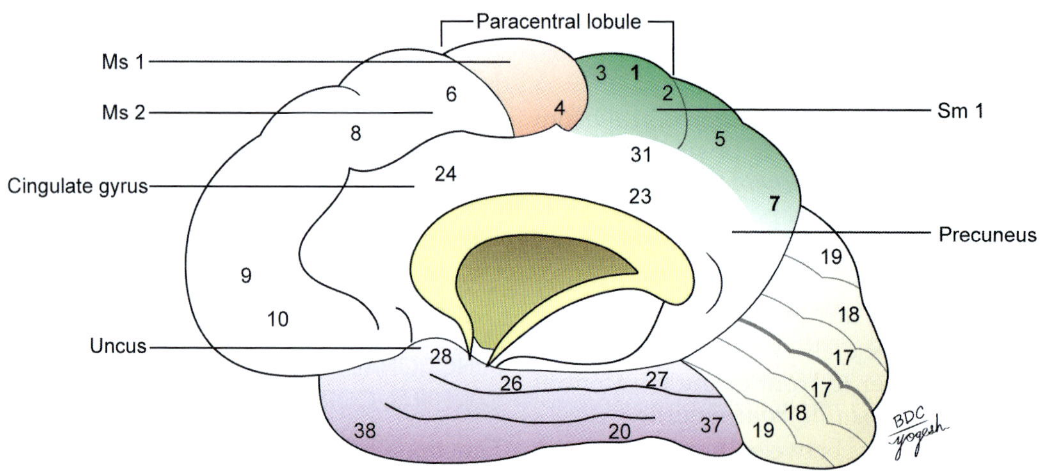

Fig. 11.8: Functional areas of the medial surface of cerebral hemisphere

TABLE 11.2: Functional areas of the cerebral cortex

Lobe	*Area*	*Area no.*	*Location*	*Function*	*Effect of lesion*
Frontal	Motor	4	Precentral gyrus and paracentral lobule	Controls voluntary activities of the opposite half of body Body represented upside down except face	Contralateral paralysis and Jacksonian fits
	Premotor	6	Posterior parts of superior, middle and inferior frontal gyri	Controls extrapyramidal system	Often mixed with pyramidal effect
	Frontal eye field	6, 8	Posterior part of middle frontal gyrus	Controls horizontal conjugate movements of the eyes	Horizontal conjugate movements are lost
	Motor speech (Broca's area)	44, 45	Pars triangularis and pars opercularis	Controls the spoken speech	Aphasia (motor)
	Prefrontal	9, 10, 11, 12	The remaining large, anterior part of frontal lobe	Controls emotions, concentration, attention initiative and judgement	Loss of orientation
Parietal	Sensory (somesthetic)	3, 1, 2	Postcentral gyrus and paracentral lobule	Perception of exteroceptive (touch, lobule pain and temperature) and proprioceptive impulses Body represented upside down except face	Loss of appreciation of the impulses received
	Sensory association	5, 7	Between sensory and visual areas	Stereognosis and sensory speech	Astereognosis and sensory aphasia
		39, 40	Inferior part of parietal lobule as angular gyrus and supramarginal gyrus	Sensory speech area Language comprehension Emotional responses	Sensory aphasia
Occipital	Visuosensory area or striate	17	In and around the postcalcarine sulcus	Reception and perception of the isolated visual impressions of colour, size, form, motion, illumination and transparency Macular area has largest representation	Homonymous hemianopia with macular sparing
	Visuopsychic area, parastriate and peristriate	18, 19	Surround the striate area	Correlation of visual impulses with past memory and recognition of objects seen, and also the depth	Visual agnosia
Temporal	Auditosensory	41, 42	Heschl's gyrus (situated within the lateral sulcus, on the superior surface of the temporal lobe)	Reception and perception of isolated auditory impressions of loudness, quality and pitch	Impaired hearing
	Auditopsychic (Wernicke's area)	22	Superior temporal gyrus of the dominant cerebral hemisphere	Correlation of auditory impressions with past memory and identification (interpretation) of the sounds heard	Auditory agnosia Sensory aphasia

Note: The inferior aspect of the supramarginal gyrus within the inferior parietal lobule of the dominant hemisphere corresponds to Wernicke's area, which extends along the posterior aspect of the superior temporal gyrus. The functionally defined Wernicke's area is not clearly delineated anatomically, but corresponds to Broca's area 22 (*Reference*: Gray's Anatomy, 42nd ed.). Some authors consider areas 39, 40 and 22 together as Wernicke's area.

Function: The primary motor area controls the muscles on the opposite side of body.

The contralateral half of the body is represented as upside down, except the face. The pharyngeal region and tongue are represented in the most ventral and lower part of precentral gyrus, followed by the face, hand, arm, trunk and thigh. The leg, foot and perineum are on the medial surface of hemisphere in the paracentral lobule.

Note: The primary motor area shows the significant ipsilateral control of most of the muscles of the head and axial muscles of the body.

The size of the cortical motor area for a particular part of the body is determined by the functional importance of the part and its need for sensitivity and intricacy of the movements of that region. The area for the face, especially the *larynx and lips*, is, therefore, disproportionately large and a large area is assigned to the hand particularly the thumb and index finger. Movements of joints are represented rather than individual muscles.

Premotor Area *(Area 6)*

This area coincides with the Brodmann's area 6 and is situated anterior to motor area in the superolateral and medial surfaces of the hemisphere (Figs 11.7 and 11.8).

Function: The premotor area contributes to motor function by its direct contribution to the pyramidal and other descending motor pathways and by its influence on the primary motor cortex.

Note: In general, the primary motor area is the cortex in which execution of movements originates and relatively simple movements are maintained. In contrast, the premotor area programmes skilled motor activity and thus directs the primary motor area in its execution.

The premotor and primary motor areas are together referred to as the ***primary somatomotor area*** (Ms1). Both these areas give origin to corticospinal and corticonuclear fibres and receive fibres from cerebellum after relay in ventral intermediate nucleus of thalamus.

Supplementary Motor Area (Ms2)

It is predominantly motor in function. This motor area is in the part of area 6 that lies on the medial surface of the hemisphere anterior to the paracentral lobule. Different parts of body are represented within this area. It differs from the main motor area in that its stimulation produces bilateral movements (Fig. 8.8). Its function is to control complex movements which require sequential organisation.

Motor Speech Area of Broca (Areas 44 and 45)

(French Neurologist, 1824–1840)

The Broca's area occupies the opercular and triangular portions of the inferior frontal gyrus corresponding to the areas 44 and 45 of Brodmann. This is present on the left side in 98% of right-handed persons. In 70% of left-handers, it is again present in the left hemisphere. Only in 30%, it is situated in the right hemisphere.

Frontal Eye Field (Areas 8)

It lies in the middle frontal gyrus just anterior to precentral gyrus. It is the lower part of area 8 of Brodmann on the lateral surface of cerebral hemisphere, extending slightly beyond that area. Electrical stimulation of this area causes deviation of both the eyes to the opposite side. This is called conjugate movements of eyes. Movements of the head and dilatation of pupil may also occur. This area is connected to the cortex of occipital lobe which is concerned with vision.

Prefrontal Cortex (Areas 9, 10, 11, 12)

Prefrontal cortex is a large area lying anterior to the precentral area. It includes the superior, middle, and inferior frontal gyri, medial frontal gyrus, orbital gyri and anterior half of the cingulate gyrus. These include Brodmann's areas 9, 10, 11 and 12. This area is connected to other areas of the cerebral cortex, corpus striatum, thalamus and hypothalamus. It is also connected to cerebellum through the pontine nuclei. It controls emotions concentration, attention, initiative and judgement. It has reciprocal connections with thalamic dorsomedial nucleus, hypothalamus, and limbic system.

CLINICAL NEUROANATOMY

- Destructive lesion of primary motor area 4 results in voluntary paresis of the affected part of body. Spastic voluntary paralysis of the opposite side of body characteristically follows, if the lesion spreads beyond area 4 or that interrupts projection fibres in the medullary centre or internal capsule. Irritative lesion of the motor area leads to focal convulsive movements of the corresponding part of body, referred to as ***Jacksonian epilepsy***.
- Lesion of supplementary motor area 6 leads to apraxia and akinesia. This is the condition that involves difficulty in performing the skilled movements once learnt, in the absence of paralysis, ataxia or sensory loss. When the disability affects writing, it is called *agraphia*.
- *Frontal eye field:* Destruction of this area causes conjugate deviation of the eyes towards the side of lesion. The patient cannot voluntarily move his eyes in the opposite direction, but this movement occurs involuntarily when he observes an object moving across the field of vision.
- *Speech area:* Lesion of Broca's area on the dominant side of hemisphere causes expressive aphasia. It is characterised by hesitant and distorted speech with relatively good comprehension.
- A lesion involving language areas *(Wernicke's area* and *Broca's area)* leads to receptive aphasia. In this condition, auditory and visual comprehension of language that is naming of objects and repetition of a sentence spoken by the examiner are all defective (Fig. 8.8).
- A lesion involving Wernicke's area and superior longitudinal fasciculus or arcuate fasciculus results in *jargon aphasia* in which speech is fluent but unintelligible jargon.
- Voluntary smile in a stroke patient will accentuate the asymmetry. A genuine smile which uses only extrapyramidal pathways, will be symmetrical and there will be no asymmetry for the duration of the smile. One needs to remember that motor cortex is required only for voluntary moment.

Sensory Areas (Figs 11.7 to 11.9)

First Somesthetic Area (Areas 3, 1, and 2)

First somesthetic (general sensory) area is also called *first somatosensory area* (Sm1). It occupies postcentral gyrus on the superolateral surface of the cerebral hemisphere and posterior part of paracentral lobule on the medial surface. It corresponds to areas 3, 1 and 2 of Brodmann.

The representation of the body in this area corresponds to that in the motor area that is contralateral half of body is represented upside down except the face.

The ventral posterior nucleus of thalamus is the main source of afferent fibres for the sensory area. This thalamic nucleus is the site of termination of all the fibres of the medial lemniscus. Most of the fibres of the spinothalamic and trigeminothalamic tracts carrying

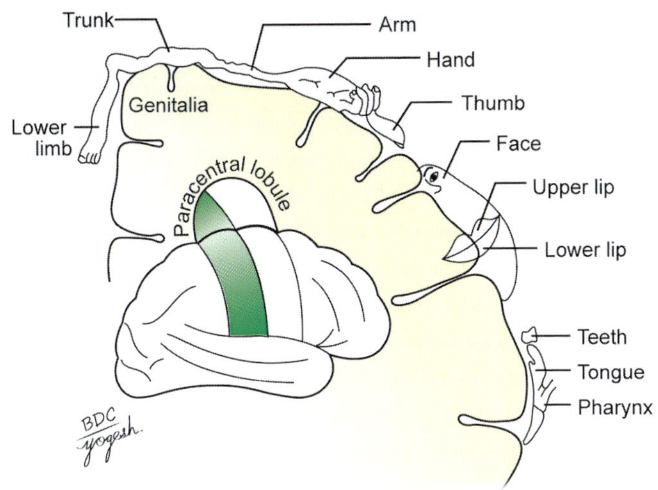

Fig. 11.9: Sensory homunculus of the postcentral gyrus

fibres for cutaneous sensibility end in anterior part of the area and those for deep sensibility end in the posterior part.

Note: The area of the cortex that receives sensations from a particular part of body is not proportional to the size of that part, but rather to the intricacy of sensations received from it. Thus, the thumb, fingers, lips and tongue have a disproportionately large representation. The different sensations, i.e. cutaneous and proprioceptive, are represented in different parts within sensory area.

Second Somesthetic Area

Second somesthetic area, also known as second *somatosensory area* (Sm2). This is situated in the superior lip of the posterior ramus of lateral sulcus with postcentral gyrus. The parts of body are represented bilaterally.

Somesthetic Association Cortex *(Areas 5 and 7)*

Somesthetic association cortex is mainly in the superior parietal lobule on the superolateral surface of the hemisphere and in the precuneus on the medial surface. It coincides with areas 5 and 7 of Brodmann. This receives afferents from first sensory area and has reciprocal connection with dorsal tier of nuclei of lateral mass of thalamus. Data pertaining to the general senses are integrated, permitting a comprehensive assessment of the characteristic of an object held in hand and its identification without visual aid.

Receptive Speech Area of Wernicke

(German Neurologist, 1848–1903)

This is also known as *sensory language area*. It consists of auditory association cortex and of adjacent parts of the inferior parietal lobule.

CLINICAL NEUROANATOMY

- First somesthetic or general sensory area (areas 3, 1 and 2 of Brodmann): When this part of cortex is the site of destructive lesion, a crude form of awareness persists for the sensation of pain, heat and cold on the opposite side of lesion. There is poor localisation of stimulus. There is loss of discriminative sensations of fine touch, movements and position of part of the body.
- Somesthetic association cortex (superior parietal lobule) areas 5 and 7 of Brodmann: A lesion in this area leads to defect in understanding the significance of sensory information, which is called ***agnosia***. A lesion that destroys a large portion of this association cortex causes tactile agnosia and ***astereognosis*** which are closely related. This is the condition when a person is unable to recognize the objects held in the hand, while the eyes are closed. He is unable to correlate the surface, texture, shape, size and weight of the object or to compare the sensations with previous experience.

Areas of Special Sensations

Vision *(Areas 17, 18 , and 19)*

The ***visual area*** is located above and below the calcarine sulcus on the medial surface of occipital lobe. It corresponds to **area 17** of Brodmann. The visual area is also called the striate area because the cortex here contains the *line of Gennari*, which is just visible to the unaided eye.

The chief source of afferent fibres to area 17 is the *lateral geniculate nucleus* of thalamus by way of geniculocalcarine tract.

Area 17 constitutes the first visual area. It is continuous both above and below with **area 18** and beyond this with **area 19** of Brodmann which are also known as ***visual association or psychovisual areas***. Since fibres of geniculocalcarine tract (optic radiation) terminate in these regions also, therefore, these areas are regarded as second and the third visual areas, respectively.

The role of the second and third visual areas includes among other complex aspects of vision, the relating of present to past visual experience, with recognition of what is seen and appreciation of its significance. The three areas are linked together by association fibres. The visual areas give efferent fibres which reach frontal eye field.

Hearing *(Areas 41, and 42)*

The ***auditory* (acoustic) *area*** lies in the temporal lobe. Most of it is concealed as it lies in that part of superior temporal gyrus which forms inferior wall of the posterior ramus of lateral sulcus. It corresponds with areas ***41 and 42 of Brodmann***.

The *medial geniculate* body of the thalamus is the principal source of fibres ending in the auditory cortex with these fibres constituting the auditory radiation. There is spatial representation in the auditory area with respect to pitch of sounds. Impulses of low frequencies impinge on anterolateral part of area and impulses of high frequencies get heard on the posteromedial part.

Cortex gets afferents from both ears. Body receives information that originates mainly in the organ of Corti of opposite side, the incomplete decussation of ascending pathways ensures a substantial input from the ear of same side as well.

The auditory radiation does not only end in first auditory area but extends to neighbouring area as well, that is known as ***auditory association area*** or second auditory area. This area lies behind the first auditory area in superior temporal gyrus. It corresponds to ***area 22*** of Brodmann on the lateral surface of superior temporal gyrus. This region of the cortex is also known as ***Wernicke's area*** and is of major importance in language functions.

Taste (Area 43)

The ***taste area*** (gustatory area) is located in dorsal wall of posterior ramus of lateral sulcus, with extension into insula and corresponds to ***area 43*** of Brodmann. It places the taste area adjacent to first sensory area of cortex for tongue and pharynx. Its location is similar to second somesthetic area.

Smell

Ends in ***pyriform lobe***.

Vestibular Area

Vestibular area is situated close to the part of postcentral gyrus concerned with sensations of face.

CLINICAL NEUROANATOMY

Special sensory areas

a. Primary visual area 17: Lesion of this area, leads to loss of vision in the visual field of the opposite side – homonymous hemianopia.
b. Auditory area:
   - Primary auditory areas 41 and 42: A unilateral lesion involving the auditory area causes diminution in the acuity of hearing in both ears and the loss is greater in the opposite ear. However, the impairment is slight because of the bilateral projection to the cortex and the deficit is difficult to detect by clinical tests.
   - Auditory association cortex or secondary area 22. In lesions of this area, interpretation of the sounds is lost.

Aphasia is a disorder of language (speech) that results from damage to that portion of the brain which are responsible for language (Wernicke's area and Broca's area). It usually occurs suddenly often as the result of a stroke or head injury. But it may develop slowly as in the case of a brain tumour.

Table 11.3 depicts summary of functions and effects of damage of lobes of brain.

Cerebral Dominance

One cerebral hemisphere dominates the other one in relation to handedness, speech, perception of language and spatial judgement. In 80–95% subjects, the left hemisphere dominates the right one. The dominant lobe contains the Broca's motor speech area. Since left hemisphere controls the right half of the body, all these subjects are right-handed. The left hemisphere is verbal speech, writing, mathematical, analytical, scientific, calculative and has direct link to consciousness (Flowchart 11.3).

Flowchart 11.3: Lateralisation of functions in the dominant and nondominant hemispheres

Cerebral dominance

Dominant left hemisphere	Nondominant right hemisphere
Verbal	Almost nonverbal
Speech	Imagination
Writing	Musical
Language	Geometrical
Mathematical	Recognition of faeces
Analytical	Creative acts of arts
Scientific	Spatial comprehension
Calculative	Religious

The right hemisphere is almost non-verbal, active in understanding geometrical figures imaginative, artistic, religious, and important for temporal synthesis and spatial comprehension. It helps in recognition of faeces, figures and appreciating music.

Localisation of speech on left side in 70% of left handed and 98% of right-handed is well known. Association of negative emotions with right prefrontal activity and of positive emotions with left prefrontal activity is also known.

Functional asymmetry in a structurally symmetrical structure is a great and ingenious way of economising on neural tissue. It practically doubles the capabilities of the brain.

Note: Mahatma Gandhi (father of the nation), Bill Clinton, Bill Gates, Amitabh Bachchan and Abhishek Bachchan, are all left-handed.

Competency:

AN64.1 Describe and identify the microanatomical features of spinal cord, cerebellum and cerebrum.

Microanatomy/histology of cerebrum is described here. For others see the appropriate chapters.

HISTOLOGY OF CEREBRUM

It is characterised by *heterotypical cortex*, i.e. histological structure differs in various regions of cerebral cortex. The outermost covering of the cerebral cortex is the pia mater which is the innermost meningeal layer. It carries capillaries to the grey matter. The cerebral cortex contains variety of cells. These are arranged in layers with one or more cell types predominant in each layer. The horizontal fibres are associated with each layer and give it a laminated appearance. From superficial to deep, the following six layers are seen (Plate 11.2):

1. *Molecular layer* consists of a few fibres and some spindle-shaped or stellate cells.
2. *Outer granular layer* contains small cells, triangular in shape, with an apex directed peripherally and the base

Plate 11.2: Histology of cerebrum

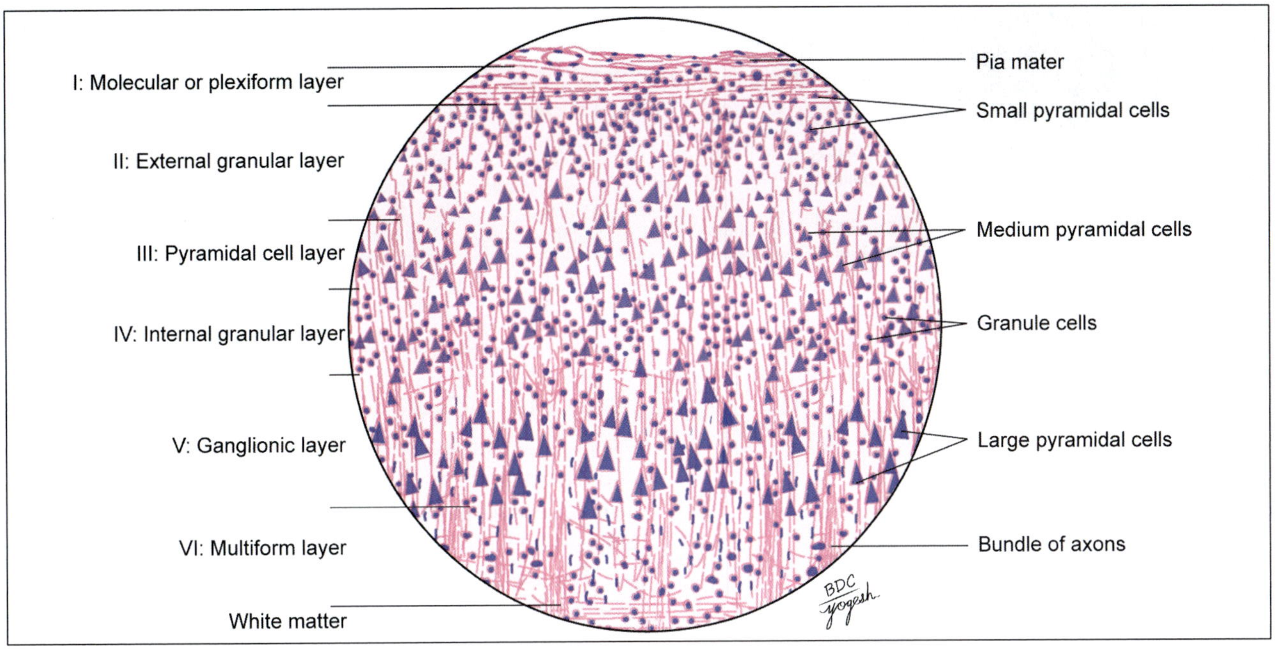

TABLE 11.3: Summary of functions and effects of damage of lobes of brain

Lobes of brain	*Functions*	*Effects of damage*
Frontal	Personality, emotional control, social behaviour, contralateral motor control, micturition, judgement thinking, planning behaviour, executive function, language production (Broca's area)	Lack of initiation, antisocial behaviour, impaired memory and incontinence
Parietal (non-dominant)	Spatial orientation, recognition of faces, appreciation of music and figures	Spatial disorientation, non-recognition of faces
Parietal (dominant)	Language, calculation, analytical, logical, and geometrical	Dyscalculia, dyslexia, apraxia (inability to do complex movements) and agnosia (inability to recognize)
Temporal (non-dominant)	Auditory perception, pitch perception, non-verbal memory, smell and balance	Reception aphasia and impaired musical skills
Temporal (dominant)	Language, verbal memory and auditory perception (Wernicke's area)	Dyslexia, verbal memory impaired and receptive aphasia
Occipital	Visual reception and interpretation	Visual loss and visual agnosia

directed inwards. The axons leave from the basal part of the cell. A few stellate cells are also seen.

3. *Outer pyramidal layer* has similar cells as outer granular layer, but the cells are distinctly larger than those of the outer granular layer.
4. *Inner granular layer* contains cells which are larger than outer pyramidal cells, but have large number of stellate cells between them.
5. *Inner pyramidal layer* contains cells which are triangular in shape and are the largest cells of the cerebral cortex, especially in the motor cortex where these are termed as the Betz cells.
6. *Fusiform layer* or *polymorphous layer* contains mainly fusiform cells with a few stellate cells. No pyramidal cells are seen in this layer.

The granular cell layers are *afferent* in connection and the pyramidal cell layers are *efferent* in nature. The pyramidal cells are more pronounced in the motor areas, whereas the granular cells are more conspicuous in the sensory areas of the brain. In between the nerve cells are the nerve fibres of these cells and capillaries. The neuroglial elements are protoplasmic astrocytes, oligodendroglia and microglia.

Competency:

AN62.4 Enumerate parts and major connections of basal ganglia/nuclei and limbic lobe. Also explain the anatomical basis of Parkinson's disease, chorea, athetosis and ballismus.

Limbic lobe/system is described in Chapter 12.

BASAL NUCLEI

The basal nuclei are subcortical and, intracerebral masses of grey matter forming important parts of the extrapyramidal system (Fig. 11.10, Flowchart 11.4).

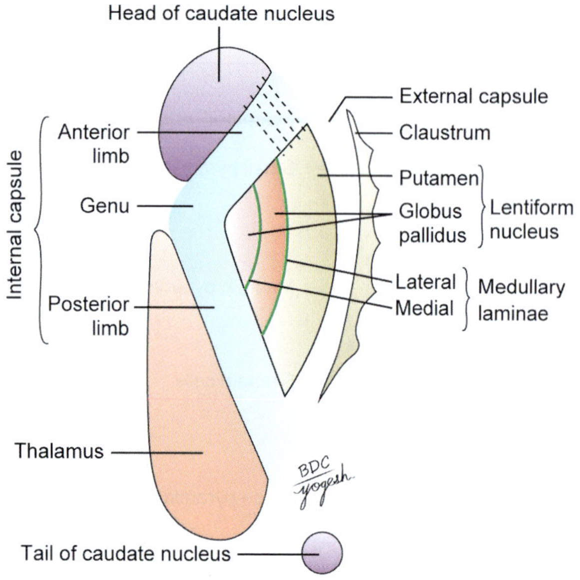

Fig. 11.10: Horizontal section through corpus striatum, thalamus and internal capsule

Flowchart 11.4: Basal ganglia

Basal ganglia

Grey matter in the basal part of cerebrum

Components
- Corpus striatum
  - – Caudate nucleus
  - – Lentiform nucleus: Globus pallidus, Putamen
- Claustrum
- Amygdaloid body

Functions
- Corpus striatum
  - Controls extrapyramidal system
- Amygdaloid body
  - Part of limbic system
- Claustrum
  - Function – not known

Components

The basal nuclei include the following (Fig. 11.10):

1. *Corpus striatum,* which is partially divided by the internal capsule into two nuclei:
   a. *Caudate nucleus.*
   b. *Lentiform nucleus.*
2. *Amygdaloid body* forms a part of the limbic system.
3. *Claustrum.*

The four nuclei (caudate, lentiform, amygdaloid and claustrum) are joined to the cortex at the anterior perforated substance.

CORPUS STRIATUM

Corpus striatum (Latin *striped body*) comprises the caudate nucleus and lentiform nucleus.

Corpus striatum is subdivided by the fibres of internal capsule into (Flowchart 11.5):

1. Caudate nucleus
2. Lentiform nucleus: It is divided into a lateral part, the *putamen,* and a medial part, the *globus pallidus.*

Note: The caudate and lentiform nuclei are interconnected by a few bands of grey matter below the anterior limb of the internal capsule. The bands give it a striped appearance, hence the name.

Flowchart 11.5: Corpus striatum

Corpus striatum

Caudate nucleus
- C-shaped mass of grey matter
- Parts: Head, body, and tail

Lentiform nucleus
- Biconvex, lens-shaped mass of grey matter
- Parts:
  - Putamen: Large, lateral
  - Globus pallidus: Small, medial
  - External medullary lamina

Functions
- Refinement of reflex and voluntary, skilled and manipulative movements
- Controls automatic associated movements
- Prevents unwanted movements
- Maintains muscle tone
- Controls emotional expression of movements

Caudate Nucleus

It is a C-shaped or comma-shaped nucleus which is surrounded by the lateral ventricle. The concavity of 'C' encloses the thalamus and the internal capsule (Fig. 11.11).

The nucleus has a head, a body, and a tail.

1. ***Head:*** The head forms the floor of the anterior horn of the lateral ventricle, and the medial wall of the anterior limb of the internal capsule. Bands of grey matter connect it to the putamen across the anterior limb of the internal capsule near the anterior perforated substance.
2. ***Body:*** The body forms the floor of the central part of the lateral ventricle, and lies medial to the posterior limb of the internal capsule. It is separated from the thalamus by the stria terminalis and the thalamostriate vein. Superiorly, it is related to the fronto-occipital bundle and the corpus callosum.
3. ***Tail:*** The tail forms the roof of the inferior horn of the lateral ventricle, and ends by joining the amygdaloid body at the temporal pole. It is related medially to the stria terminalis, laterally to the tapetum, and superiorly to the sublentiform part of the internal capsule and to the globus pallidus.

Lentiform Nucleus

This is a large, lens-shaped (biconvex) nucleus, forming the lateral boundary of the internal capsule. It lies beneath the insula and the claustrum.

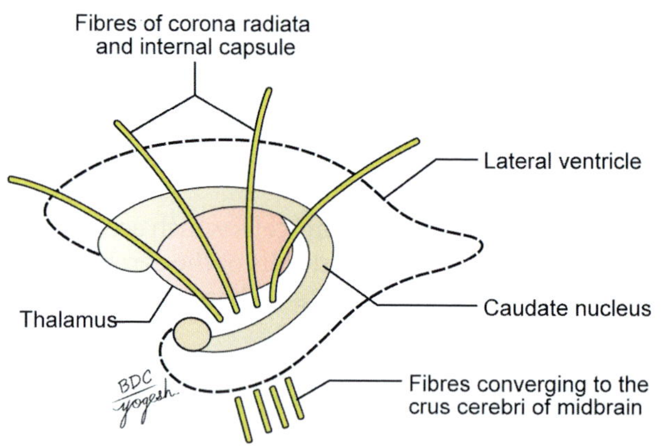

Fig. 11.11: Relations of caudate nucleus to lateral ventricle, thalamus and internal capsule seen in lateral view

The lentiform nucleus has three surfaces:

1. The *lateral surface* is convex. It is related to the external capsule – the claustrum, the extreme capsule, insula, and is grooved by the *lateral striate arteries*.
2. The *medial surface* is more convex. It is related to the internal capsule – the caudate nucleus and the thalamus.
3. The *inferior surface* is related to the sublentiform part of the internal capsule which separates it from the optic tract, the tail of the caudate nucleus, and the inferior horn of the lateral ventricle. The surface is grooved by the anterior commissure just behind the anterior perforated substance.

The lentiform nucleus is divided into two parts by a thin lamina of white matter.

The larger lateral part is called the *putamen (*Latin *to cut)*. Structurally, it is similar to the caudate nucleus and contains small cells.

The smaller medial part is called the *globus pallidus*. It is made up of large (motor) cells.

Morphological Divisions of Corpus Striatum

1. The *paleostriatum* is the older and primitive part. It is represented by the globus pallidus (pallidum).
2. The *neostriatum* is more recent in development. It is represented by the caudate nucleus and the putamen of the lentiform nucleus. The neostriatum is often called the striatum.

Connections of Corpus Striatum

The caudate nucleus and putamen are afferent nuclei, while the globus pallidus is the efferent nucleus, of the corpus striatum (Fig. 11.12). The connections are shown in Table 11.4.

Functions of Corpus Striatum

The corpus striatum performs important role in the extrapyramidal system. It performs the following functions:

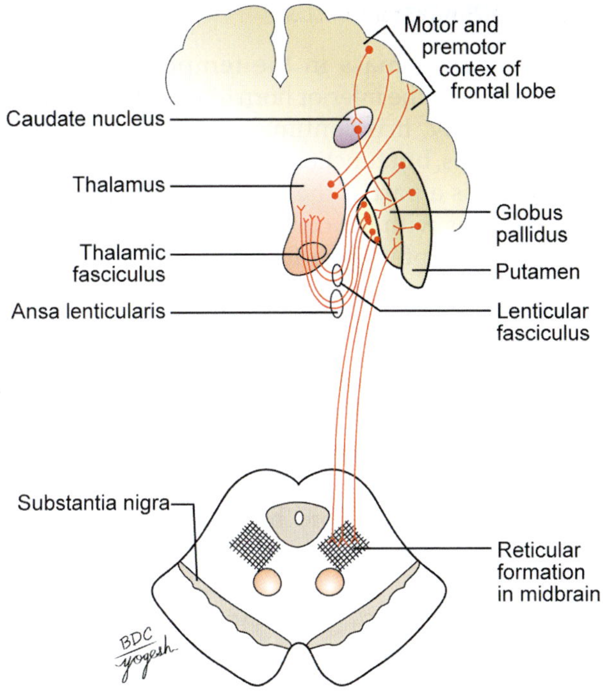

Fig. 11.12: Connections of corpus striatum

1. Refinement of reflex and voluntary movements.
2. Refinement of skilled and manipulative movements of the body. For example, threading a needle.
3. Controls automatic associated movements such as swinging of arms during walking.
4. Prevents unwanted movements.
5. Maintains muscle tone.
6. Controls emotional expression of movements.

CLAUSTRUM

It is saucer-shaped nucleus situated between the putamen and the insula, with which it is coextensive. Inferiorly, it is thickest and continuous with the anterior perforated substance. Its connections and functions are not known.

TABLE 11.4: Connections of the corpus striatum

Nucleus	*Afferents*	*Efferents*
A. Caudate nucleus and putamen	• Corticostriate fibres from cerebral cortex • Thalamostriate fibres • Nigrostriate fibres from substantia nigra	• Striatopallidal fibres to globus pallidus • Few fibres to thalamus and substantia nigra
B. Globus pallidus	• Most of the fibres from neostriatum (caudate nucleus + putamen) • Few fibres from – Substantia nigra – Thalamus and subthalamus	Efferent fibres to thalamus, hypothalamus, subthalamus, red nucleus, olivary nucleus, substantia nigra, and reticular nuclei through 1. Ansa lenticularis 2. Fasciculus lenticularis 3. Subthalamic fasciculus

Note:

1. ***Lenticular fasciculus*** *(fasciculus lenticularis)*: It carries efferent fibre from the globus pallidus. It passes through the posterior limb of internal capsule. They pass superior to the subthalamic nucleus as lentiform fasciculus and terminates in the thalamus.
2. ***Ansa lenticularis:*** Some efferent fibres from globus pallidus curve around the inferior aspects of posterior limb of internal capsule and form a loop called ansa lenticularis. Its fibres terminate in thalamus, substantia nigra, red nucleus, reticular nuclei, and inferior olivary nucleus.
3. ***Thalamic fasciculus:*** Lenticular fasciculus + Thalamic fibres of ansa lenticularis.
4. ***Subthalamic fasciculus:*** These are fibres connecting globus pallidus and subthalamic nuclei (medial and lateral geniculate bodies).

AMYGDALOID BODY

This is a nuclear mass in the temporal lobe, lying anterosuperior to the inferior horn of the lateral ventricle. Topographically, it is continuous with the tail of the caudate nucleus, but functionally, it is related to the stria terminalis. It is a part of the limbic system (Fig. 11.13). It is continuous with the cortex of the uncus, the limen insulae and the anterior perforated substance.

Afferents: From the olfactory tract.

Efferents: It gives rise to the stria terminalis which ends in the anterior commissure, the anterior perforated substance and in hypothalamic nuclei.

Functions: Emotional control. Controls smell related sexual behavior.

Damage to amygdaloid body if bilateral causes increase in sexual activity and reduced fear.

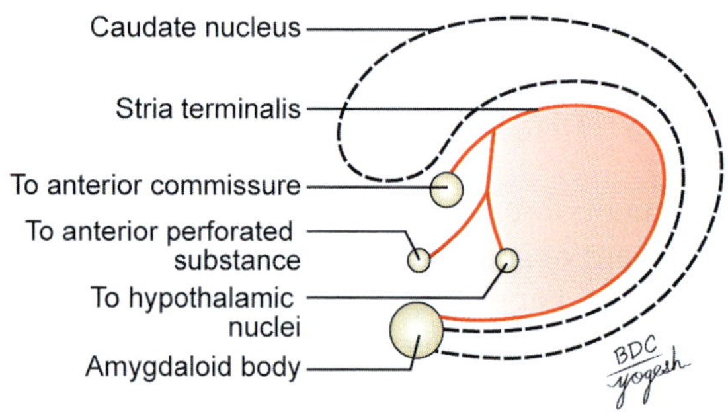

Fig. 11.13: Connections of amygdaloid body

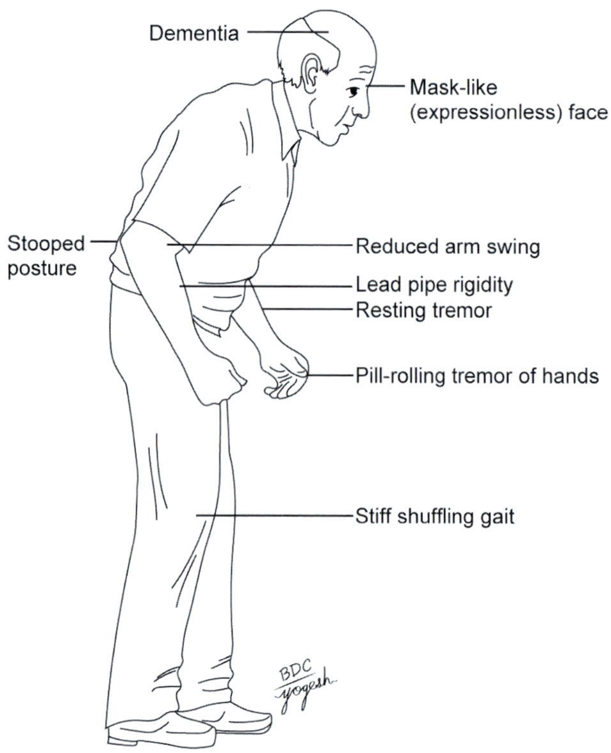

Fig. 11.14: Posture in parkinsonism

CLINICAL NEUROANATOMY

Parkinsonism: Lesions of corpus striatum lead to parkinsonism (Fig. 11.14). Its features are:

a. Hypertonicity or lead pipe rigidity.
b. Loss of automatic associated movements and also of facial expression.
c. Involuntary movements like tremors, choreiform movements, athetoid movements.
d. Continuous writhing movements of trunk and limbs may continue even in sleep. Voluntary movements may be impossible.

L-dopa (a precursor of dopamine) is used as a replacement therapy in parkinsonism because dopamine, the normal neurotransmitter in the striatum, is reduced in these cases. The Nigrostriate fibres are considered important in the genesis of parkinsonism tremor, since its neurons utilize dopamine in the neurotransmission.

Chorea: Chorea means dancing. Chorea is form of involuntary movement characterised by fine random movements of hands and feet. These movements are rather disorganised. This occurs due to disease of caudate nucleus.

Athetosis: It is a form of movement which is slow repetitive and writhing in nature. It is due to lesion of putamen.

Ballismus: This is characterised by irregular movements of trunk, girdles and both the limbs. It is due to disease of subthalamic nucleus.

Neurosurgically, pallidectomy and thalamodectomy have been used with success to control the contralateral tremors in different types of disease of corpus striatum.

Competency:

AN62.3 Describe the white matter of cerebrum. Also describe the effects of damage to corpus callosum and different parts of internal capsule.

DISSECTION

Raise the lower border of the insula, stripping a thin layer of grey matter situated deep to the white matter of insula. This grey matter is known as the claustrum. As the insula is gradually raised, the external capsule and on a deeper plane, a fan-shaped layer of white matter, the corona radiata, are identifiable. Fibres or corona radiata pass on a deeper plane than that of superior longitudinal fasciculus.

To explore the lentiform nucleus, strip the external capsule and identify rounded lentiform nucleus. Dissect the striate branches of the middle cerebral artery on the lateral surface of the lentiform nucleus.

Remove the genu and rostrum of corpus callosum from the cerebral hemisphere, identify the head of the caudate nucleus and the anterior part of the corona radiata emerging from between the caudate and the lentiform nuclei. Identify the anterior commissure and trace its fibres reaching till the temporal lobe.

Internal Capsule

To expose the internal capsule, remove the lentiform nucleus as it forms the lateral boundary of the internal capsule. It is difficult to separate as many fibres of internal capsule enter the lentiform nucleus. Some fibres form two medullary laminae and divide the lentiform nucleus into outer dark part – the putamen and two paler inner parts – the globus pallidus. Putamen is continuous with the caudate nucleus. Trace the continuity of the corona radiata with the internal capsule and of the internal capsule with the crus cerebri. The latter part is visible after stripping the optic tract from the lateral side of the internal capsule.

WHITE MATTER OF CEREBRUM

The white matter of the cerebrum consists chiefly of myelinated fibres which connect various parts of the cortex to one another and also to the other parts of the CNS.

TYPES OF FIBRES

The cerebrum contains three types of white fibres (Fig. 11.15):

1. ***Association fibres*** – connect one area with another area of same cerebral hemisphere.
2. ***Commissural fibres*** – connect the corresponding areas of two cerebral hemispheres.
3. ***Projection fibres*** – connect the cerebral cortex with subcortical part of nervous system.

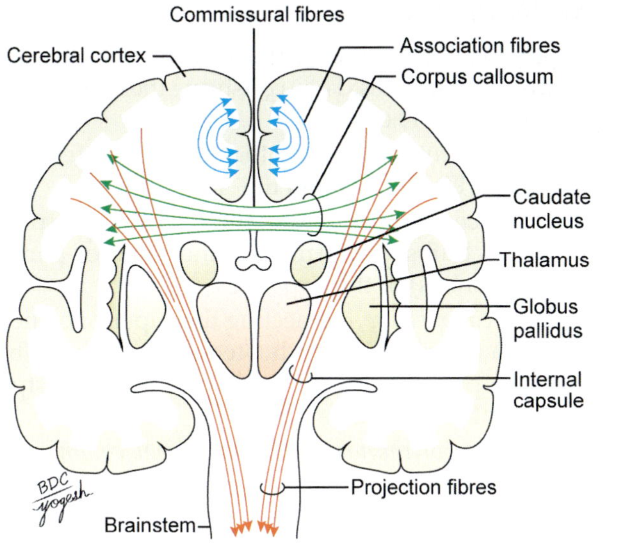

Fig. 11.15: White fibres of cerebrum (coronal section of the brain)

Flowchart 11.6: White fibres of cerebrum

White fibres of cerebrum

Association fibres	***Commissural fibres***	***Projection fibres***
Connect areas of same cerebral hemispheres Types A. Short/ arcuate: B. Long - Uncinate fasciculus - Superior longitudinal fasciculus - Inferior longitudinal fasciculus - Cingulum - Fronto-occipital fasciculus	Connect corresponding areas of right and left cerebral hemispheres For example: Corpus callosum Anterior commissure Hippocampal commissure Posterior commissure Habenular commissure	Connect cerebral cortex with subcortical centres For example: Corona radiata Internal capsule Fimbria Fornix

Association (Arcuate) Fibres

These are the fibres that connect different cortical areas of the same hemisphere. These are subdivided into the following two types (Fig. 11.16 and Flowchart 11.6).

Short Association Fibres

These fibres connect adjacent gyri.

Long Association Fibres

These fibres connect more widely separated gyri. Some examples are:

1. *Uncinate fasciculus,* connecting the temporal pole to the motor speech area and the orbital cortex.
2. *Cingulum,* connecting the cingulate gyrus to the parahippocampal gyrus seen on the medial surface.
3. *Superior longitudinal fasciculus,* connecting the frontal lobe to occipital and temporal lobes.
4. *Inferior longitudinal fasciculus,* connecting the occipital and temporal lobes.
5. *Fronto-occipital fasciculi* seen on the medial surface.

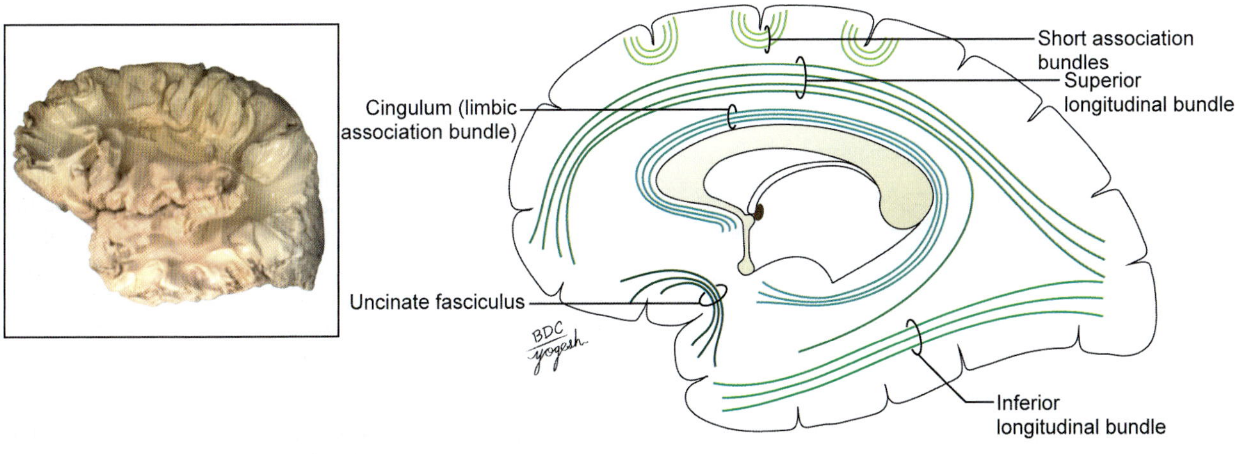

Fig. 11.16: Association fibres of cerebrum

Commissural Fibres

These are the fibres which connect corresponding parts of the two hemispheres. They constitute the commissures of the cerebrum. They are:

1. *Corpus callosum* connecting the cerebral cortex of the two sides (Figs 11.17a and b).
2. *Anterior commissure,* connecting the archipallia (olfactory bulbs, piriform area and anterior parts of temporal lobes) of the two sides.
3. *Posterior commissure,* connecting the superior colliculi, and also transmitting corticotectal fibres and fibres from the pretectal nucleus to the Edinger-Westphal nucleus of the opposite side.
4. *Commissure of the fornix (hippocampal commissure),* connecting the crura of the fornix and thus the hippocampal formations of the two sides.
5. *Habenular commissure,* connecting the habenular nuclei.
6. *Hypothalamic commissures,* including the anterior hypothalamic commissure of Ganser, the ventral supraoptic commissure of Gudden and the dorsal supraoptic commissure of Meynert.

Projection Fibres

They interconnect cerebral cortex with subcortical centres. They include the *corticofugal fibres* which originate in cerebral cortex and go to subcortical centres and the *corticopetal fibres* which reach the cerebral cortex from subcortical centres.

Examples:

1. Corona radiata
2. Internal capsule
3. Fimbria
4. Fornix.

Note: The descending fibres of the lobes of cerebrum converge to form the 'corona radiata' and continue as internal capsule.

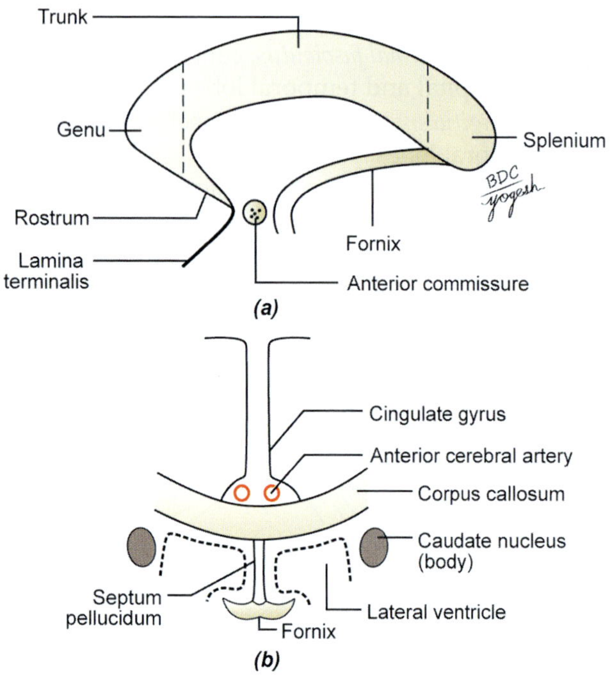

Figs 11.17a and b: (a) Parts of corpus callosum and (b) coronal section of the trunk of corpus callosum showing its relations

DISSECTION

Scrape the grey matter between adjacent gyri till the white matter connecting the adjacent gyri is visible. This will expose the short association fibres. Identify the cingulate gyrus on the medial surface of the left hemisphere. Scrape the grey matter of this gyrus till a band of white matter – the cingulum is exposed. Define the extent of cingulum from the anterior end of corpus callosum, around its convex trunk and splenium into the parahippocampal gyrus.

Similarly, scrape the cortex between temporal pole, motor speech area and the orbital cortex to expose uncinate fasciculus. Also expose superior longitudinal fasciculus joining the frontal lobe to the occipital and temporal lobes. Lastly, scrape the grey matter between occipital and temporal lobes to expose the inferior longitudinal fasciculus.

Identify the various parts of the corpus callosum. Remove the fibres of the cingulum and identify the superficial fibres of the genu of corpus callosum passing into the medial aspect of hemisphere. Such fibres of the two sides form the forceps minor.

Expose the band of fibres passing from splenium of corpus callosum towards the superior part of occipital lobe. Trace the fibres of tapetum arising from the trunk and splenium of corpus callosum curving to reach the inferior parts of the occipital and temporal lobes.

Identify the anterior commissure lying just anterior to column of fornix and the interventricular foramen. Examine the posterior commissure situated dorsal to the upper part of aqueduct and inferior to the root of the pineal body. Look for habenular commissure present at the root of the pineal body. Lastly, identify the commissure of the fornix and the hypothalamic commissures.

Lift up a strip of superficial fibres of the genu of corpus callosum and tear these laterally. Identify the intersectioning fibres of corpus callosum and those of the vertically disposed fibres of the corona radiata.

CORPUS CALLOSUM

The corpus callosum is the largest commissure of the brain. It connects the two cerebral hemispheres. Since it is the neopallial commissure, it attains enormous size in man (10 cm long, 2.5 cm wide). It contains 150–200 million fibres (axons).

The corpus callosum connects all parts of the cerebral cortex of the two sides, except the lower and anterior parts of the temporal lobes which are connected by the anterior commissure (Figs 11.17a and b and Flowchart 11.7).

Parts of Corpus Callosum

1. ***Genu:*** It is the anterior end. It lies 4 cm behind the frontal pole. It is related anteriorly to the anterior cerebral arteries, and posteriorly to the anterior horn of the lateral ventricle.
2. ***Rostrum:*** It is directed downwards and backwards from the genu, and ends by joining the lamina

Flowchart 11.7: Corpus callosum

Corpus callosum

Commisural fibres
Connects right and left
cerebral hemispheres

Size and shape
- L: 10 cm
- Breadth: 2.5 cm
- Connects cerebral hemispheres
- C-shaped
- Concave downward

Parts
- Rostrum
- Genu
- Body (trunk)
- Splenium

Clinical
- Congenital absence of corpus callosum
- ↓
- Split brain syndrome

terminalis, in front of the anterior commissure. It is related superiorly to the anterior horn of the lateral ventricle, and inferiorly to the indusium griseum and the longitudinal striae.

3. ***Trunk or body:*** It is the middle part, between the genu and the splenium.
   a. Its *superior surface* is convex from before backwards and concave from side-to-side. It is related to the anterior cerebral arteries and to the lower border of the falx cerebri. It is overlapped by the cingulate gyrus and is covered by the indusium griseum and the longitudinal striae.
   b. The *inferior surface* is concave from before backwards and convex from side-to-side. It provides attachment to the septum pellucidum and the fornix, and forms the roof of the central part of the lateral ventricle.
4. ***Splenium:*** It is the posterior end forming the thickest part of the corpus callosum. It lies 6 cm in front of the occipital pole. Its *inferior surface* is related to the tela choroidea of the third ventricle – the pulvinar, the pineal body, and the tectum of the midbrain. The *superior surface* is related to the inferior sagittal sinus and the falx cerebri. *Posteriorly*, it is related to the great cerebral vein, the straight sinus and the free margin on the tentorium cerebelli.

Fibres of Corpus Callosum

1. *Rostrum* connects the orbital surfaces of the two frontal lobes.
2. *Forceps minor* is made up of fibres of the genu that connect the two frontal lobes (Fig. 11.18).
3. *Forceps major* is made up of fibres of the splenium connecting the two occipital lobes.
4. *Tapetum* is formed by some fibres from the trunk and splenium of the corpus callosum. The tapetum forms the roof and lateral wall of the posterior horn, and the lateral wall of the inferior horn of the lateral ventricle.

Functional Significance

The corpus callosum helps in coordinating activities of the two hemispheres.

Note: ***Indusium griseum*** is a thin layer of grey matter that covers the superior convex surface of corpus callosum. The pair of ***medial and lateral longitudinal stria*** (white fibres) lie within the indusium griseum.

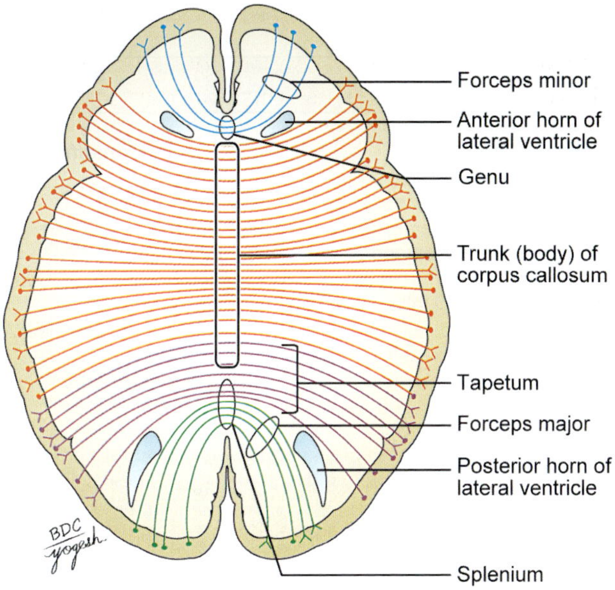

Fig. 11.18: Fibres of corpus callosum

Forceps minor are fork-like commissural fibres of genu of corpus callosum that connect the either side of frontal lobes.

Tapetum: These are the fibres of corpus callosum that form the roof and lateral wall of the posterior horn of lateral ventricle and lateral wall of the inferior horn. These fibres do not intersect the fibres of corona radiata.

Forceps major are fork-like commissural fibres of corpus callosum that connect the occipital lobes.

Bulb of the posterior horn are the fibres of forceps major that bulge in the medial wall of the posterior horn of lateral ventricle.

CLINICAL NEUROANATOMY

Split-brain syndrome: In the congenital absence of corpus callosum, the two cerebral hemispheres work separate and patient behaves as he/she has two separate brains. This condition is called *split-brain syndrome*.

INTERNAL CAPSULE

The internal capsule is a large band of fibres, situated in the inferomedial part of each cerebral hemisphere.

Shape

In horizontal sections of the brain, it appears V-shaped with its concavity directed laterally. The concavity is occupied by the lentiform nucleus (Fig. 11.19 and Flowchart 11.8).

Relations

Medially: Head of caudate nucleus and thalamus.

Laterally: Lentiform nucleus.

Continuation

The internal capsule contains fibres going to and coming from the cerebral cortex. It can be compared to a narrow

Flowchart 11.8: Internal capsule

Internal capsule

Projection fibres

Continuation
- Upward as corona radiata
- Below as crus cerebri

Parts
- V-shaped
- Anterior limb
- Genu
- Posterior limb
- Retrolentiform part
- Sublentiform part

Constituent fibres

Motor
- Corticopontine: Frontopontine, parietopontine, temporopontine, occipitopontine
- Pyramidal: Corticonuclear, corticospinal
- Extrapyramidal fibres

Sensory
- Anterior thalamic radiation
- Superior thalamic radiation
- Inferior thalamic radiation
- Posterior thalamic radiation

Blood supply
- Medial and lateral branches of MCA
- Striate branches of ACA
- Cortical branches of anterior choroidal artery
- Few direct branches from ICA
- Central branches of posterior communicating artery
- Posterolateral central branches of PCA

Clinical integration:

Lesion of artery of cerebral haemorrhage (Charcot's artery) → damage to posterior limb → paralysis of opposite half of body and face

Lesion of recurrent artery of Huebner → damage to genu and anterior limb of internal capsule → paralysis of face and upper limb on opposite side

Thrombosis of anterior choroidal artery → damage to posterior limb, sublentiform and retrolentiform parts → visual (hemiplegia) and auditory defects

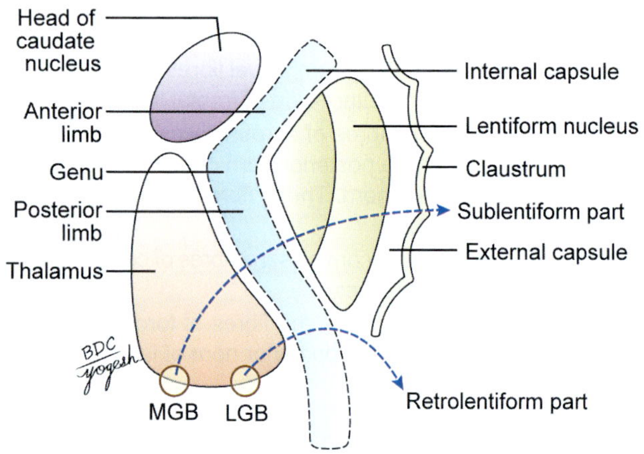

Fig. 11.19: Parts of internal capsule as seen in horizontal section

gate where the fibres are densely crowded. Small lesions of the capsule can give rise to widespread derangements of the body.

Corona radiata: The fibres of internal capsule fan out cranially and form corona radiata (radiating fibres like sunrays).

Crus cerebri: The fibre of internal capsule approximates inferiorly to form crus cerebri of midbrain.

Parts

The internal capsule is divided into the following parts:

a. *Anterior limb* lies between the head of the caudate nucleus and the lentiform nucleus.
b. *Genu* is the bend between the anterior and posterior limbs.
c. *Posterior limb* lies between the thalamus and the lentiform nucleus.
d. *Sublentiform part* lies below the lentiform nucleus. It can be seen in a coronal section, whereas the rest of the parts are seen in a horizontal section.
e. *Retrolentiform part* lies behind the lentiform nucleus.

Fibres of Internal Capsule (Table 11.5)

Motor Fibres

1. *Corticopontine fibres*
   - Frontopontine fibres from frontal lobe to pontine nuclei.
   - Parietopontine fibres from parietal lobe pontine nuclei.
   - Occipitopontine fibres from occipital lobe to pontine nuclei.
   - Temporopontine fibres from temporal lobe to pontine nuclei.
2. *Pyramidal fibres*
   - Corticonuclear fibres from cerebral cortex to contralateral motor nuclei of IIIrd, IVth, Vth to XIIth cranial nerves.
   - Corticospinal fibres from cerebral cortex to contralateral anterior horn cells of spinal cord.
3. *Extrapyramidal fibres* from cerebral cortex to subcortical nucleus such as red nucleus, substantia nigra, reticular nuclei, olivary nucleus, and so on.

Sensory Fibres (Thalamocortical Fibres)

The most of the sensory fibres received by thalamocortical fibres. They form thalamic radiation as follows:

1. *Anterior thalamic radiation* from anterior and dorsomedial nucleus of thalamus to the frontal lobe.
2. *Superior thalamic radiation* from ventral group of thalamic nuclei to sensory cortex of frontal and parietal lobes.
3. *Inferior thalamic radiation* from medial geniculate body to the primary auditory area of temporal lobe as *auditory radiation*.
4. *Posterior thalamic radiation* from lateral geniculate body to the primary visual area (area 17) as *optic radiation*.

Constituent fibres: The fibres of internal capsule are shown in Figs 11.20 and 11.21.

TABLE 11.5: Fibres in the internal capsule

Part	*Descending tracts*	*Ascending tracts*	*Arterial supply*
Anterior limb (Fig. 8.29)	Frontopontine fibres (a part of the corticopontocerebellar pathway)	Anterior thalamic radiation (fibres from anterior and medial nuclei of thalamus)	1. Recurrent branch of anterior cerebral 2. Direct branches from anterior cerebral
Genu	Corticonuclear fibres (a part of the pyramidal tract going to motor nuclei of cranial nerves and forming their supranuclear pathway)	Anterior part of the superior thalamic radiation (fibres from posterior ventral nucleus of thalamus)	1. Direct branches from internal carotid 2. Posterior communicating
Posterior limb	1. Corticospinal tract (pyramidal tract for the upper limb, trunk and lower limb) 2. Corticopontine fibres 3. Corticorubral fibres	1. Superior thalamic radiation 2. Fibres from globus pallidus to subthalamic nucleus	1. Lateral striate branches of middle cerebral 2. Medial striate branches of middle cerebral 3. Anterior choroidal
Sublentiform part	1. Parietopontine and temporopontine fibres 2. Fibres between temporal lobe and thalamus	1. Auditory radiation 2. Fibres connecting thalamus to temporal lobe	1. Branches of posterior cerebral 2. Anterior choroidal
Retrolentiform part	1. Parietopontine and occipitopontine fibres 2. Fibres from occipital cortex to superior colliculus and pretectal region	Posterior thalamic radiation made up of: 1. Mainly optic radiation 2. Partly fibres connecting thalamus to the parietal and occipital lobes	Branches of posterior cerebral

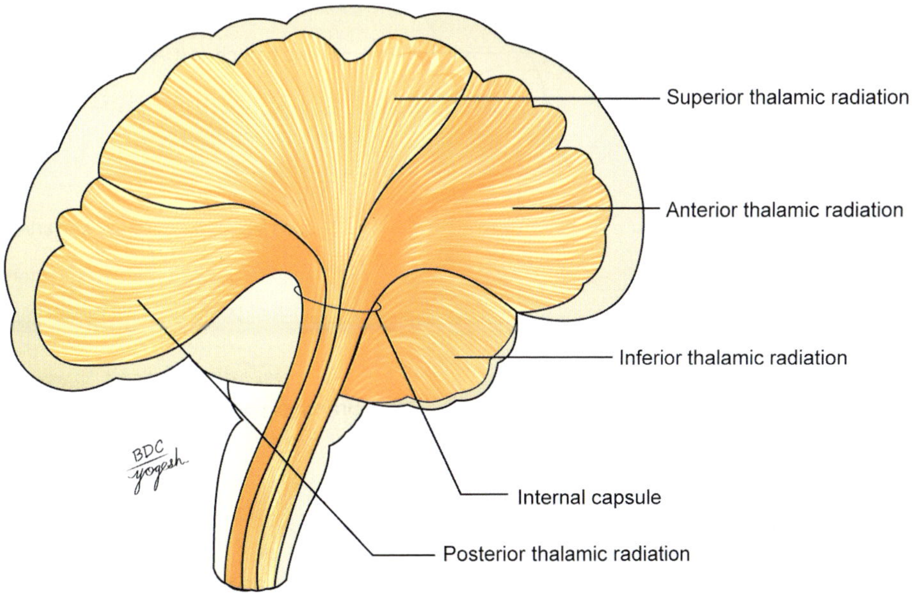

Fig. 11.20: Fibres of various parts of internal capsule

Blood Supply

The internal capsule gives passages to large number of fibres through a small zone. Hence, its vascular lesion affects large area of body. The internal capsule is supplied by the following arteries (Fig. 11.22):

1. Medial and lateral branches of middle cerebral artery.
2. Striate branches of anterior cerebral artery.
3. Cortical branches of anterior choroidal artery.
4. Few direct branches from internal carotid artery.
5. Central branches of the posterior communicating artery.
6. Posterolateral central branches of posterior cerebral artery.

Charcot's artery of cerebral haemorrhage is one of the lateral striate branches of the middle cerebral artery. It is a larger branch and more frequently ruptured.

Recurrent artery of Huebner is one of the striate branches of anterior cerebral artery which is large and takes the recurrent course.

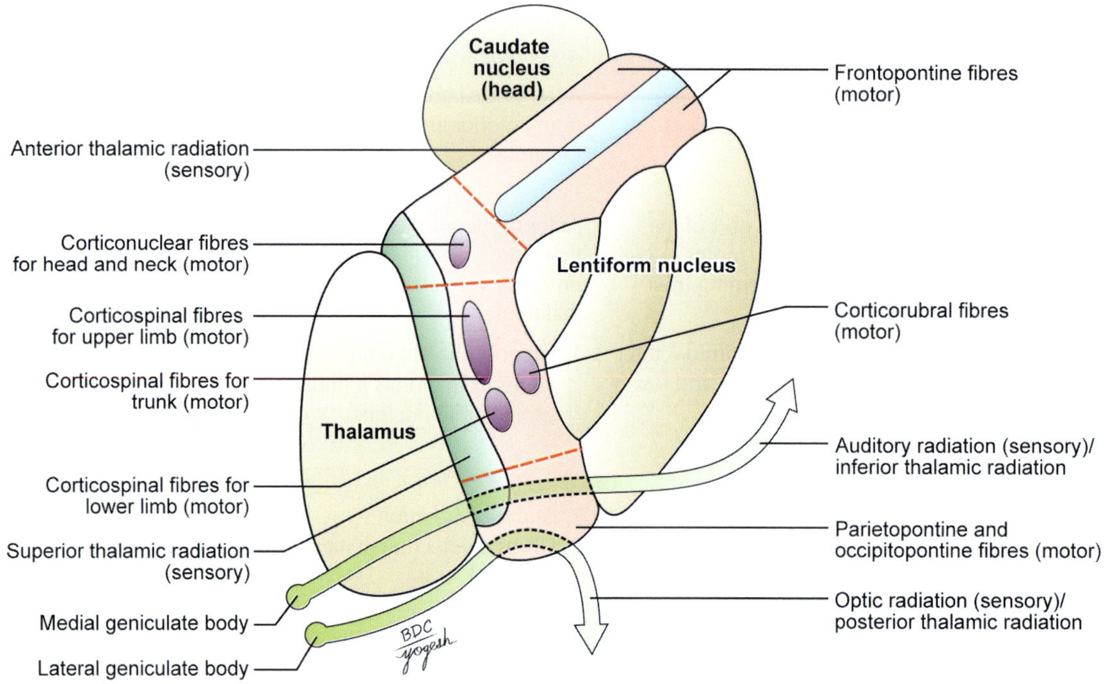

Fig. 11.21: Fibre components of internal capsule

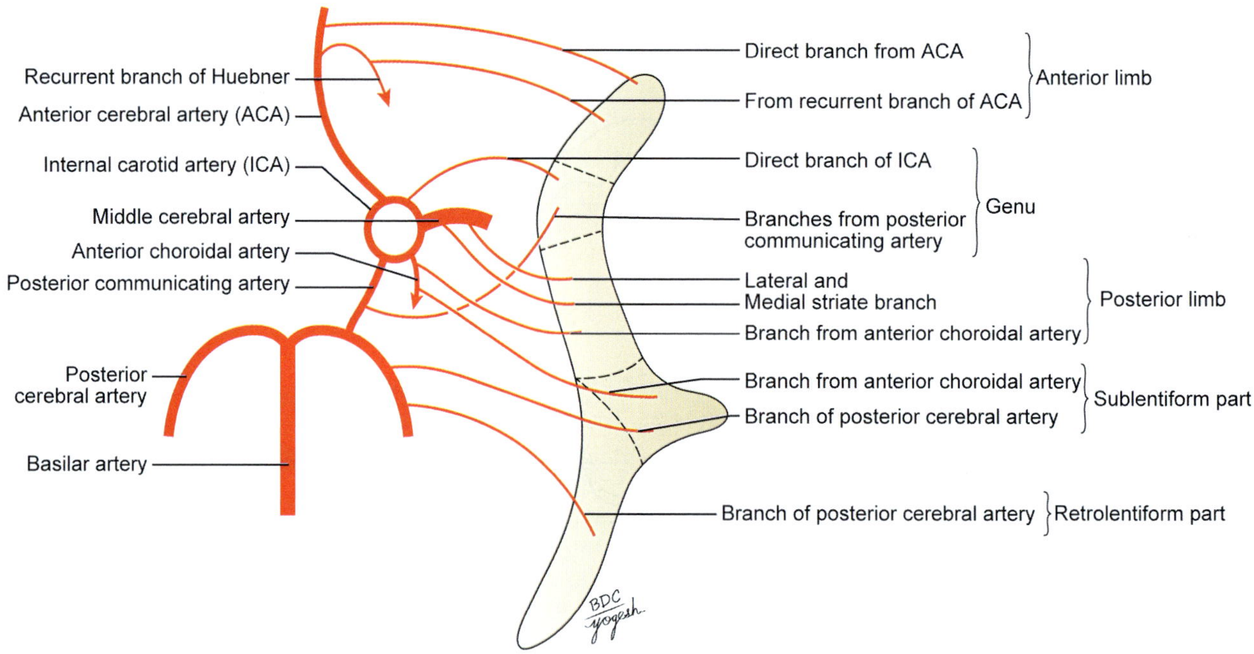

Fig. 11.22: Arteries supplying the internal capsule

CLINICAL NEUROANATOMY

- ***Lesion of internal capsule:*** A vascular lesion of internal capsule is common. It involves rupture of vessels which results in haemorrhage or occlusion (necrosis). It occurs commonly in the medial and lateral branches of the middle cerebral artery. Effects lesion of internal capsule which results in upper motor neuron type of paralysis of the opposite half of body and face.
- ***Specific lesions***
  a. Lesion of artery of cerebral haemorrhage (Charcot's artery) → damage to the posterior limb → paralysis of opposite half of body and face (common cause of hemiplegia) (Fig. 11.23).
  b. Lesion of recurrent artery of Huebner → damage to genu and anterior limb of internal capsule → paralysis of face and upper limb on the opposite side.
  c. Thrombosis of anterior choroidal artery → damage to posterior limb, sublentiform and retrolentiform parts → visual (hemianopia) and auditory defects.

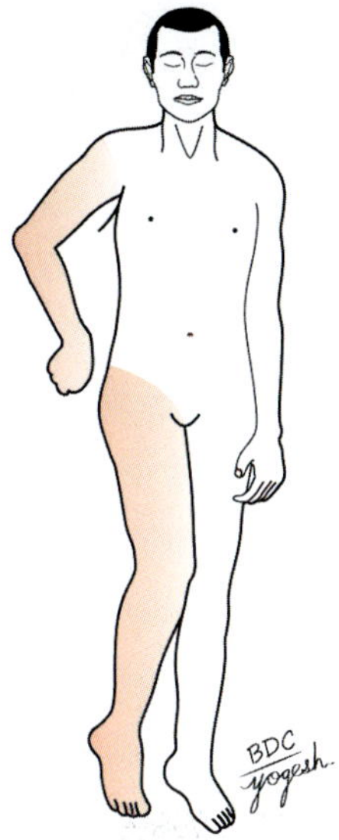

Fig. 11.23: Posture in right-sided hemiplegia

VIDEO

Video 4.8 **Cerebrum:** Superolateral surface, Inferior surface, Medial surface, Brodmann areas, White matter of brain.

Facts to Remember

- Cerebrum receives sensations from the opposite side of body. It controls the movements of the opposite side of body, a few structures are controlled by both sides.
- Body is represented upside down, only the face and area of vocalization are represented straight.
- Lateral sulcus has three limbs: Anterior horizontal, ascending, and posterior.
- Heschl's gyrus is anterior transverse temporal gyrus which is hidden by posterior ramus of lateral sulcus.
- Insula is the fifth lobe of the cerebral cortex.
- Paracentral lobule has the highest cortical centre of micturition.
- Areas 44 and 45 are Broca's area.
- Basal nuclei disorder produces parkinsonism.
- Corpus callosum is the largest bundle of commissural fibres.
- Internal capsule is the most typical example of projection fibres. Its posterior limb is supplied by lateral striate arteries. These are end arteries. Blockage or haemorrhage of these arteries causes upper motor neuron type of paralysis on the opposite side of the body.

BDC's Anatomy *e*-book

1. Types of sulci
2. Connections of motor area
3. Some functions of cerebrum
4. Human speech
5. Ageing changes in cerebrum
6. Further reading
7. Viva voce questions

Chapter

12

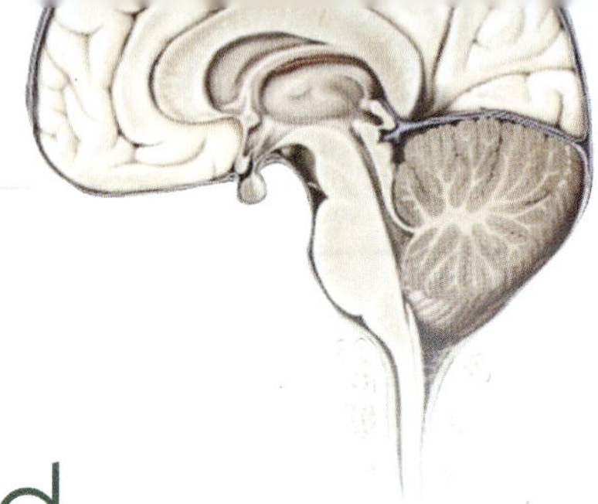

Lateral Ventricle and Limbic System

Competency:

AN63.1 Describe and demonstrate parts, boundaries and features of lateral ventricle.

LATERAL VENTRICLE

The lateral ventricles are two irregular cavities situated one in each cerebral hemisphere. Its capacity is about 7–10 ml (Figs 12.1a and b and 12.2 and Flowchart 12.1).

Communications

Each lateral ventricle communicates with the third ventricle through an interventricular foramen (foramen of Monro).

Contents

1. Cerebrospinal fluid
2. Choroid plexus.

PARTS OF LATERAL VENTRICLE

Each lateral ventricle consists of:

1. A central part
2. Three horns: Anterior, posterior and inferior (Figs 12.3a and b).

Central Part

This part of the lateral ventricle extends from the interventricular foramen in front to the splenium of the corpus callosum behind.

Boundaries

Roof: It is formed by the undersurface of the corpus callosum (Figs 12.4a and b).

Floor: It is formed (from lateral to medial side) by:

1. Body of caudate nucleus
2. Stria terminalis
3. Thalamostriate vein
4. Lateral portion of the upper surface of the thalamus
5. Choroid plexus
6. Upper surface of symmetric half of body of fornix.

Medial wall: It is formed by:

1. Septum pellucidum
2. Body of fornix.

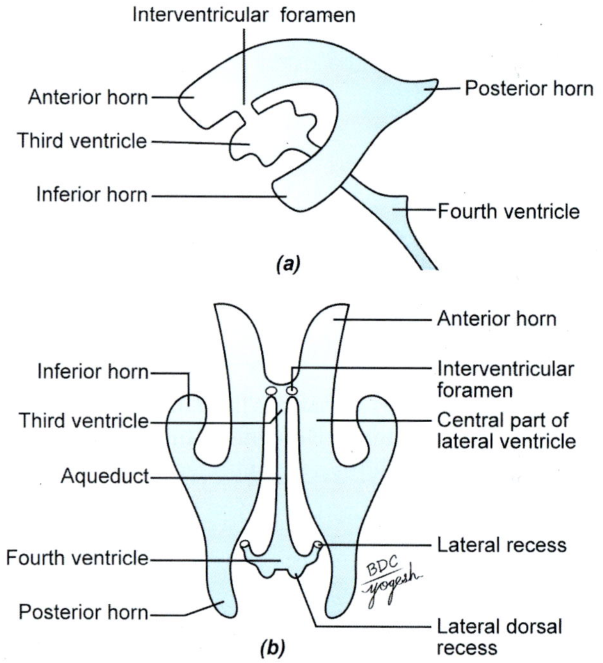

Figs 12.1a and b: Ventricles of the brain: (a) Lateral view and (b) superior view

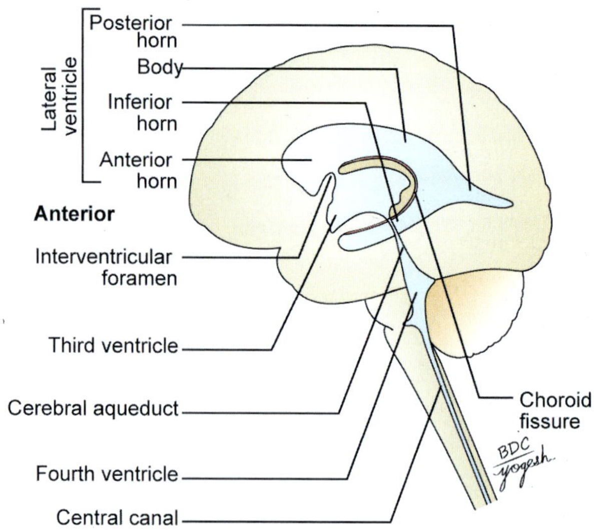

Fig. 12.2: Ventricle seen from the lateral surface

Flowchart 12.1: Lateral ventricle

Lateral ventricle

C-shaped cavity, Capacity: 7–10 ml

Contents: CSF, choroid plexus

Communicates with 3rd ventricle through interventricular foramen

Body
- Extent: From interventricular foramen to splenium
- Shape: Triangular
- Roof: Corpus callosum
- Medial wall: Septum pellucidum
- Floor:
  - Caudate nucleus
  - Stria terminalis
  - Thalamostriate vein
  - Thalamus
  - Choroid plexus
  - Fornix

Anterior horn
- Extent: From interventricular foramen to genu of corpus callosum
- Shape: Triangular
- Roof: Body of corpus callosum
- Floor: Rostrum, Head of caudate nucleus
- Medial wall: Septum pellucidum
- Lateral wall: Head of caudate nucleus
- Anterior wall: Genu of corpus callosum

Posterior horn
- Extent: Behind the splenium of corpus callosum
- Shape: Triangular
- Roof: Tapetum of corpus callosum
- Lateral wall: Tapetum
- Medial wall:
  - Bulb of posterior horn
  - Calcar avis

Inferior horn
- Extent: Inferiorly in temporal lobe
- Shape: Transverse slit
- Roof: Tapetum of corpus callosum, Tail of caudate nucleus, stria terminalis, amygdaloid body
- Floor:
  - Collateral eminance
  - Hippocampus with alveus

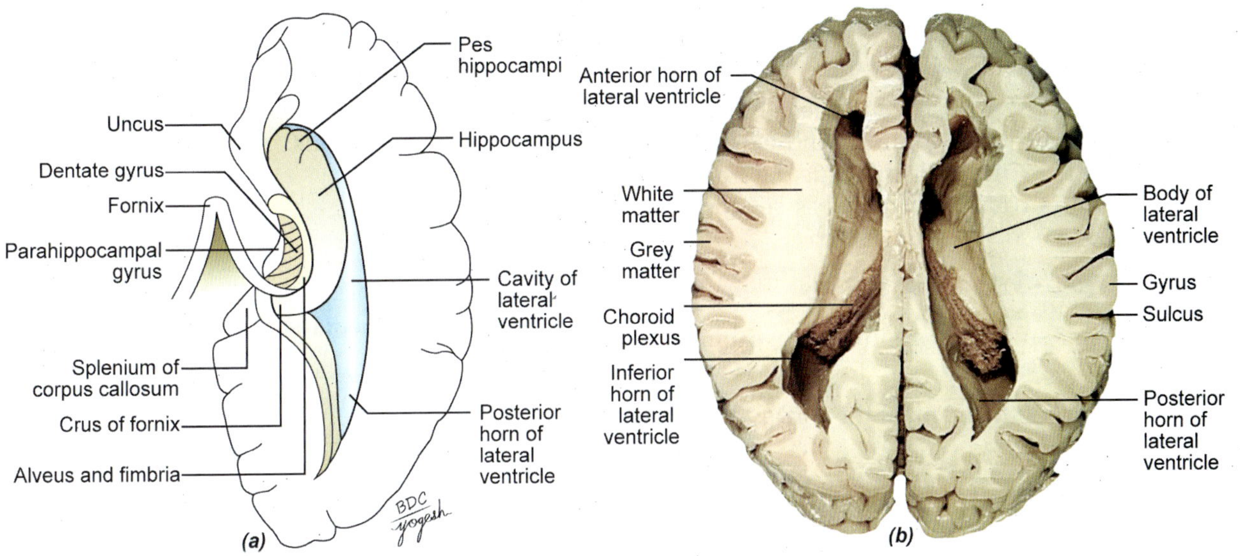

Figs 12.3a and b: Cavity of lateral ventricle including its anterior horn, body, inferior and posterior horns

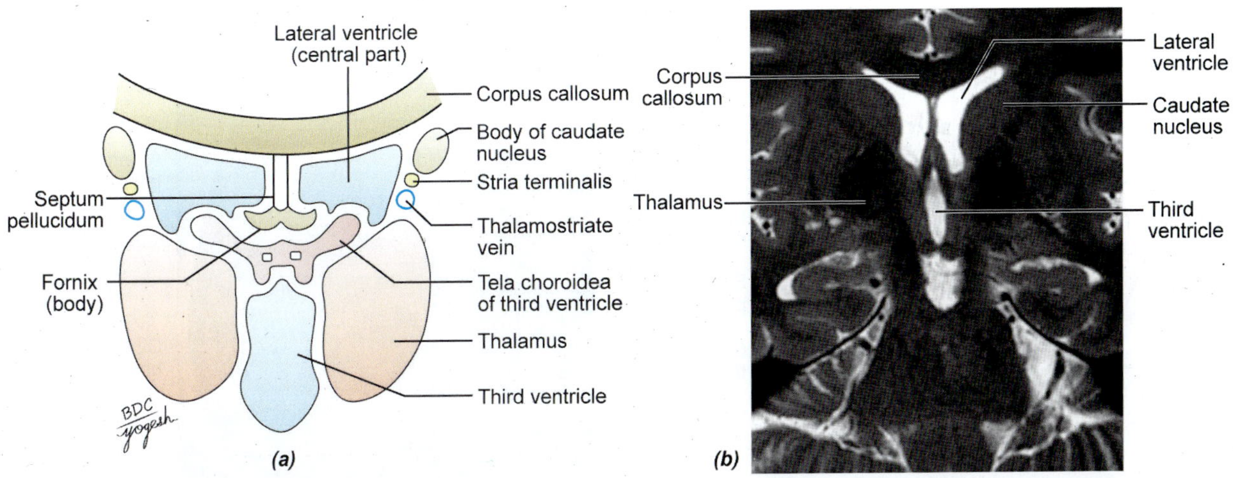

Figs 12.4a and b: (a) Boundaries of third ventricle and central part of lateral ventricle (coronal section) and (b) MRI showing third ventricle and part of lateral ventricle

Choroid Fissure

The line along which the choroid plexus invaginates into the lateral ventricle is called the choroid fissure. It is a C-shaped slit in the medial wall of the cerebral hemisphere. It starts at the interventricular foramen (above and in front) and passes around the thalamus and cerebral peduncle to the uncus (in the temporal lobe). Thus, it is present only in relation to the central part and inferior horn of the lateral ventricle. Its convex margin is bounded by the fornix (body and crus), the fimbria and the hippocampus, and the concave margin is bounded by the thalamus (superior and posterior surfaces), the tail of the caudate nucleus and the stria terminalis. At the fissure, the pia mater and ependyma come into contact with each other and both are invaginated into the ventricle by the choroid plexus.

In the central part of lateral ventricle, the choroid fissure is a narrow gap between the edge of the fornix and the upper surface of the thalamus. The gap is invaginated by the choroid plexus.

Anterior Horn

This is the part of the lateral ventricle which lies in front of the interventricular foramen and extends into the frontal lobe. It is directed forwards, laterally and downwards, and is triangular on cross-section (Figs 12.5a and b).

Boundaries

Anterior: Posterior surface of genu and rostrum of the corpus callosum.

Roof: Anterior part of the trunk of the corpus callosum.

Floor

1. Head of the caudate nucleus.
2. Upper surface of the rostrum of the corpus callosum.

Medial

1. Septum pellucidum
2. Column of fornix.

Posterior Horn

This is the part of the lateral ventricle which lies behind the splenium of the corpus callosum and extends into the occipital lobe. It is directed backwards and medially (Fig. 12.6).

Boundaries

Floor and medial wall

1. Bulb of the posterior horn raised by the forceps major.
2. Calcar avis raised by the anterior part of the calcarine sulcus.

Roof and lateral wall: Tapetum fibres of optic radiation.

Inferior Horn

This is the largest horn of the lateral ventricle. It begins at the junction of the central part with the posterior horn of the lateral ventricle; and extends into the temporal lobe (Fig. 12.7).

Boundaries

Roof and lateral wall

1. Chiefly the tapetum
2. Tail of caudate nucleus
3. Stria terminalis
4. Amygdaloid body.

Floor

1. Collateral eminence raised by the collateral sulcus.
2. Hippocampus, medially.

In the inferior horn, the line of ependymal invagination by the choroid plexus (i.e. the choroid fissure) lies between the stria terminalis and the fimbria.

CLINICAL NEUROANATOMY

For visualisation of lateral ventricle, computerised axial tomography (CT), scanning and magnetic resonance imaging (MRI) are useful.

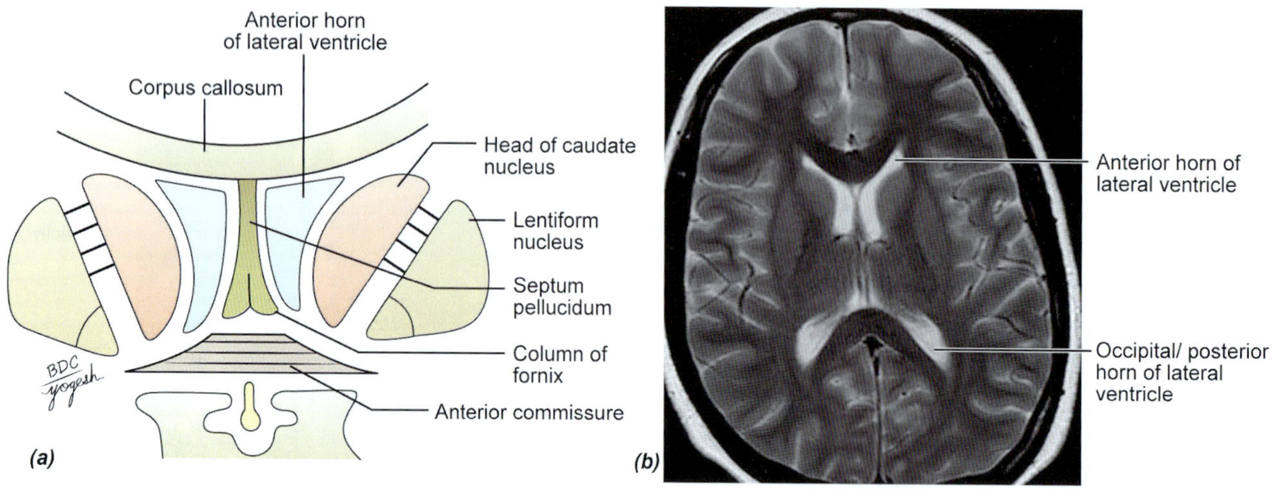

Figs 12.5a and b: (a) Boundaries of anterior horn of lateral ventricle (coronal section) and (b) MRI of anterior and occipital horns of lateral ventricles

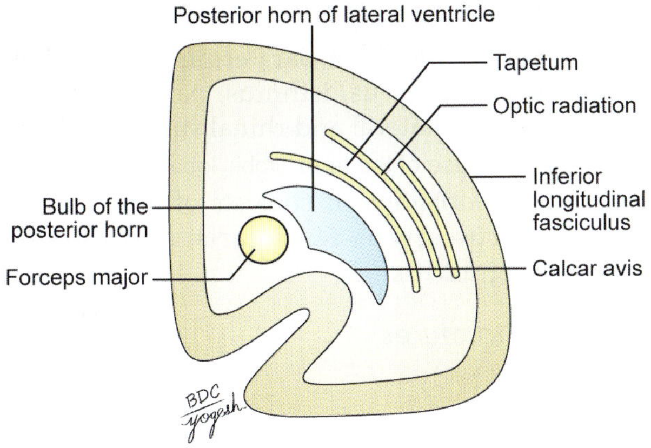

Fig. 12.6: Boundaries of posterior horn of lateral ventricle (coronal section)

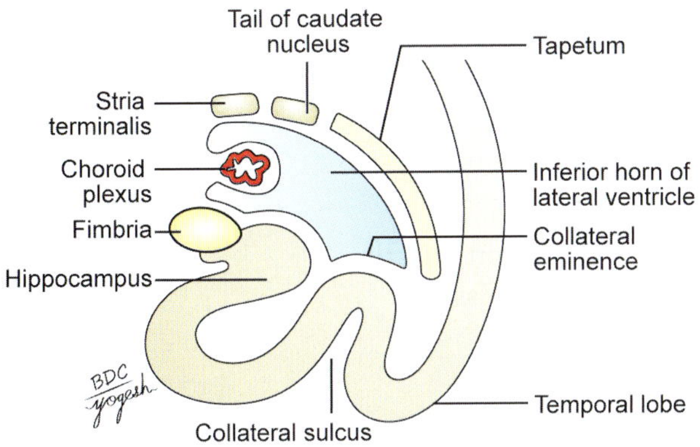

Fig. 12.7: Boundaries of inferior horn of lateral ventricle (coronal section)

DISSECTION

Take the right hemisphere and put the tip of the knife at the interventricular foramen. Give a vertical incision through the fornix, septum pellucidum, body of corpus callosum, the medial surface of the hemisphere till the superomedial border (Fig. 12.8a).

Turn the brain so that superolateral surface points towards you. Continue the previous incision on this surface for 2 cm. Carry the incision posteriorly and then curve it downwards till the end of the posterior ramus of the lateral sulcus (Fig. 12.8b).

Expose the insula by depressing the temporal lobe. Cut through the medial part of the gyri situated on the superior surface of the temporal lobe till the stem of the lateral sulcus (Fig. 12.8c).

Now try to separate the frontal lobe from the temporal lobe, and open up the stem of the lateral sulcus. Put the knife in the anterior part of stem of the lateral sulcus and extend the incision medially to the inferior part of stem of the lateral sulcus. Keep on opening the cut while making it and identify the choroid plexus entering the inferior horn of the lateral ventricle from its medial side.

Now brain is easily separable into an upper frontal part and a lower occipitotemporal part. Lift the fornix from the thalamus, separating the fornix from the choroid plexus. Identify the choroidal branches of the posterior cerebral artery.

Identify structures in all horns of lateral ventricle with the help of the two parts, i.e. frontal and occipitotemporal parts of the cerebral hemisphere.

Expose the anterior column of fornix by scraping the ependyma of anterior part of third ventricle. Trace the anterior column of fornix till the mammillary body. Trace another bundle, the mammillothalamic tract till the anterior nucleus of the thalamus.

Competency:

AN62.4 Enumerate parts and major connections of basal ganglia and limbic lobe.

LIMBIC SYSTEM

Limbic system (*limbus* = ring, *limbic* = border) is a part of cortical and subcortical structures that performs the primary maintenance of the organism, that is, food and sex.

Rhinencephalon (*smell brain*) is the previous name of limbic system. It is associated with sense of smell and smaller in size in humans.

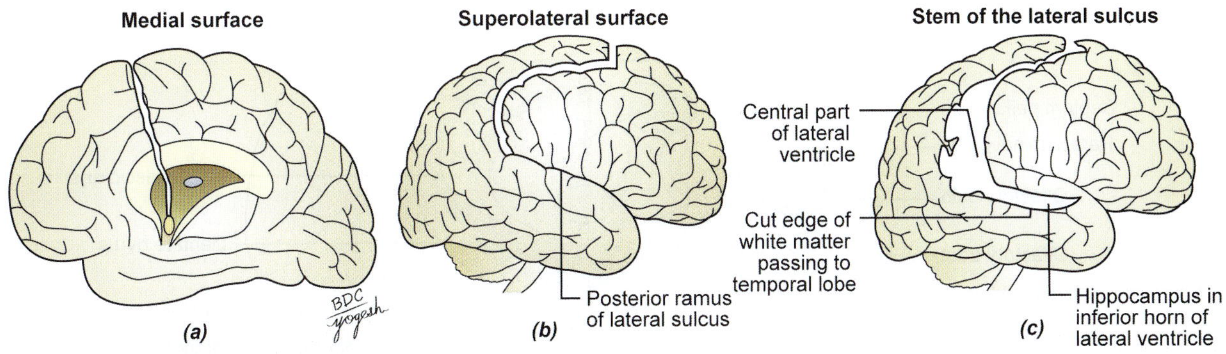

Figs 12.8a to c: (a) The first incision to be made in the dissection to expose the lateral ventricle, (b) the second part of the incision to be made in the dissection to expose the lateral ventricle, and (c) the third part of the incision to complete the exposure of the lateral ventricle

The ***limbic cortex*** is allocortex, hence consists of three neuronal layers. The transition zone (3 to 6 neuronal layers) is called *juxta-allocortex* that lies between allocortex and neocortex. The neocortex consists of six neuronal layers.

Functions of Limbic System

1. Emotional reactions
2. Integration of olfactory, visceral, and somatic impulses
3. Learning and retention of recent memory.

Emotional reactions, that are essential for maintenance of self and species, include:

1. Procuring, storing, and eating food
2. Sex
3. Rearing of young
4. Other emotions: Fear, rage, defence reactions, production of salivation and nausea on perception of smell
5. Visceral responses based on emotions.

Thus, limbic system is called *visceral brain.*

Components of Limbic System

The limbic system consists of many cortical and subcortical areas (Fig. 12.10, Flowchart 12.2). Hypothalamus is major control headquarter.

Cortical Area

1. *Limbic lobe*: It consists of paraterminal (subcallosal) gyrus, cingulate gyrus, isthmus, parahippocampal gyrus, uncus, collateral and rhinal sulci (Fig. 12.9). (*Note*: Currently use of the term 'limbic lobe' is decreased).
2. *Hippocampal formation*: It consists of hippocampus, dentate gyrus, gyrus fasciolaris, and indusium griseum (Fig. 12.10).

Subcortical Structures

1. Amygdaloid body
2. Septal nuclei
3. Olfactory areas
4. Hypothalamus – main headquarter of limbic system
5. Anterior nucleus of thalamus.

Fibres of Limbic System

They include:

1. Fornix
2. Mammillothalamic tract
3. Stria medullaris thalami
4. Stria terminalis
5. Medial forebrain bundle
6. Anterior commissure

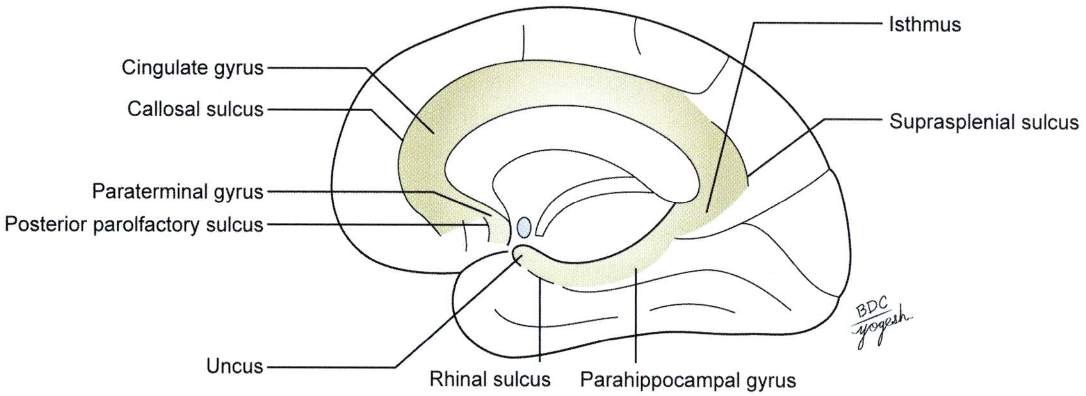

Fig. 12.9: Limbic lobe (medial surface of the right cerebral hemisphere)

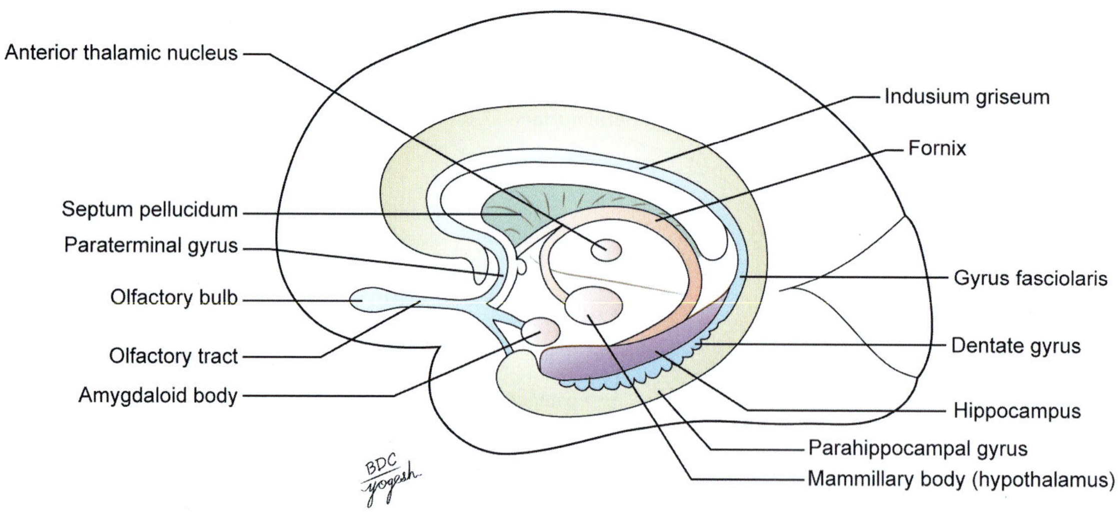

Fig. 12.10: Components of hippocampal formation

Flowchart 12.2: Limbic system: Components

Limbic system: Components

- ***Cortical area***
  - ***Limbic lobe***
    - Paraterminal gyrus
    - Cingulate gyrus
    - Isthmus
    - Parahippocampal gyrus
    - Uncus
  - ***Hippocampal formation***
    - Hippocampus
    - Dentate gyrus
    - Subiculum
    - Indusium griseum
    - Medial and lateral longitudinal stria
- ***Subcortical structures***
  - Amygdaloid body
  - Septal nuclei
  - Olfactory areas
  - Hypothalamus
  - Anterior nucleus of thalamus
- ***Fibres***
  - Fornix
  - Mammillothalamic tract
  - Stria medullaris thalami
  - Stria terminalis
  - Medial forebrain bundle
  - Anterior commissure
  - Cingulum
  - Diagonal band of Broca
  - Papez circuit

7. Cingulum
8. Diagonal band of Broca
9. Papez circuit.

Areas Concerned with Sense of Smell

The limbic system performs its function based on the sense of smell and other sensory stimuli (Fig. 12.11).

1. The *olfactory nerve* receives sensory input from olfactory mucosa. The *olfactory bulb* is a small oval structure that is situated above the cribriform plate of ethmoid. The *olfactory tract* is a narrow band of white fibres that passes backwards from the olfactory bulb to the anterior perforated substance.
2. ***Olfactory trigone*** is flattened posterior end of olfactory tract. It divides into medial, lateral, and intermediate olfactory stria.
   a. *Medial olfactory stria* continues in the paraterminal gyrus which lies in front of lamina terminalis.
   b. *Lateral olfactory stria* runs laterally and continues into the *limen insulae*. It turns medially to form *gyrus semilunaris* (periamygdaloid area).
   c. *Intermediate olfactory stria* is occasionally present. It ends as *olfactory tubercle* in the *anterior perforated substance*.
   d. *Medial and lateral olfactory gyri* are the thin layers of grey matter that cover the medial and lateral olfactory stria.

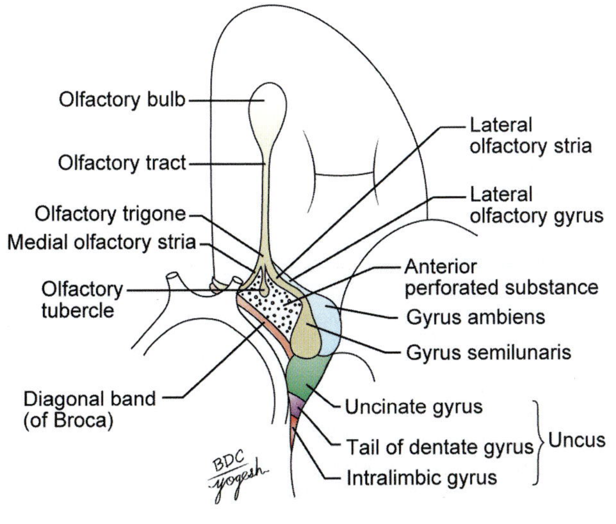

Fig. 12.11: Areas concerned with sense of smell

3. The ***anterior perforated substance*** is a small, depressed area of grey matter. It is perforated by central branches of the anterior and middle cerebral arteries.
4. ***Limen insulae*** is a small ridge connecting the anterior perforated substance with the apex of insula.
5. ***Parahippocampal gyrus*** lies on the tentorial surface of cerebral hemisphere. It lies medial to the collateral sulcus. Posteriorly, it is continuous with the *isthmus* and *lingual gyrus*. It has centre for taste and smell. ***Uncus*** is the anterior 2.5 cm of the parahippocampal gyrus. It is hook-like. *Rhinal notch* separates the uncus from the temporal pole. Uncus lies just behind the anterior perforated substance.
6. ***Primary olfactory area*** is responsible for reception and perception of smell. It includes lateral olfactory gyrus, gyrus ambiens, gyrus semilunaris, limen insulae, uncus and dorsomedial part of amygdaloid body. The ***secondary olfactory gyrus*** or *entorhinal area* performs the olfactory association. It includes the anterior part of parahippocampal gyrus. It is called area 28. The ***isthmus*** connects the cingulate gyrus with the parahippocampal gyrus. It lies behind the splenium of corpus callosum.
7. ***Septal area and septal nuclei*** is considered as pleasure zone. It consists of:
   a. ***Paraterminal gyrus*** is a narrow strip of cortex that lies along the anterior surface of lamina terminalis.
   b. ***Paraolfactory (subcallosal) gyrus*** is a narrow lamina on the medial surface cerebral hemisphere in front of lamina terminalis. It is continuous around the genu of corpus callosum with indusium griseum (*supracallosal gyrus*).
   c. ***Paraolfactory area (subcallosal area)*** is a small triangular area on the medial surface of cerebral hemisphere. It lies anterior to the subcallosal gyrus. Inferiorly, it is continuous with *olfactory trigone*.

Amygdaloid Body

It is almond-shaped mass of grey matter that lies in the anterior part of parahippocampal gyrus. It lies above the tip of the inferior horn of lateral ventricle, beneath the lentiform nucleus (Flowchart 12.3). Posteriorly, it is continuous with tail of caudate nucleus and stria terminalis.

Flowchart 12.3: Amygdaloid body

Amygdaloid body

Definition	*Connections*	*Functions*
Almond-shaped Grey matter in the anterior part of parahippocampal gyrus, above the tip of inferior horn of lateral ventricle	Afferent: Primary olfactory area Efferent: Stria terminalis - Septal area - Anterior region of thalamus - Stria medullaris thalami to habenular nucleus	Controls somatic responses of internal needs Controls smell-mediated sexual behaviour

Lesion of amygdaloid body→ ↓Fear, ↑Sexual activity

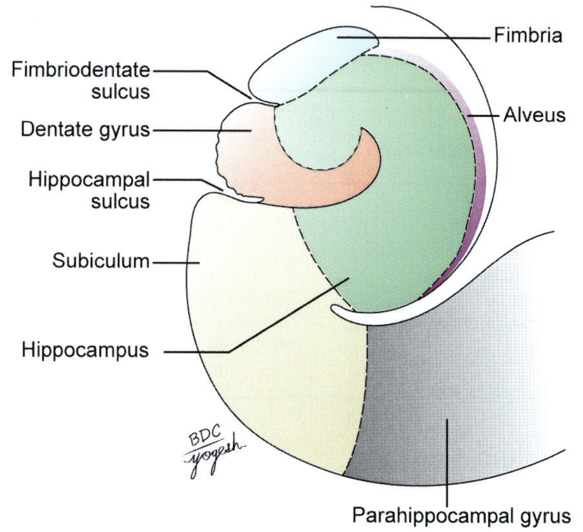

Fig. 12.12: Hippocampal formation (coronal section of right cerebral hemisphere, posterior view)

Connections

Afferent: From primary olfactory area.

Efferent: Stria terminalis – the efferent fibres of amygdaloid body form stria terminalis. It takes a C-shaped course along with caudate nucleus.

Termination: Stria terminalis ends in septal area and anterior region of thalamus. *Stria medullaris thalami* – these are some fibres of stria terminalis that run backwards and end in the habenular nucleus.

Functions

1. Controls the somatic responses of internal needs
2. Controls the smell-mediated sexual behaviour.

Hippocampal Formation

The hippocampal formation is a part of limbic system. It consists of (Plate 12.1, Figs 12.12 and 12.13):

1. ***Hippocampus*** is C-shaped grey matter (resembles seahorse or rams' horn). Hence, called *Ammon's horn* (mythology – Ammon was Egyptian deity with ram's head). It is located in the floor of inferior horn of lateral ventricle. ***Pes hippocampus*** is an anterior end of hippocampus with 2–3 digit-like ridges (similar to animals' paw, *pes* = foot). The ***alveus*** is thin layer of white matter that covers the ventricular surface of hippocampus. These are efferent fibres of hippocampus. The efferent fibres of hippocampus from alveus posteriorly these fibres converge to form ***fimbria of hippocampus***. It is a flattened band of white matter. It lies superior to the dentate gyrus. The fibres of fimbria of hippocampus continue posteriorly as ***crus of fornix***.
2. ***Dentate gyrus*** is a narrow crenated, toothed strip of grey matter. It lies on the upper surface of parahippocampal gyrus. Posteriorly, it is continuous with gyrus fasciolaris through indusium griseum. The dentate gyrus runs medially across the inferior surface of uncus. Here, it forms the ***tail of dentate gyrus***.
3. ***Subiculum*** lies between the hippocampus proper and entorhinal area at the inferomedial part of the cerebral hemisphere. It is a transition zone (3 to 6 neuronal layers) and hence called juxta-allocortex.
4. ***Indusium griseum*** (*supracallosal gyrus*) is a thin layer of grey matter that covers the superior surface of

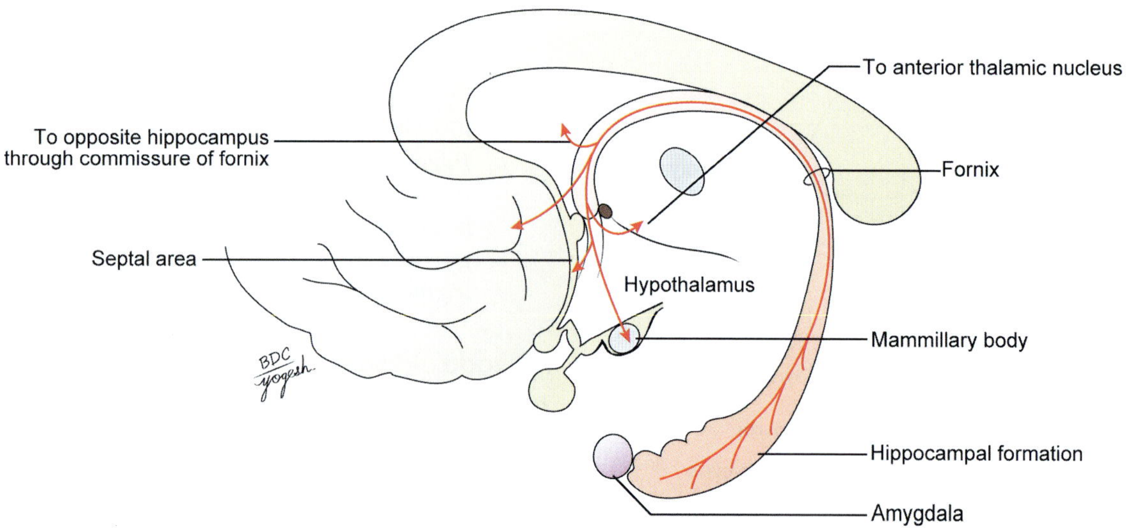

Fig. 12.13: Connection of hippocampus

Plate 12.1: Hippocampal formation (coronal section of right cerebral hemisphere)

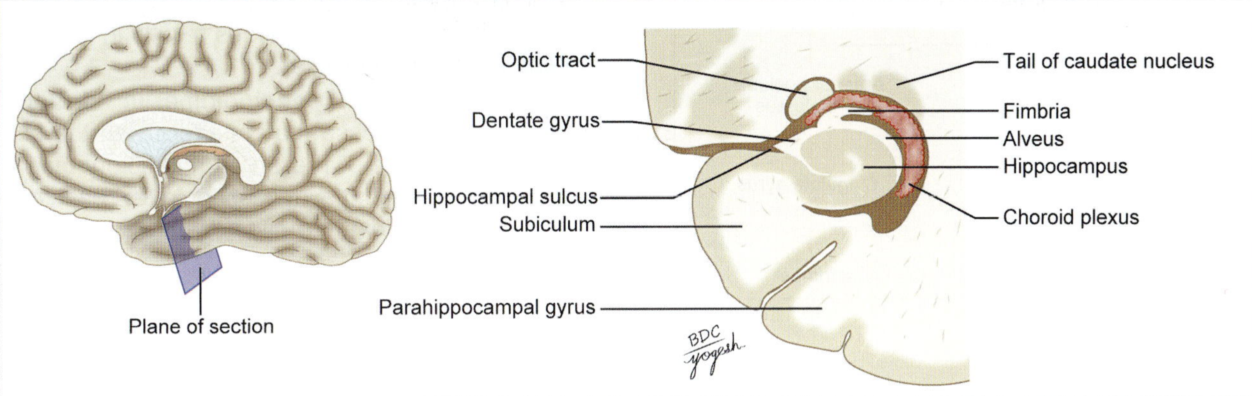

corpus callosum. Anteriorly, it is continuous with paraterminal gyrus and posteriorly with gyrus fasciolaris.

5. ***Medial and lateral longitudinal stria*** are two thin longitudinal strands of white fibres on each side. They are embedded in indusium griseum.

Functions

1. Physiologically, a part of limbic system.
2. Controls endocrine and visceral functions and emotional status
3. Recent memory.

Connection of hippocampus

- *Afferent*: From entorhinal area
- *Efferent*: Through fornix → to opposite hippocampus, septal area, anterior hypothalamic regions, mammillary body.

Fornix

The fornix is an arched bundle of projection fibres from hippocampus to the mammillary body (Fig. 12.14 and Flowchart 12.4).

Formation

The fornix made-up of efferent fibres of hippocampus. Axon of pyramidal cells of hippocampus → alveus (thin sheet of white matter covering ventricular surface of hippocampus) → fimbria (flat band) → crus of fornix.

1. *Crus of fornix*: Curves upwards behind the thalamus.
2. *Body of fornix*: Both the crura (right and left) converge in the midline to form the body of fornix. It lies above the roof of third ventricle and below the splenium and body of corpus callosum.
3. *Commissure of fornix*: Few fibres of crura decussate just posterior to the body of fornix as commissure of fornix (hippocampal commissure).
4. *Anterior column of fornix*: Anteriorly, the body of fornix divides downwards to the anterior columns. Each anterior column curves downwards to the anterior commissure. It extends through the hypothalamus and ends in the mammillary body. Its few fibres terminate into septal areas.

Functions: The fornix is efferent tract of hippocampus.

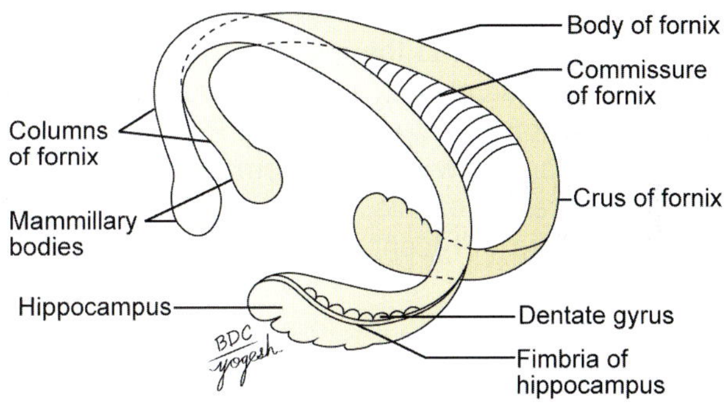

Fig. 12.14: Fornix (left lateral view with posterior oblique tilt)

Flowchart 12.4: Fornix

Fornix

Definition	*Parts*	*Function*	*Lesion*
Projection fibres of hippocampus to mammillary body	Crus of fornix Body Commissure Anterior column	Form efferent tract of hippocampus	Bilateral lesion of fornix ↓ Acute amnestic syndrome

Papez Circuit

It is an intraneuronal communication of limbic system that forms the basis for emotional experiences [*James Wenceslas Papez, American neuroanatomist, 1883–1958*] (Flowchart 12.5).

Components

1. Hippocampal formation
2. Fornix
3. Mammillary body
4. Anterior nucleus of thalamus
5. Cingulate gyrus
6. Entorhinal cortex.

Functions

The papez circuit plays an import role in emotion and consolidation of memory [short-term → long-term memory].

Flowchart 12.5: Papez circuit

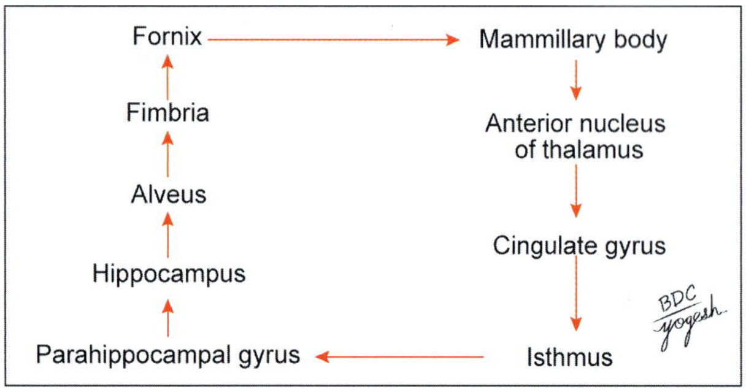

CLINICAL NEUROANATOMY

- Hippocampus can be regarded as the cortical centre for autonomic reflexes. Hippocampal-amygdala complex is related to the memory of recent events. Lesions of this complex are associated with a loss of memory for recent events only. Patient is unable to commit any new facts to memory and does not remember recent events. The lesion of hippocampus results in loss of recent memory and psychomotor epilepsy.
- A bilateral damage to the fornix causes inability in consolidation of short-term memory into long-term memory. This is called ***acute amnestic syndrome***.
- Bilateral damage to amygdaloid body → reduction in fear and increase in sexual activity. A lesion that affects the uncus and amygdaloid body may cause, '***uncinate fits***' characterised by an imaginary disagreeable odour, by movements of lips and tongue, and often by a 'dreamy state'.
- Destruction of olfactory nerves results in loss of the sense of smell (anosmia).
- A tumour, usually a meningioma, in the floor of anterior cranial fossa may interfere with the sense of smell because of pressure on olfactory bulb and the olfactory tract. It is necessary to test each nostril separately because the olfactory loss is likely to be unilateral.

VIDEO

Video 4.9 Ventricles of Brain

Facts to Remember

- Lateral ventricle is the largest ventricle of the brain.
- The right and left lateral ventricles communicate with the single third ventricle through the interventricular foramen.
- Limbic system comprises connections of fornix and Papez circuits. These are mostly present on the flat medial surface of cerebral hemisphere.

BDC's Anatomy *e*-book

1. Further reading
2. Viva voce questions

Chapter

13

Some Neural Pathways and Reticular Formation

SOME NEURAL PATHWAYS

The descending tracts controls the activity of the body through the pyramidal and extrapyramidal tracts (For details, Chapter 5).

The ascending tracts carry the sensory input to the central nervous system. They carry the following sensations:

1. Pain and temperature sensation
2. Fine touch and conscious proprioception
3. Unconscious proprioception.

The special sensory pathways carry the olfactory, light, auditory, and taste sensations.

Pyramidal Tracts

For the pyramidal tract, see the descriptions given in Chapter 5. This is a descending tract, extending from the cerebral cortex to various motor nuclei of the cranial nerves as corticobulbar tracts and spinal nerves as corticospinal tracts. It constitutes the upper motor neuron in the motor pathway from the cortex to voluntary muscles. Corticonuclear fibres reach the nuclei of cranial nerves (Fig. 13.1).

Before termination, all fibres of the pyramidal tract cross to opposite side. They terminate, mostly through an interneuron, in the motor nuclei of cranial nerves and in relation to the anterior horn cells of the spinal cord. The fibres which terminate in the motor nuclei of the cranial nerves collectively form the corticonuclear tract.

CLINICAL NEUROANATOMY

Effects of lesion of the pyramidal tract: Lesions above the level of decussation cause contralateral paralysis, while lesions below the decussation cause ipsilateral paralysis. It is an upper motor neuron type of paralysis which is characterised by the following:

a. Loss of the power of voluntary movements.
b. Clasp-knife type of rigidity (hypertonia).
c. Tendon reflexes are exaggerated.
d. Superficial reflexes are lost.
e. Babinski's sign is positive.
f. Reaction of degeneration is absent.

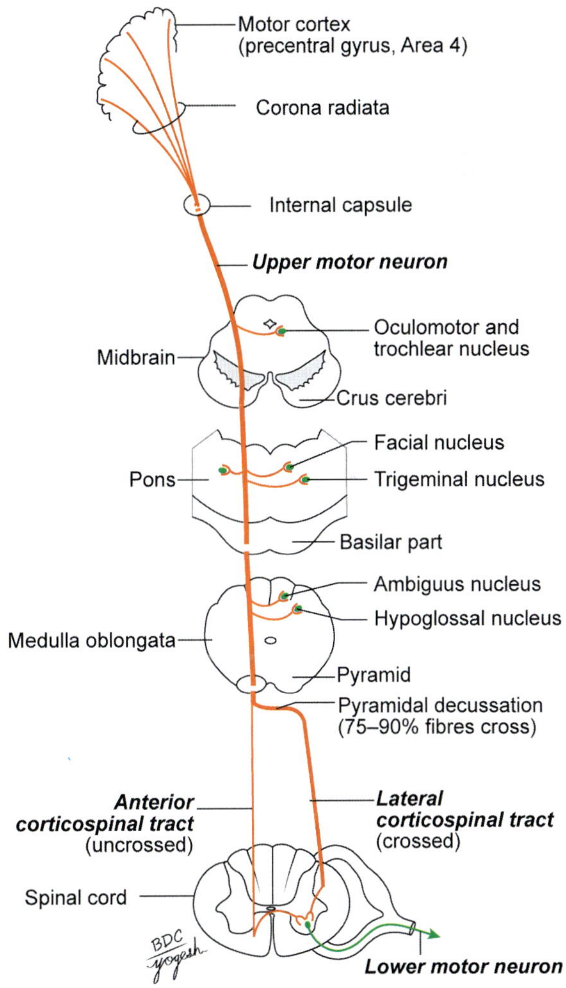

Fig. 13.1: Pathway of pyramidal fibres

Pathway of Pain and Temperature

These sensations are carried from the opposite half of the body and face by the lateral spinothalamic tract and the trigeminal nerve respectively. For details *see* Chapter 5. It consists of three order neurons (Figs 13.2a and b).

For the lateral spinothalamic tract:

1. First order neurons are located in the dorsal root ganglia.
2. Second order neurons are located in the grey matter of the spinal cord. Their axons form the lateral spino-

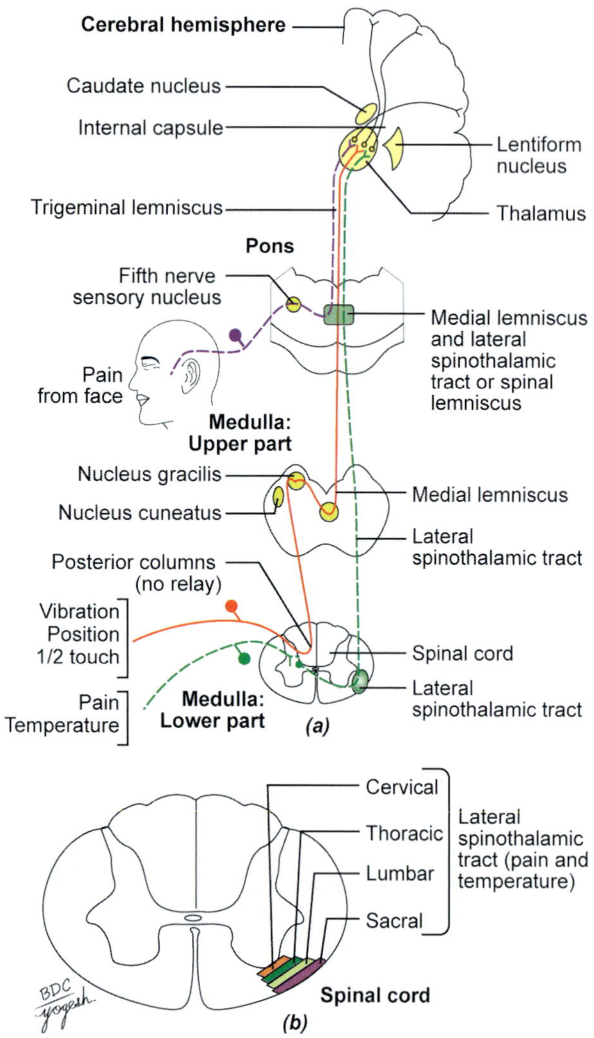

Figs 13.2a and b: Pathway of: (a) Posterior column and (b) pain and temperature impulses

thalamic tract and later the spinal lemniscus in the brainstem.

3. Third order neuron lies in the ventral posterolateral nucleus of the thalamus. Fibres arising in this nucleus pass through the internal capsule and the corona radiata to reach the somatosensory areas 3, 1, 2 of cerebral cortex.

For face, head and neck: The first order neurons lie in the trigeminal ganglion. They form spinal tract of trigeminal nerve in the brainstem. The second order neurons lie in the spinal nucleus of trigeminal nerve. Their crossed axons form trigeminothalamic tract. The third order neurons lie in the ventral posteromedial nucleus of the thalamus. Fibres arising in this nucleus pass through the internal capsule and the corona radiata to reach the somatosensory areas 3, 1, 2 of cerebral cortex.

Pathway of Fine Touch, Proprioceptive (Kinaesthetic) Impulses—Position, Movement, Vibration

These sensations are carried from the opposite half of the body and face by the fasciculus gracilis and the fasciculus cuneatus and the trigeminal nerve respectively. For details *see* Chapter 5. It consists of three order neurons.

For the lateral spinothalamic tract:

1. First order neuron is located in the dorsal root ganglia. Their axons ascend in the spinal cord as the fasciculus gracilis and the fasciculus cuneatus in the dorsal white column.
2. Second order neuron is located in the nucleus gracilis or nucleus cuneatus in the medulla oblongata. Their axons cross to form internal arcuate fibres which further ascend as the medial lemniscus in the brainstem.
3. Third order neuron lies in the ventral posterolateral nucleus of the thalamus. Fibres arising in this nucleus pass through the internal capsule and the corona radiata to reach the somatosensory areas 3, 1, 2 of cerebral cortex.

For face, head and neck: The first order neurons lie in the trigeminal ganglion. The second order neurons lie in the mesencephalic nucleus of trigeminal nerve in the midbrain. Their crossed axons reach thalamus. The third order neurons lie in the ventral posteromedial nucleus of the thalamus. Fibres arising in this nucleus pass through the internal capsule and the corona radiata to reach the somatosensory areas 3, 1, 2 of cerebral cortex.

Pathway of Crude Touch and Pressure

These sensations are carried from the opposite half of the body and face by the anterior spinothalamic tract and the trigeminal nerve respectively. For details *see* Chapter 5.

For the anterior spinothalamic tract:

1. First order neurons are located in the dorsal root ganglia.
2. Second order neurons are located in the grey matter of the spinal cord. Their axons form the anterior spinothalamic tract and later the spinal lemniscus in the brainstem.
3. Remaining pathway is similar to lateral spinothalamic tract.

For face, head and neck: The first order neurons lie in the trigeminal ganglion. They form spinal tract of trigeminal nerve in the brainstem. The second order neurons lie in the spinal nucleus of trigeminal nerve. Their crossed axons form trigeminothalamic tract. The third order neurons lie in the ventral posteromedial nucleus of the thalamus. Fibres arising in this nucleus pass through the internal capsule and the corona radiata to reach the somatosensory areas 3, 1, 2 of cerebral cortex.

Pathway of Unconscious Proprioceptive Impulses

These impulses end in the cerebellum.

1. The first neuron has been described above.
2. The *second neuron* fibres are represented by three tracts—the posterior and anterior spinocerebellar tracts (from the lower limb and trunk) and the cuneocerebellar tract (posterior external arcuate fibres) from the upper limb.

The *posterior spinocerebellar tract* contains ipsilateral fibres arising in dorsal (thoracic) nucleus of the spinal cord. It enters the ipsilateral cerebellar hemisphere through the inferior cerebellar peduncle.

The *anterior spinocerebellar tract* is made up mainly of crossed fibres arising from the spinal grey matter (posterior grey column). The fibres ascend to the upper part of pons and then turn down into the superior cerebellar peduncle to reach the cerebellum of same side.

The *cuneocerebellar tract (posterior external arcuate fibres)* is functionally similar to the posterior spinocerebellar tract. It arises from the accessory (external) cuneate nucleus which receives afferents from the fasciculus cuneatus. The tract enters the ipsilateral cerebellar hemisphere through the inferior cerebellar peduncle.

Taste Pathway

1. The taste from anterior two-thirds of tongue except from vallate papillae is carried by chorda tympani branch of facial nerve till the geniculate ganglion. The central processes go to the tractus solitarius in the medulla (Fig. 13.3).
2. Taste from posterior one-third of tongue including the vallate papillae is carried by cranial nerve IX till the inferior ganglion. The central processes also reach the tractus solitarius.
3. Taste from the posterior most part of tongue and epiglottis travels through vagus nerve till the inferior ganglion of vagus. These central processes also reach tractus solitarius.
4. After a relay in tractus solitarius, the solitariothalamic tract is formed which becomes a part of trigeminal lemniscus and reaches the ventroposteromedial nucleus of thalamus of opposite side. Another relay here takes the fibres to lowest part of postcentral gyrus, which is the area for taste.

Visual Pathway and Auditory Pathways

These are described in Chapter 6.

RETICULAR FORMATION

The reticular formation is a diffuse (ill-defined) mass of grey matter with intermingled nerve fibres. It extends throughout the brainstem (Plate 13.1 and Fig. 13.4).

Plate 13.1: Location of reticular formation in the brainstem

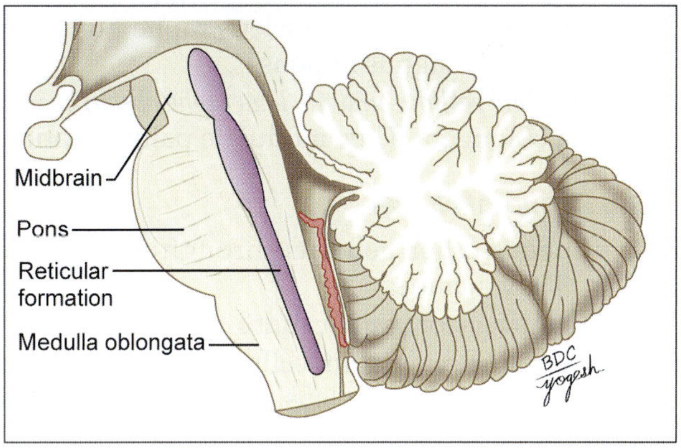

Functions

1. *Arousal*: Reticular formation maintains the state of consciousness (ascending reticular activating system).
2. Controls *autonomic reflex centers* of brainstem – regulation of respiration, heart rate and blood pressure.
3. Regulation of endocrine, visceral and emotional responses.
4. Influences motor activity through extrapyramidal connections.
5. Modulates sensory inputs, especially pain.

Reticular Nuclei

The neurons of reticular formation form bilaterally the following three longitudinal nuclei as follows:

1. *Raphe nuclei*
2. *Magnocellular or medial column*
3. *Parvocellular or lateral column*
4. The paramedian nuclei are also present that lie in pons and medulla.

Raphe Nuclei

They lie in the paramedian position. They produce serotonin. They include:

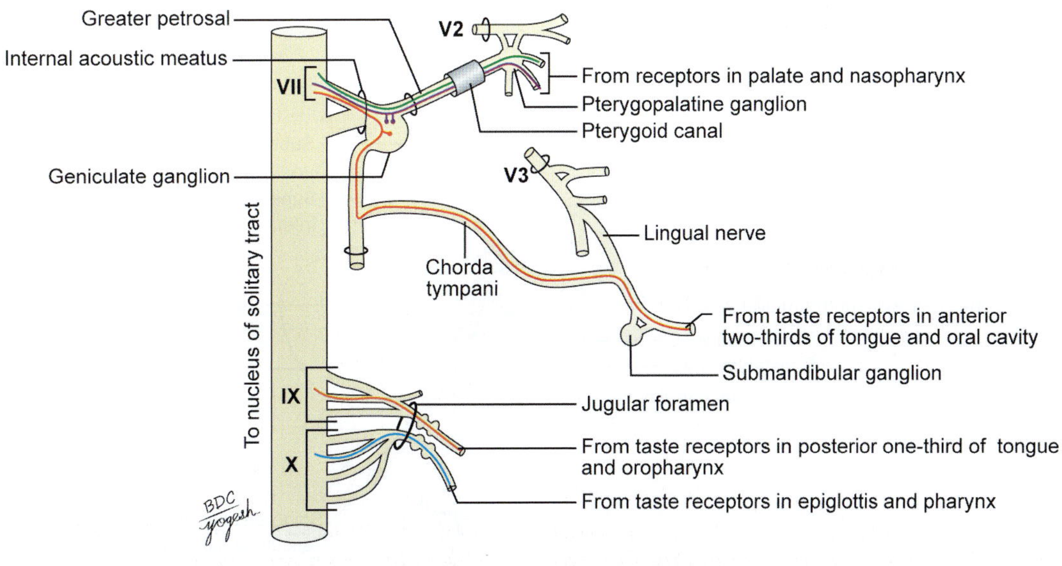

Fig. 13.3: Taste pathway

1. *Dorsal raphe nucleus* and *dorsal tegmental nucleus* in the midbrain. They form pain controlling pathway.
2. Superior central nucleus, nucleus raphe pontis, and nucleus raphe magnus in pons.
3. *Nucleus raphe pallidus and nucleus raphe obscurus* in the medulla oblongata. They modulate pain sensation.

Medial Group of Nuclei

They influence other neurons through polysynaptic pathway. They include:
1. Pontine nuclei – oral and caudal
2. Medullary nuclei – gigantocellular reticular nucleus, and ventral reticular nucleus.

Lateral Group of Nuclei

They receive information of ascending tracts and give efferent to medial group of nuclei. They include:
1. In midbrain: Cuneiform nucleus, parabrachial nucleus, and pedunculopontine nucleus.
2. In pons: Parabrachial nucleus, pedunculopontine nucleus, and parvocellular nucleus.
3. In medulla: Parvocellular nucleus.

Connections

Reticular formation receives almost all sensory and motor information and influences most of the body responses based on this input. They receive afferents from spinoreticular fibres, visual inputs by tectoreticular fibres, auditory inputs by tectoreticular fibres, olfactory inputs by descending fibres from limbic system, fibres from cerebrum, corpus striatum, cerebral cortex and contralateral reticular and cranial nerve nuclei (Fig. 13.5).

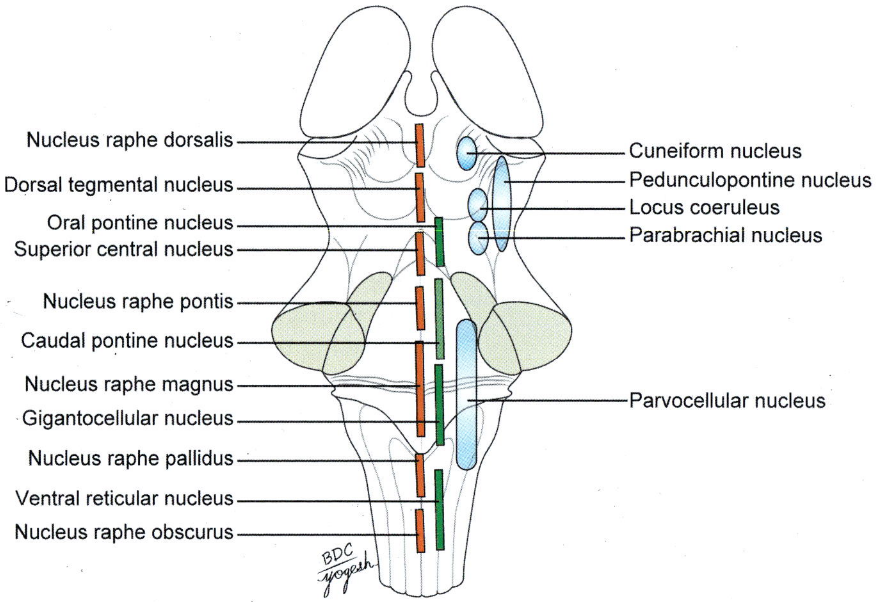

Fig. 13.4: Schematic diagram to show the reticular nuclei in the brainstem (posterior view of brainstem) *Note*: Paramedian group of nuclei are not shown

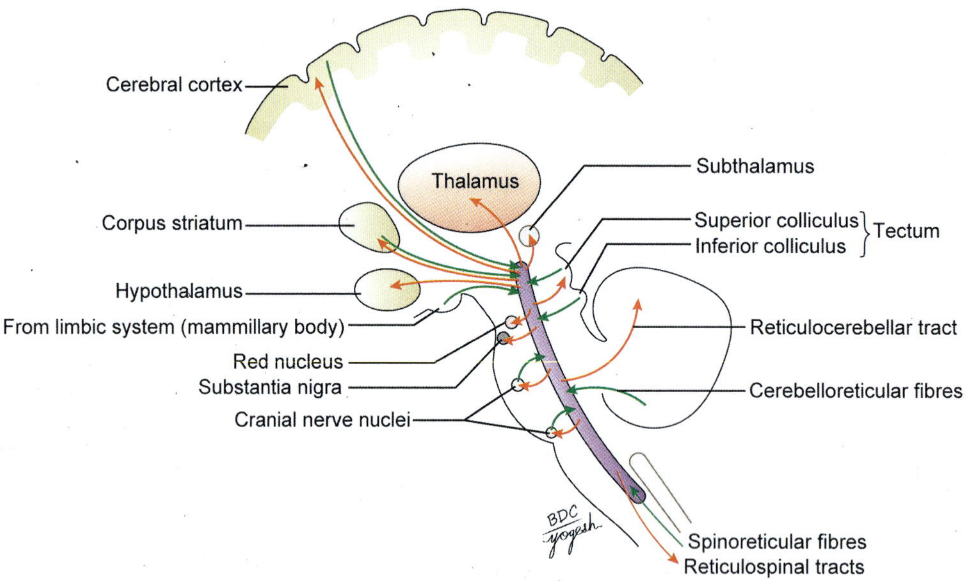

Fig. 13.5: Major connections of reticular formation

These nuclei give rise to the reticulospinal tracts, reticulobulbar tract, reticulocerebellar tract. They also give rise to efferent fibres to the red nucleus, substantia nigra and tectum of midbrain, subthalamus, thalamus, hypothalamus, corpus striatum, and the cerebral cortex (Fig. 13.5).

Ascending Reticular Activating System (ARAS)

It is also called reticular activating system (RAS). It is responsible for wakefulness and alertness.

The ascending fibres of all sensory tracts of spinal cord and cranial nerve give collaterals to the reticular formation. The efferent fibres from this reticular formation project to the cerebral cortex through thalamus. It stimulates wide area of cerebral cortex, and the individual becomes alert.

CLINICAL NEUROANATOMY

- *Coma*: Bilateral lesion of RAS causes coma (state of unconscious). In coma patients, the powerful sensory stimuli fail to cause arousal.
- *Sleep*: Decreased activity of RAS induces sleep.
- *Drug-effect on RAS*: General anaesthetics and tranquilizing drugs cause suppression of RAS.
- Severe damage to RAS may cause loss of consciousness, coma and even death.

Facts to Remember

- Corticonuclear fibres give fibres to cranial nerve nuclei.
- The corticonuclear fibres of one side of cortex reach VII nerve nucleus of both sides which supply the muscles of upper half of face on both sides. It also gives fibres to nucleus of VII and supply to lower half of facial muscles only on the contralateral side.
- Unconscious impulses reach ipsilateral cerebellum, while conscious impulses reach the contralateral cerebrum.
- Anterior spinothalamic tract carrying crude touch and pressure joins the medial lemniscus during its upward journey through the brainstem. Thus, medial lemniscus carries conscious proprioceptive sensations, i.e. movement, vibration and position including whole touch and pressure to the thalamus.
- Nucleus of tractus solitarius receives impulses of taste through chorda tympani, branch of VII from most of anterior two-thirds of tongue; through glossopharyngeal from circumvallate papillae and posterior one-third of tongue. It also receives impulses from posteriormost part of tongue and vallecula via internal laryngeal branch of vagus nerve.

BDC's Anatomy *e*-book

1. Functions of reticular system
2. Action of drugs on reticular system
3. Viva voce questions

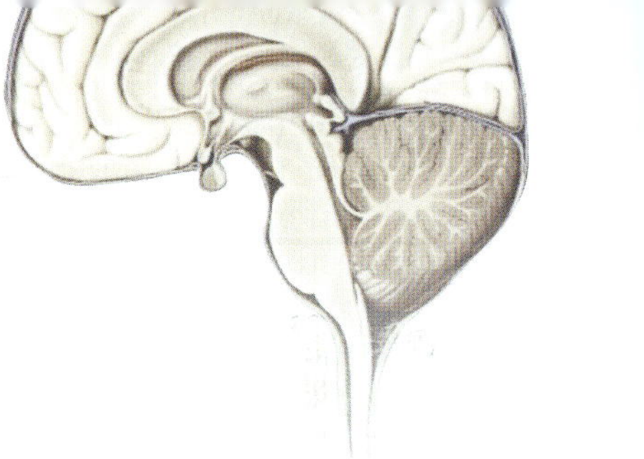

Chapter

14

Blood Supply of Brain

The nervous tissue is too delicate to bear anoxia beyond three minutes. The blood supply to nervous tissue per unit tissue is maximum in the body. It shows the importance of the grey matter. The blood supply may be erratic due to haemorrhage, thrombosis or embolism of the arteries supplying the nervous tissue. Further the arteries are 'end arteries' once these reach the deeper level.

ARTERIES OF BRAIN

Two vertebral and two internal carotid arteries carry the total arterial supply to the brain (Figs 14.1 and 14.2).

VERTEBRAL ARTERIES

The vertebral artery on each side is a branch of first part of subclavian artery. Its course is divided into four parts:

- 1st part lies from its origin to the foramen transversarium of 6th cervical vertebra.
- 2nd part courses through foramen transversaria of 6th to 1st cervical vertebrae (Plate 14.1).
- 3rd part lies on the posterior arch of atlas vertebra in the suboccipital triangle.
- 4th part of the vertebral artery enters the cranium through foramen magnum under the free margin of posterior atlanto-occipital membrane.

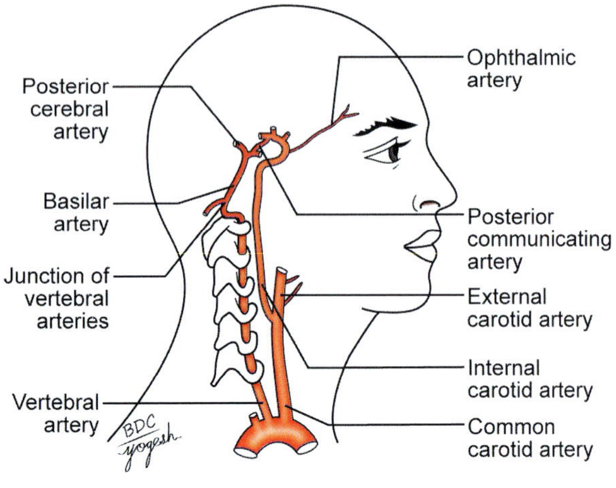

Fig. 14.1: Carotid and vertebral arteries

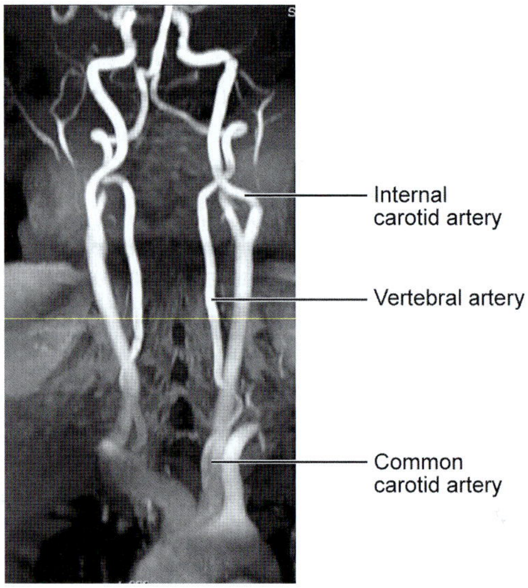

Fig. 14.2: MRI of the arteries of brain

It enters the subarachnoid space in the upper part of vertebral canal after piercing the dura mater and arachnoid mater. Then it curves round the ventrolateral aspect of the medulla oblongata between the rootlets of hypoglossal nerve, to unite with its fellow at the lower border of pons and forms the median basilar artery.

Intracranial Branches of Vertebral Artery

1. Posterior spinal artery
2. Posterior inferior cerebellar artery
3. Anterior spinal artery
4. Medullary branches
5. Meningeal branches.

Note:

1. *Posterior spinal artery* is the first intracranial branch. It passes inferiorly on the spinal medulla among dorsal roots of spinal nerves.
2. *Posterior inferior cerebellar artery* is the largest branch which arises from vertebral artery after it pierces the meninges. It pursues a tortuous course, passes between rootlets of hypoglossal, vagus and glossopharyngeal nerves; supplies almost lateral half of medulla as far as the lower border of pons, reaches its posterior aspect between the thin roof of cavity of fourth ventricle and cerebellum, gives a choroidal branch to

Plate 14.1: Branches of vertebral and basilar arteries (anterior view of brainstem)

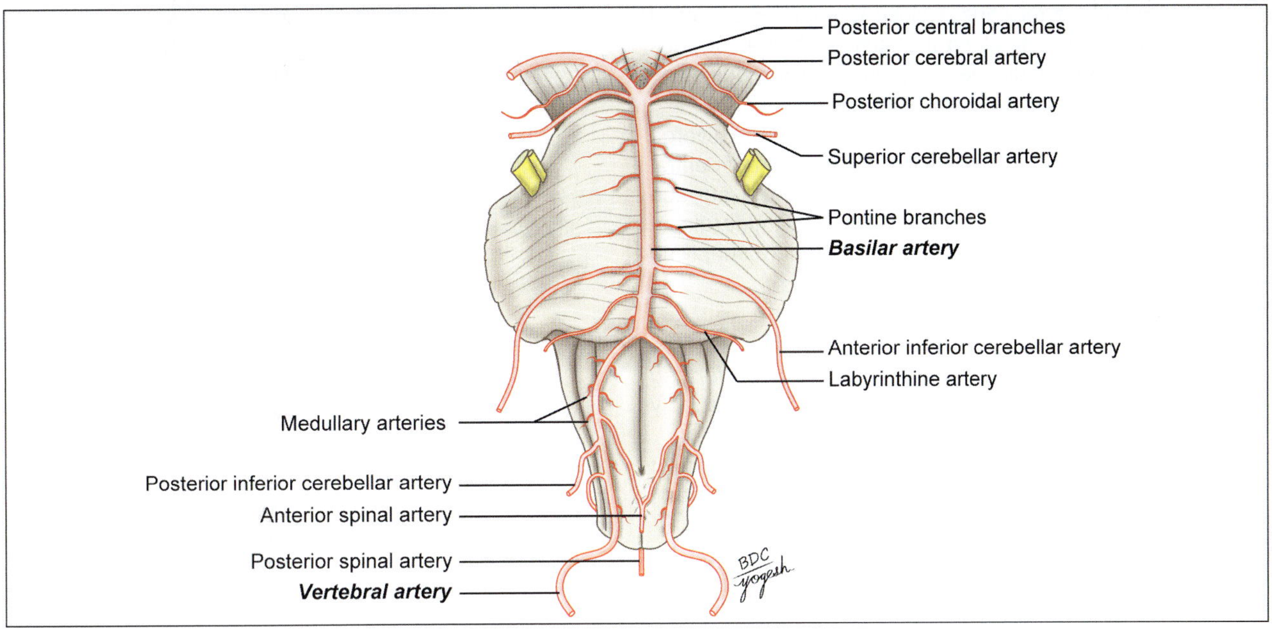

the choroid plexus of 4th ventricle and turns downwards on the cerebellum supplying it.

3. *Anterior spinal artery* is formed by the union of a branch from each vertebral artery on ventral surface of medulla oblongata close to the pons. It supplies the median part of medulla oblongata and continues inferiorly throughout the length of spinal medulla/cord.
4. *Medullary branches*: As vertebral artery ascends along medulla oblongata, it gives number of branches to the medulla oblongata.
5. *Meningeal branches* of vertebral artery supply the meninges.

BASILAR ARTERY

It is formed by the union of two vertebral arteries at the lower border of pons. It lies in the median groove of pons in *cisterna pontis* and at the upper border of pons ends by dividing into two posterior cerebral arteries (Plate 14.1 and Figs 14.3a and b).

Branches

1. Pontine branches
2. Anterior inferior cerebellar artery
3. Labyrinthine artery
4. Superior cerebellar artery
5. Posterior cerebral artery
   a. Posterior central branches
   b. Posterior choroid artery
   c. Cortical branches: Temporal, parieto-occipital, occipital, calcarine branches.

Note:

1. *Anterior inferior cerebellar artery* arises at the lower border of pons, and passes laterally, supplying the sixth, seventh and eighth cranial nerves. It then loops over the flocculus of cerebellum and supplies anteroinferior aspect of cerebellum.
2. *Labyrinthine artery* accompanies the vestibulocochlear nerve and enters the internal auditory meatus to supply the internal ear. It is an end artery.

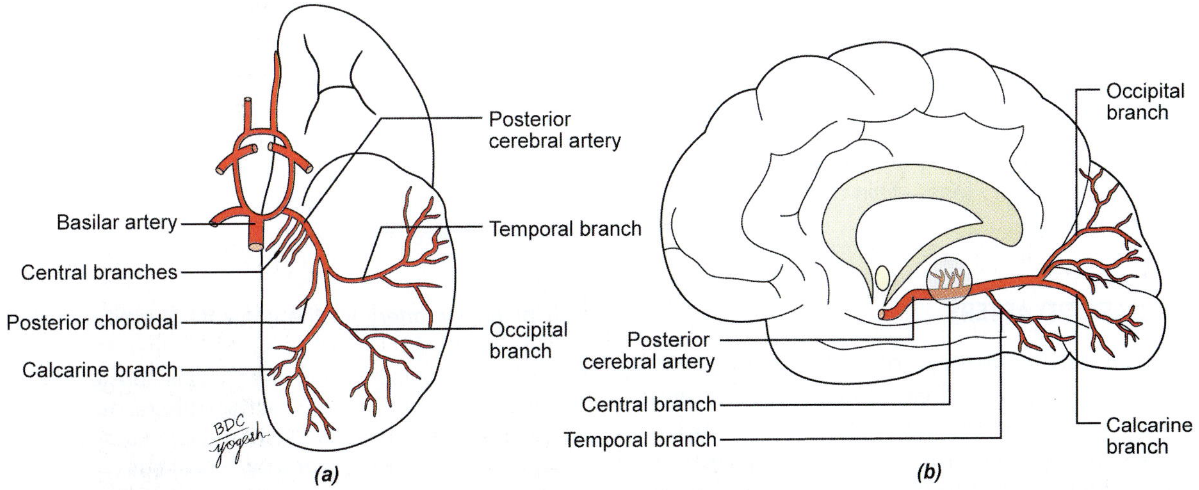

Figs 14.3a and b: Posterior cerebral artery on: (a) Inferior surface of left cerebral hemisphere and (b) medial surface of right cerebral hemisphere

3. *Pontine branches* are numerous slender branches that pierce the pons both in the medial and lateral parts.
4. *Superior cerebellar artery* arises close to superior border of pons. It winds posteriorly along the superior border of pons and middle cerebellar peduncle, supplying both. It sends many branches to the superior surface of cerebellum.
5. *Two terminal branches – posterior cerebral branches* diverge at upper border of pons*:* These give rise to number of central (posteromedial group) branches into the ventral surface of midbrain and then curve posterolateral to midbrain at inferomedial surface of corresponding hemisphere supplying it with cortical branches.

   Branches of posterior cerebral arteries

   a. *Posteromedial central branches* pierce ventral surface of base of brain, thus forming the *posterior perforated substance* in the interpeduncular fossa. These supply midbrain and caudal part of diencephalon.
   b. *Posterior choroidal artery* arises on the lateral aspect of central branches, supplies choroid plexus of the lateral ventricle and the third ventricle.
   c. *Cortical branches,* namely temporal branches, parietooccipital branch and occipital branch to cerebral cortex.

CLINICAL NEUROANATOMY

- Thrombosis of posterior cerebral artery results in homonymous hemianopia on the opposite side.
- Thrombosis of superior cerebellar artery results in:
  a. Cerebellum: Disturbed gait, limb ataxia (Fig. 14.4).
  b. Brainstem: Ipsilateral Horner's syndrome. Contralateral sensory loss—pain and temperature (including face).
- Damage to anterior inferior cerebellar artery results in (Fig. 14.5):
  a. Cerebellum: Ipsilateral limb ataxia.
  b. Brainstem: Ipsilateral Horner's syndrome.
  Sensory loss—pain and temperature of face.
  Facial weakness and paralysis of lateral gaze.
  Contralateral sensory loss—pain and temperature of limbs and trunk.
- Thrombosis of posterior inferior cerebellar artery causes damage as given in Fig. 14.6:
  a. Cerebellum: Dysarthria, ipsilateral limb ataxia, vertigo and nystagmus (due to damage to vestibulofloccular connections).
  b. Brainstem: Ipsilateral Horner's syndrome.
  Sensory loss—pain and temperature of face.
  Pharyngeal and laryngeal paralysis.
  Contralateral sensory loss—pain and temperature of limbs and trunk.

INTERNAL CAROTID ARTERY

Each internal carotid artery enters the cranial cavity after traversing the carotid canal and superior aspect of foramen lacerum. It then courses through the cavernous sinus, pierces the dural roof of sinus and ends immediately lateral to optic chiasma and inferior to anterior perforated substance and divides into middle and anterior cerebral arteries.

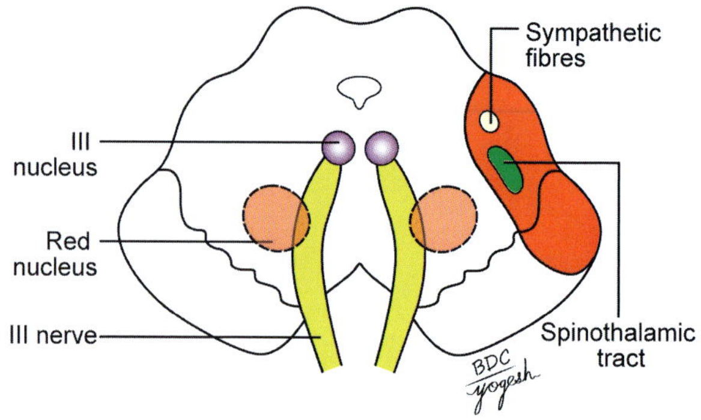

Fig. 14.4: Effects due to thrombosis of superior cerebellar artery

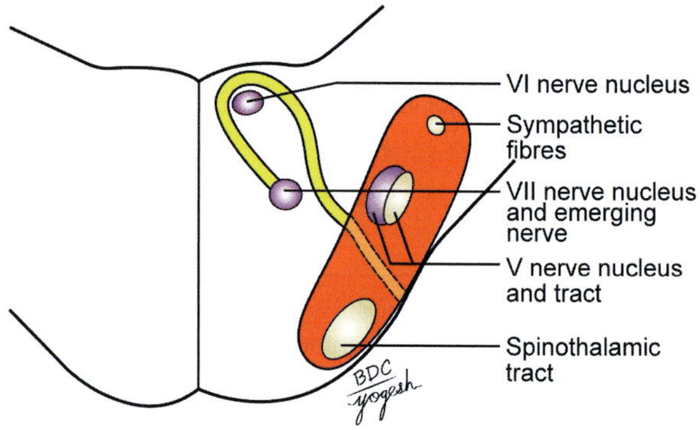

Fig. 14.5: Effects due to damage to anterior inferior cerebellar artery

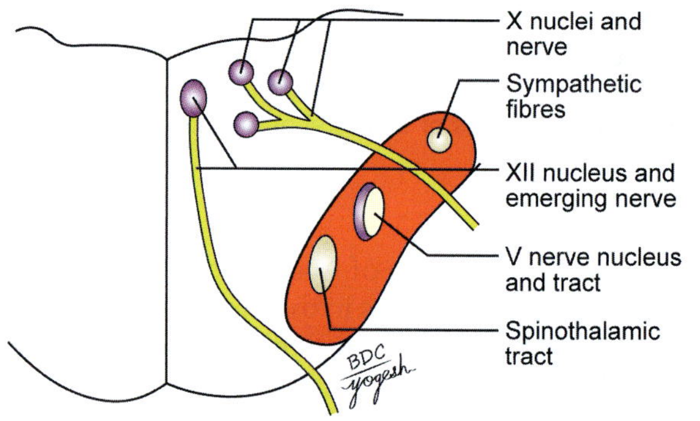

Fig. 14.6: Effects due to thrombosis of posterior inferior cerebellar artery

Branches

1. Ophthalmic artery
2. Anterior choroidal artery
3. Posterior communicating artery
4. Anterior cerebral artery
5. Middle cerebral artery.

Note:
1. *Ophthalmic artery* for the contents of orbit (For details, *see* Chapter 13, *BD Chaurasia's Human Anatomy, Volume 3*).
2. *Posterior communicating artery* passes posteriorly across the crus cerebri to join the posterior cerebral artery and helps to complete the arterial circle. It gives branches to the crus cerebri, optic tract, hypophysis and hypothalamus.
3. *Anterior choroidal artery* passes posterolaterally, supplies crus cerebri and turns laterally to the medial aspect of temporal lobe to supply choroid plexus of inferior horn of lateral ventricle.

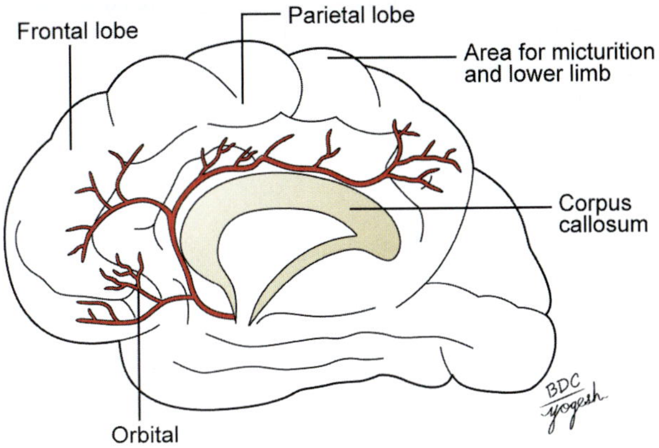

Fig. 14.7: Medial surface of right cerebral hemisphere with anterior cerebral artery

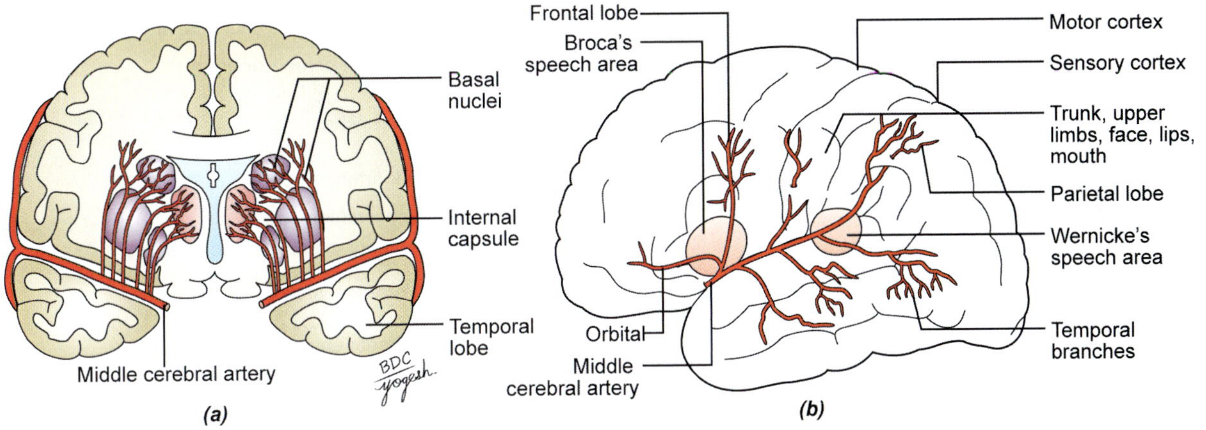

Figs 14.8a and b: (a) Deep branches of middle cerebral artery and (b) cortical branches of middle cerebral artery

4. *Anterior cerebral artery* is a terminal branch of internal carotid artery and runs above the optic nerve to follow the curve of corpus callosum. Close to its origin, this artery is joined by anterior communicating artery. Anteromedial central branches of anterior cerebral artery supply part of internal capsule and the basal nuclei. Cortical branches supply the medial surface of hemisphere by giving: Orbital, frontal, and parietal branches (Fig. 14.7).
5. *Middle cerebral artery* is the larger terminal branch of internal carotid artery that lies in line with the internal carotid artery (Figs 14.8a and b). It runs laterally in the stem of lateral sulcus. It gives off *deep or perforating branches* which supply anterior limb of internal capsule and part of basal nuclei. The artery then passes out to the lateral surface of hemisphere at the insula of the lateral sulcus. It ends by giving cortical branches to: Temporal lobe, frontal lobe, and parietal lobe.

Competency:
AN62.6 Describe and identify formation, branches and major areas of distribution of circle of Willis.

CIRCULUS ARTERIOSUS OR CIRCLE OF WILLIS

It is a hexagonal arterial circle, situated at the base of brain in the interpeduncular fossa (Figs 14.9 to 14.11).

Formation

- *Anteriorly*: Anterior communicating artery joining the two anterior cerebral arteries

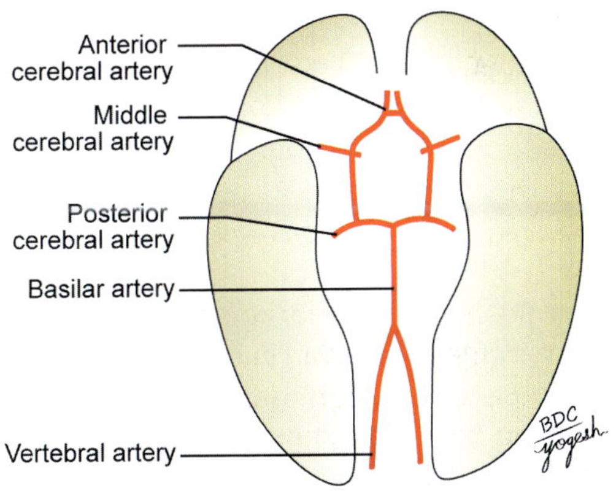

Fig. 14.9: Arteries seen on the inferior surface of brain

- *Anterolaterally*: Anterior cerebral arteries
- *Laterally*: Internal carotid arteries
- *Posterolaterally*: Posterior communicating arteries
- *Posteriorly*: Posterior cerebral arteries.

Note: Middle cerebral artery is not forming the circle of Willis.

Functional Significance

The circulus arteriosus attempts to equalize the flow of blood to different parts of brain and provides a collateral circulation in the event of obstruction to one of its components. There is hardly any mixing of bloodstreams on right and left sides of the circulus arteriosus.

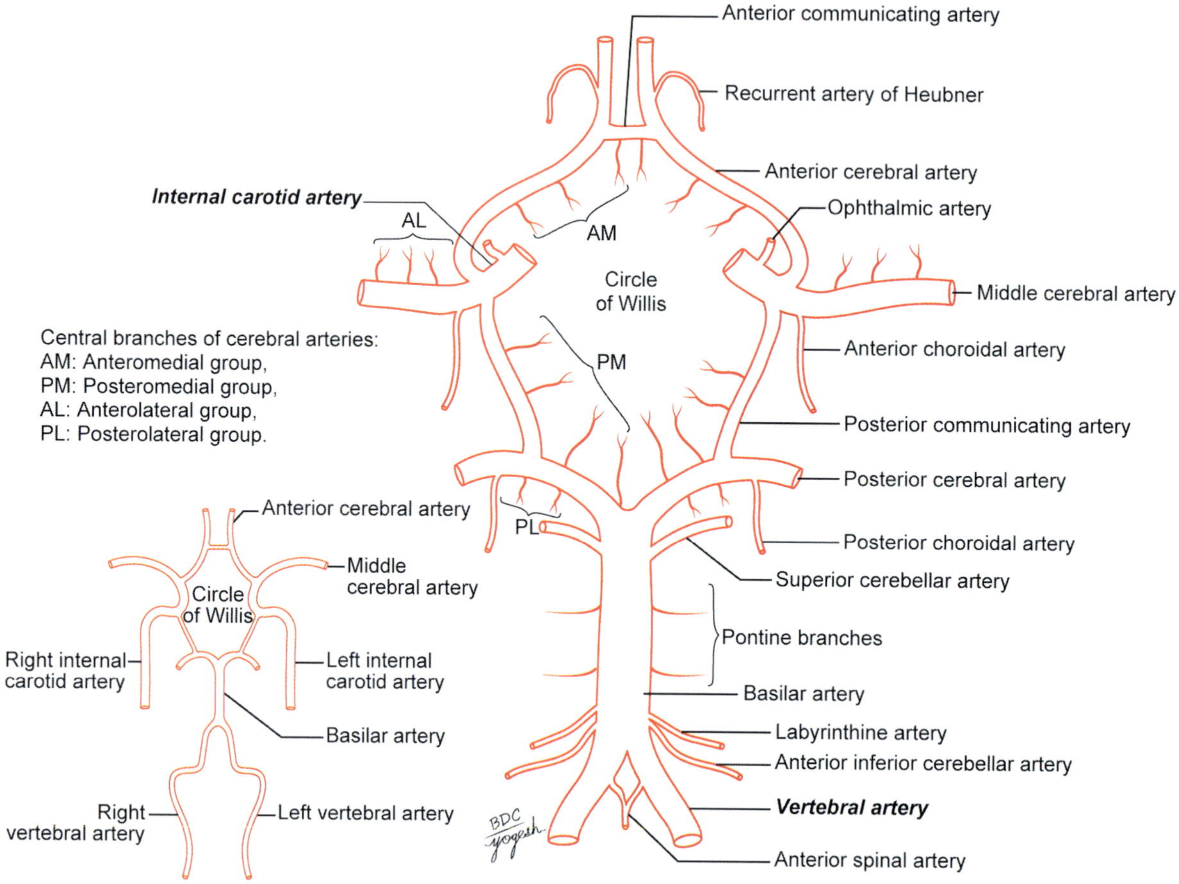

Fig. 14.10: Circle of Willis and the branches of arteries supplying the brain

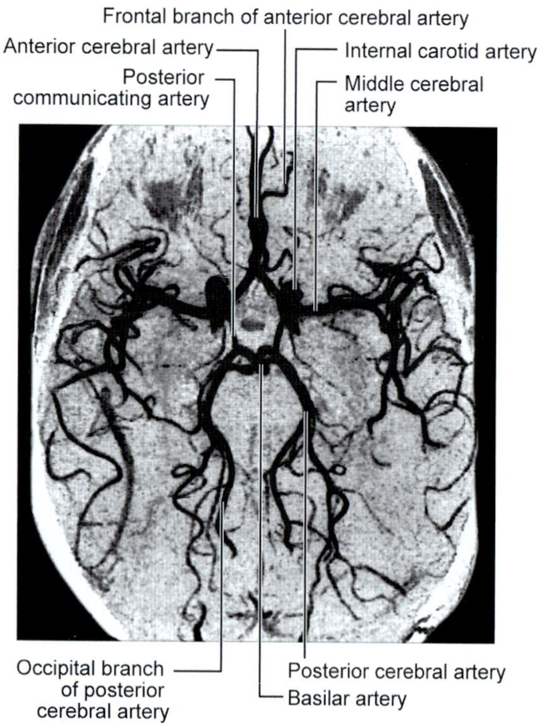

Fig. 14.11: Magnetic resonance angiogram of the cerebral blood vessels

Branches

The branches of the circulus arteriosus are cortical, central and choroidal.

1. Cortical branches run on the surface of cerebral hemispheres (Table 14.1).
2. Central branches perforate the white matter to supply thalamus, basal ganglia, and internal capsule. These are grouped as follows:
   - Anteromedial group
   - Two anterolateral groups
   - Posteromedial group
   - Two posterolateral groups.
3. Choroidal branches supply the choroid plexuses of the various ventricles. These are:
   - Anterior choroidal is a branch of internal carotid artery.
   - Posterior choroidal is a branch of posterior cerebral artery.

[*Mnemonics:* ***Cell is Clearly Circulating:*** **C** – Cortical branches; **C** – Central branches; **C** – Choroidal branches]

Important arteries of the brain are shown in Table 14.1.

Note:
The cortical branches anastomose freely and if these get blocked, they give rise to small infarcts.

The central branches do not anastomose and if these get blocked, they give rise to large infarcts.

Central Branches

1. *Anteromedial (AM) group* arises as one group from both anterior cerebral and anterior communicating arteries. These enter the medial most part of anterior perforated substance to supply anterior part of lentiform nucleus and head of caudate nucleus.

TABLE 14.1: Important arteries of brain

Artery	*Origin*	*Course*	*Cortical branches*
Middle cerebral	Largest and direct continuation of ICA	In the lateral sulcus and on the insula	1. Orbital 2. Frontal 3. Parietal 4. Temporal
Anterior cerebral	Smaller terminal branch of ICA	Follow the curve of the corpus callosum. Two arteries are connected by the anterior communicating artery	1. Orbital 2. Frontal 3. Parietal, including paracentral artery
Posterior cerebral	Terminal branch of basilar artery	Winds around cerebral peduncle to reach the tentorial surface of cerebrum	1. Temporal 2. Occipital 3. Parieto-occipital

The branch to head of caudate nucleus is called recurrent artery of Heubner. It also supplies rostral part of internal capsule.

2. *Anterolateral group* arises in two groups—one group from each middle cerebral artery. These pierce the anterior perforated substance and supply the corpus striatum and the internal capsule. These branches are called lateral striate arteries. One of the lateral striate branches is larger than the others and is called Charcot's artery of cerebral haemorrhage.
3. *The posteromedial (PM) group* arises as *one group* from posterior communicating and posterior cerebral arteries. These supply tuberoinfundibular and mammillary regions of hypothalamus, subthalamus, anterior and medial parts of thalamus, medial part of tegmentum and crus cerebri of midbrain.
4. *Posterolateral (PL) group* arises as *two groups* from the lateral parts of each posterior cerebral artery. These supply caudal part of thalamus.

Choroidal Branches

1. The anterior choroidal is a branch of internal carotid artery. It supplies blood to choroid plexus of inferior horn of lateral ventricle.
2. Posterior choroidal artery arises from posterior cerebral artery to give branches for the choroid plexus of rest of lateral ventricle including third ventricle.
3. Posterior inferior cerebellar artery supplies the choroid plexus of the fourth ventricle.

ARTERIAL SUPPLY OF DIFFERENT AREAS

Cerebral cortex is supplied by branches from all three arteries (Figs 14.12a to c).

Superolateral surface: This surface is mostly supplied by middle cerebral. Areas *not* supplied by this artery are as under:

i. A strip of about 2 cm wide along the superomedial border extending from frontal pole to the parieto-occipital sulcus is supplied by anterior cerebral artery.
ii. Area of occipital lobe is supplied by posterior cerebral artery.
iii. Inferior temporal gyrus excluding the part of the temporal pole is also supplied by posterior cerebral artery.
iv. Rest of the big area is supplied by middle cerebral artery.

Medial and tentorial surfaces: The main artery here is the anterior cerebral. The medial aspects of the occipital lobe, temporal lobe except area around temporal pole is supplied by posterior cerebral artery. Temporal pole area gets nourished by middle cerebral artery.

Inferior surface: Medial one-third of orbital surface is supplied by anterior cerebral, while lateral two-thirds, including the temporal pole area and anterior most part of tentorial surface is vascularised by middle cerebral artery. Rest of the tentorial surface is supplied by the posterior cerebral artery.

Cerebral Cortex

Cerebral cortex is supplied by branches of all three cerebral arteries. All the three surfaces receive branches from all three arteries.

Middle cerebral is main artery on superolateral surface.

Anterior cerebral artery is chief artery on medial surface.

Posterior cerebral is the principal artery on inferior surface.

Cerebellum

The little brain is supplied by the following arteries (Fig. 14.13):

1. Superior cerebellar
2. Anterior inferior cerebellar
3. Posterior inferior cerebellar.

BLOOD–BRAIN BARRIER (BBB)

The constituents of CSF are not exactly the same as those of extracellular fluid (ECF) elsewhere in the body. Many large molecular substances hardly pass from blood to CSF or interstitial fluids of brain even though these can pass to ECF of the body, thereby reflecting the existence of BBB (Fig. 14.14).

Components

The existence of a 'blood–brain barrier' (BBB or haematoencephalic barrier) is because the endothelial cells of brain capillaries are held to each other by tight junctions. The BBB is formed by structures between the blood and nerve cells of brain. The blood in the lumen of the capillary is separated from the neurons by:

a. Capillary endothelium
b. Basement membrane of endothelium

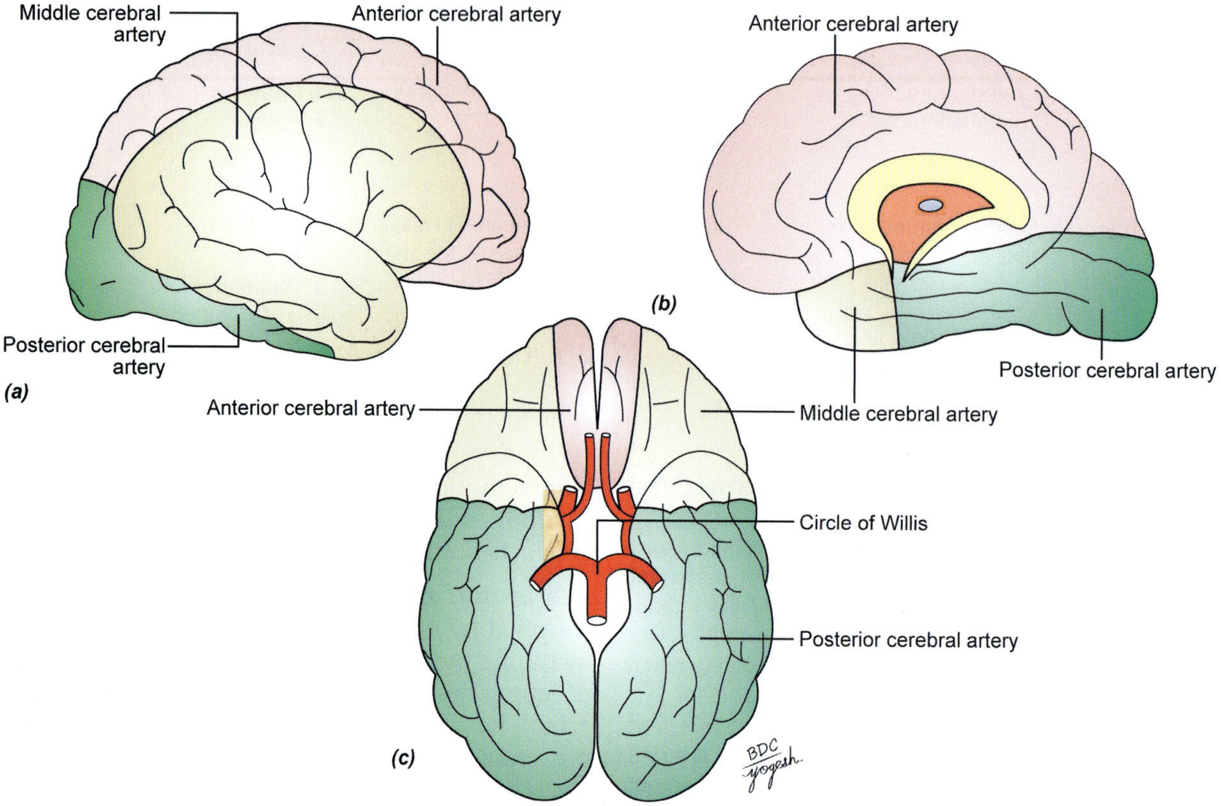

Figs 14.12a to c: Arterial supply of cerebral hemisphere: (a) Superolateral surface, (b) medial and tentorial surfaces, and (c) inferior surface

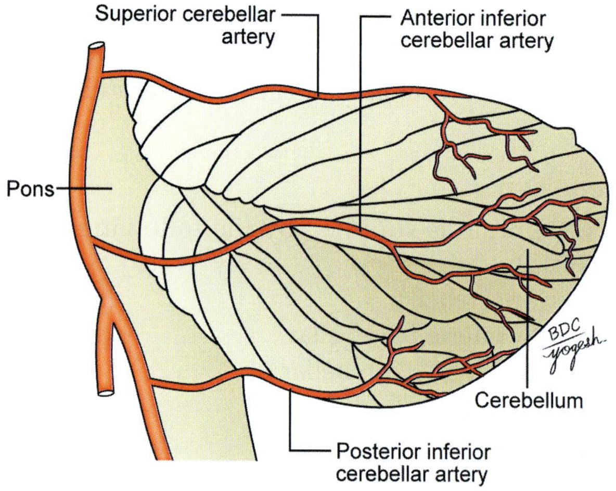

Fig. 14.13: Arterial supply of cerebellum

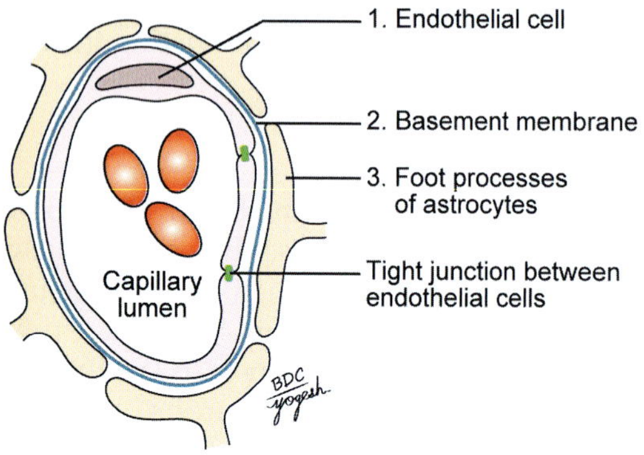

Fig. 14.14: Blood–brain barrier

c. Intimately applied to the capillaries, there are numerous processes of astrocytes and it has been estimated that these processes cover about 80% of the capillary surface.

Functions of Blood–Brain Barrier

1. To modulate entry of metabolic substrates, notably glucose.
2. It allows entry of gases, water, electrolytes, amino acids and lipid-soluble substances.
3. It restricts entry of macromolecules, i.e. lipid insoluble substances and thus blocks entry of toxins as either these are bound to the plasma albumin or their solubilities are inappropriate.
4. It blocks entry of transmitters from blood, notably of epinephrine.
5. The drugs like penicillin, noradrenaline and thiopentone cannot cross it.
6. Some drugs like atropine, chloramphenicol, tetracycline and sulphas cross the barrier easily.
7. Its other important function is to pump ions—notably potassium into and out of the blood.
8. Entry of hormones is restricted to certain places only, so that normal biological rhythm of the body is maintained.

Note: Some areas of brain are devoid of blood–brain barrier. These include pineal body, hypophysis cerebri, choroid plexuses and area postrema in fourth ventricle of brain. BBB exists in newborn but is more permeable to certain substances than it is in adult.

PERIVASCULAR SPACES

1. The ***perivascular spaces (Virchow-Robin)*** are extensions of subarachnoid space around vessels penetrating the brain surface. The spaces taper progressively. Although these are inward extensions in anatomical sense. The subarachnoid and perivascular spaces are separated by a thin layer of pia mater. The flow of extracellular fluid is outward into the subarachnoid space.

   The perivascular spaces are involved in autoregulation of brain arterioles which regulates the blood supply to tissues.
2. The chief internal source of autoregulation is the adjustment of arterial muscle tone in response to intraluminal pressure changes. Cerebral blood flow remains at 60–70 ml/100 g/min during systemic blood pressure; changes ranging from 80 to 180 mm Hg. This is achieved by a direct myogenic response to distension produced by rising intraluminal pressure.
3. The H^+ ion concentration in the perivascular space is the chief external source of autoregulation of cerebral blood vessels. A rising H^+ (usually following hypercapnia—excess plasma CO_2) travels along perivascular space from the capillary bed and it inhibits vascular muscle, perhaps by reducing ionized calcium level. On the other hand, hypocapnia causes vasoconstriction.

CLINICAL NEUROANATOMY

- Thrombosis of lateral striate branches of middle cerebral artery causes motor and sensory loss to most of the opposite side of body.
- Hemiplegia is a common condition. It is an upper motor neuron type of paralysis of one-half of the body, including the face. It is usually due to an internal capsule lesion caused by thrombosis of one of the lateral striate branches of middle cerebral artery (cerebral thrombosis) (Fig. 14.15). One of the lateral striate branches is most frequently ruptured (cerebral haemorrhage); it is known as ***Charcot's artery of cerebral haemorrhage***. This lesion also produces hemiplegia with deep coma, and is ultimately fatal.
- Thrombosis of Heubner's recurrent branch of the anterior cerebral artery causes contralateral upper limb monoplegia.
- Occlusion of anterior cerebral artery proximal to the anterior communicating artery is normally well tolerated because of the cross flow.
- Distal occlusion of anterior cerebral artery results in weakness and cortical sensory loss in the contralateral lower limb with associated incontinence (Figs 14.16a and b). This artery supplies the area of lower limb and perineum.
- Thrombosis of the paracentral artery (terminal cortical branch of the anterior cerebral artery) causes contralateral lower limb monoplegia.

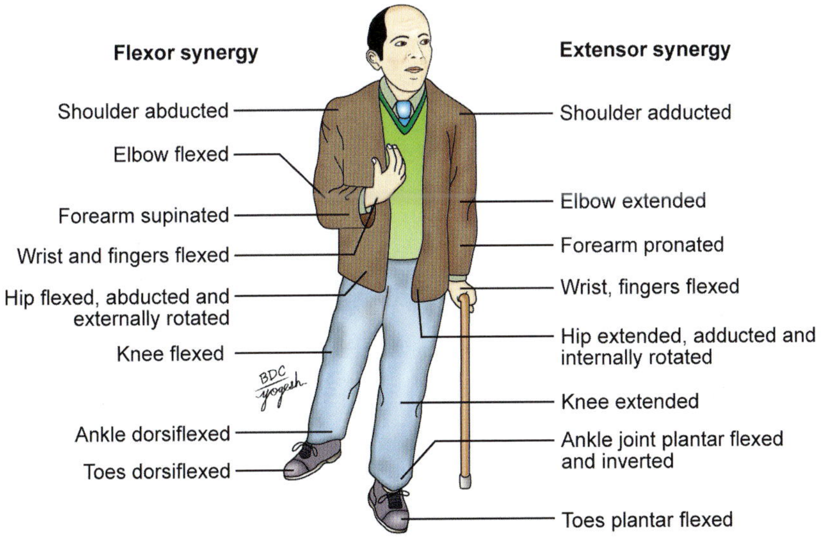

Fig. 14.15: Posture of hemiplegic person

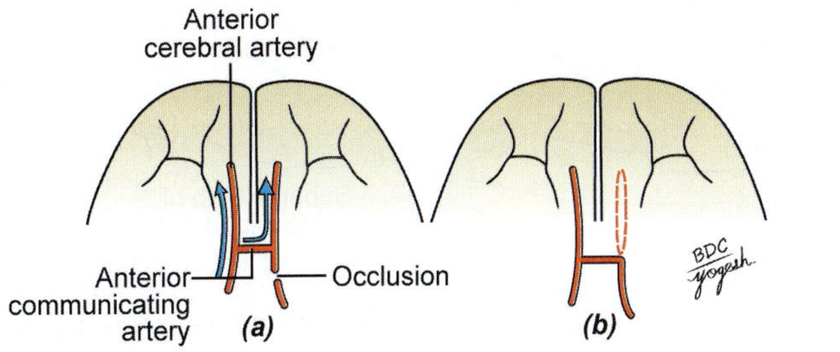

Figs 14.16a and b: Effects of occlusion of anterior cerebral artery

VEINS OF THE BRAIN

Characteristics of the Veins of Brain

1. The walls are devoid of muscle.
2. The veins have no valves.
3. To maintain patency, some of them open into the cranial venous sinuses against the direction of blood flow in the sinus, e.g. the superior cerebral veins draining into the superior sagittal sinus.

Groups of Veins (Figs 14.17 to 14.19)

External Cerebral Veins

1. ***Superior cerebral veins:*** These are 6 to 12 in number. They drain the superolateral surface of the hemisphere. They terminate in the superior sagittal sinus.
2. ***Superficial middle cerebral vein:*** This drains the area around the posterior ramus of the lateral sulcus. It terminates in the cavernous sinus, or at times into the sphenoparietal sinus. Through the superior and inferior anastomotic veins, it communicates with the superior sagittal and transverse sinuses. It also communicates with the deep middle cerebral vein.
3. ***Deep middle cerebral vein:*** This drains the surface of the insula and terminates in the basal vein.
4. ***Inferior cerebral veins:*** These are several in number. They are divided into orbital and tentorial veins. The orbital veins terminate in the superior cerebral veins or in the superior sagittal sinus. The tentorial veins terminate in the cavernous or any other surrounding sinus.
5. ***Anterior cerebral veins:*** These are small veins which drain the corpus callosum and the anterior part of the medial surface of the hemisphere. They terminate in the basal vein (Fig. 14.19).

Internal Cerebral Veins

There is one vein on each side. It is formed by the union of the thalamostriate and choroidal veins at the apex of the tela choroidea of the third ventricle. The right and left veins run posteriorly parallel to each other in the tela choroidea, and unite together to form the great cerebral vein below the splenium of the corpus callosum (Fig. 14.20). Great cerebral vein joins with inferior sagittal sinus to form straight sinus which forms left transverse sinus. It continues as left sigmoid sinus to continue as internal jugular vein on left side.

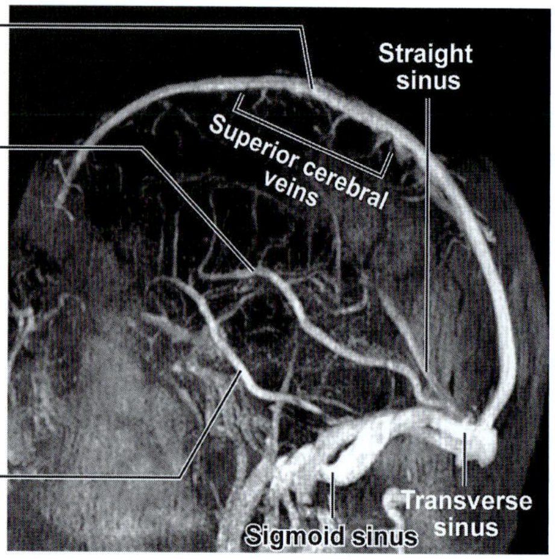

Fig. 14.18: MRI of veins of brain

Terminal Veins

1. ***Great cerebral vein of Galen:*** This is a single median vein. It is formed by union of the two internal cerebral veins. It terminates in the straight sinus. Its tributaries include the basal veins, and veins from the pineal body, the colliculi, the cerebellum and the adjoining part of the occipital lobes of the cerebrum.
2. ***Basal vein:*** There is one vein on each side. It is formed at the anterior perforated substance by the union of the deep middle cerebral vein, the anterior cerebral veins, and the striate veins. It runs posteriorly, winds round the cerebral peduncle, and terminates by joining the great cerebral vein. Its tributaries include (apart from the veins forming it) small veins from the cerebral peduncle, interpeduncular structures, the tectum of the midbrain, and the parahippocampal gyrus.
3. Ultimately, all veins drain into the various cranial venous sinuses which, in turn, drain into the internal jugular vein.

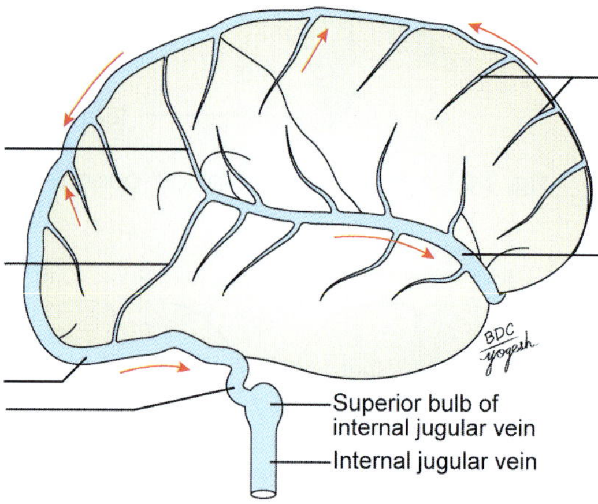

Fig. 14.17: Veins on the superolateral surface of the cerebral hemisphere (right lateral view, red arrows indicate direction of blood flow)

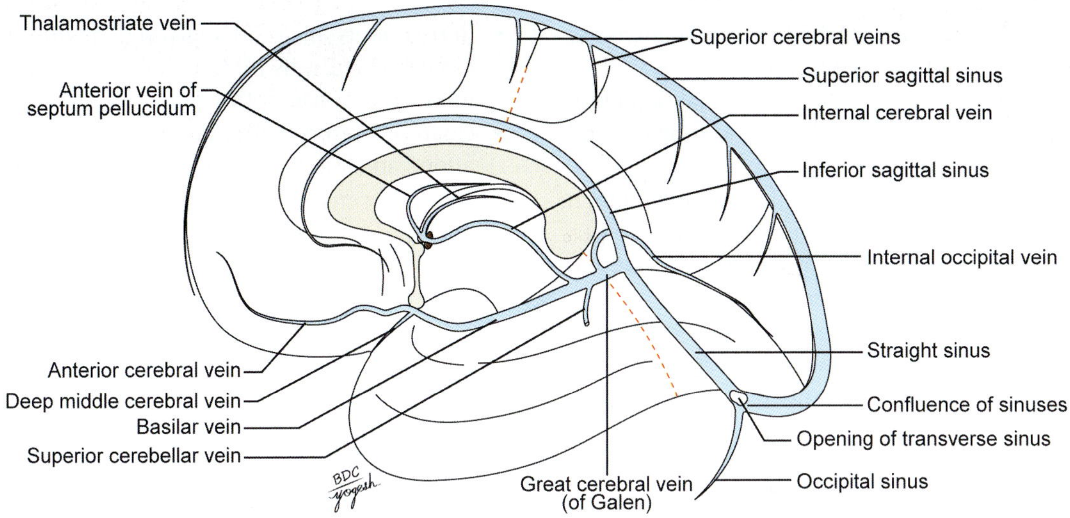

Fig. 14.19: Veins on the medial surface of right cerebral hemisphere

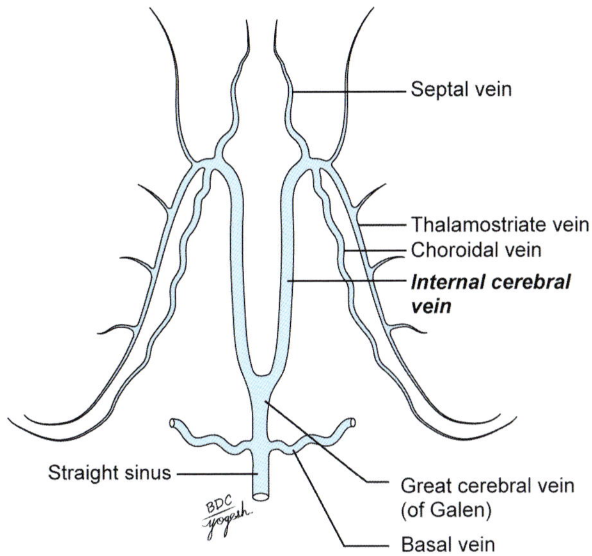

Fig. 14.20: Internal cerebral veins

BLOOD SUPPLY OF THE BRAINSTEM

Midbrain: The midbrain is supplied by branches from the posterior cerebral arteries, including their central branches, both posteromedial and posterolateral.

Pons: The pons is supplied by the pontine branches of basilar artery.

Medulla: The medulla is supplied by:

a. The medullary branches of the vertebral artery.
b. Branches from the posterior inferior cerebellar artery.

The veins of the brainstem drain into neighbouring venous sinuses.

CLINICAL NEUROANATOMY

- ***Anastomotic and end arteries***: In the circle of Willis, the blood in the three communicating arteries is normally static. Following occlusion of one of the three large arteries contributing to the circle, the other two compensate more or less completely, via communicating arteries. With occlusion of one internal carotid, the other internal carotid may perfuse both anterior cerebral arteries. With occlusion of basilar, each posterior cerebral artery may be perfused by the internal carotid of its own side.

  Further anastomosis occurs between cortical branches of cerebral arteries, prior to perforation of the branches into brain substance. Once the cortical and central branches perforate, they become end arteries hardly communicating at capillary level.
- ***Cerebral vascular disease*** is quite common in old age and manifest in different ways.
  a. Haemorrhage—cortical or subcortical
  b. Thrombosis
  c. Embolism.
- Hypertensive encephalopathy is a manifestation of sustained elevation of diastolic blood pressure in the form of multiple diffuse small lesions distributed all over, result in a variegated picture of the circle of Willis (***Berry's aneurysm***).
- The arteries of the brain are supplied with sympathetic nerves which run onto them from carotid and vertebral plexuses. They are extremely sensitive to injury and readily react by passing into prolonged spasms. This by itself may be sufficient to cause damage to brain tissue since even the least sensitive neurons cannot withstand absolute loss of blood supply for a period more than 3–7 minutes.

VIDEO

Video 4.11 **Blood Supply of Brain**

Facts to Remember

- Posterior inferior cerebellar artery is the largest branch of vertebral artery. It supplies posterolateral part of medulla oblongata, lower part of pons, inferior surface of cerebellum including choroidal branches to 4th ventricle.

- Posterior cerebral arteries are the terminal branches of the basilar artery and supply the visual cortex.
- Middle cerebral artery is the larger terminal branch of internal carotid and supplies most of the superolateral surface of the cerebral cortex.
- Anterior cerebral artery is the smaller terminal branch of the internal carotid artery. It runs along the corpus callosum supplying maximum area on the medial surface of the cerebral hemisphere.
- Two lobes of the cerebellum are supplied by 3 pairs of cerebellar arteries. These are superior cerebellar, anterior inferior cerebellar and posterior inferior cerebellar arteries.
- Carotid siphon is the hair-pin bend of the internal carotid artery within the cranial cavity.
- Berry aneurysms is a localized dilatation of arteries of circle of Willis. Its rupture is the commonest cause of intracerebral haemorrhage.
- Charcot's artery is the largest lateral (lenticulostriate artery) and known as a artery of cerebral haemorrhage.
- Artery of cerebral thrombosis is the anterior choroidal artery.

BDC's Anatomy *e*-book

1. Anterior Spinal Artery Syndrome
2. Further reading
3. Viva voce questions.

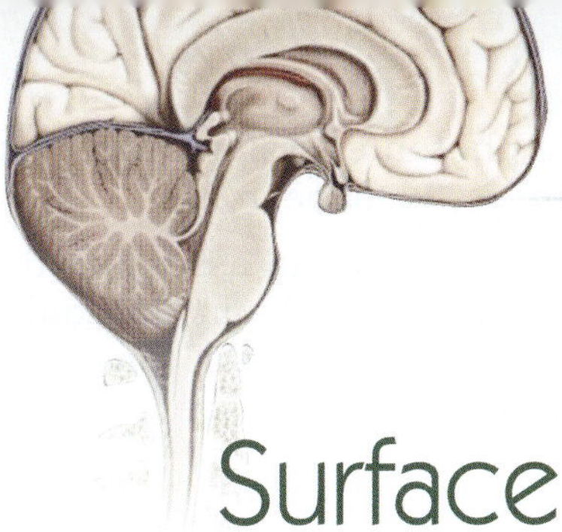

Chapter

15

Surface Marking and Radiological Anatomy of Nervous System

SURFACE MARKING

The surface anatomy of brain is important in clinical examination for assessing the location of injury and for planning and performing neurosurgery.

Borders of Cerebral Hemisphere

Mark the following points (Fig. 15.1):

Point 1: Just superolateral to inion

Point 2: Just superolateral to nasion

Point 3: At the zygomatic process of frontal bone

Point 4: At pterion

Point 5: At the middle of the upper border of zygomatic arch.

For superomedial border: Join points 1 and 2 by a paramedian line.

For superciliary border: Join points 2 and 3 by upward arched line and extend this line to point 4.

For inferolateral border: Join points 4 and 5 with curved line (convex forward) and then join points 1 and 5 by upward convex line, passing above the external acoustic meatus.

Sulci of Cerebrum

Central sulcus

Mark the following points (Fig. 15.2):

Point 1: At 1.2 cm behind the midpoint of the line joining the nasion with the inion.

Point 2: At 7.5 cm above preauricular point.

For *central sulcus*, draw S-shaped line from point 1 to point 2 running downward and forward making on the angle of 70° with the median plane.

Lateral sulcus

Mark the following points (Fig. 15.3):

Point A: At pterion

Point B: 2 cm below the parietal eminence.

For *lateral sulcus*, point A represents sylvian point and it represents the *stem of the lateral sulcus*.

For the *posterior ramus of the lateral sulcus*, mark 7 cm long line by joining points A and B.

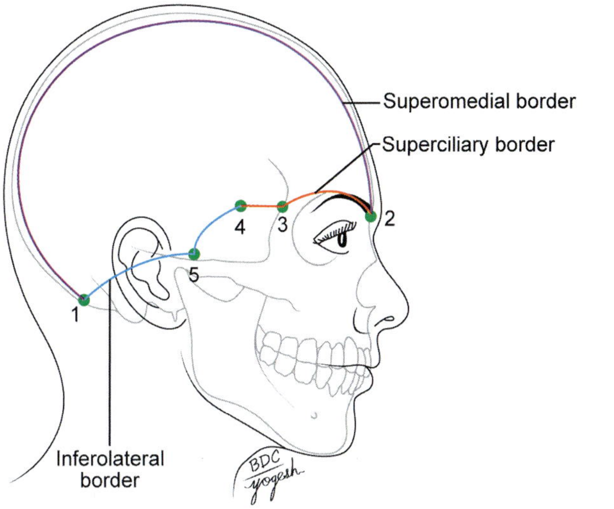

Fig. 15.1: Surface marking of the borders of cerebral hemisphere

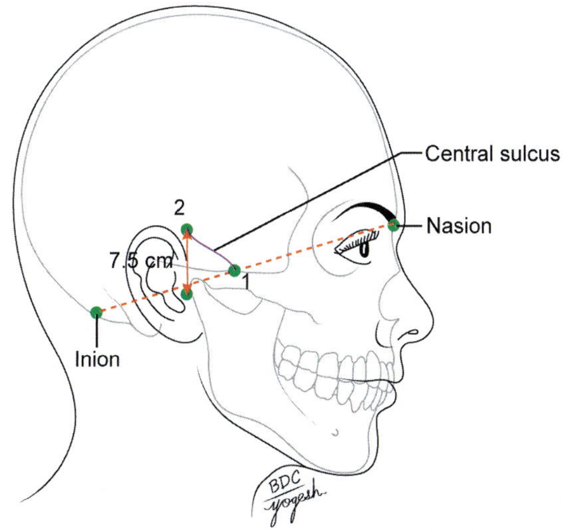

Fig. 15.2: Surface marking of the central sulcus

Functional Areas of Cerebrum (Fig. 15.4)

1. *Motor area:* It is marked by 1 cm wide strip in front of the posterior ramus of lateral sulcus (finger broad).
2. *Sensory area:* It is marked by 1 cm wide strip behind the posterior ramus of lateral sulcus.

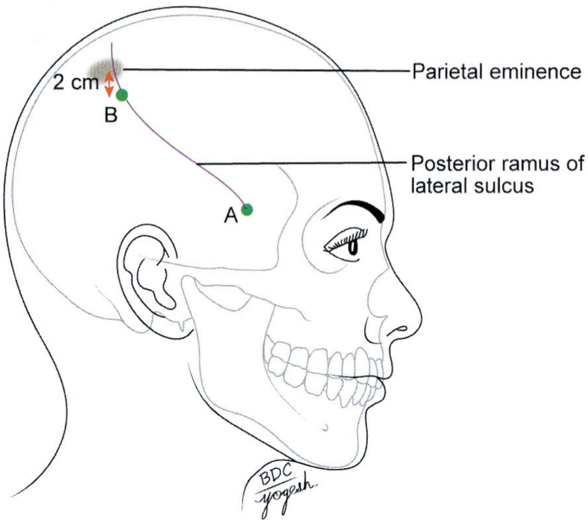

Fig. 15.3: Surface marking of the posterior ramus of lateral sulcus (right lateral view)

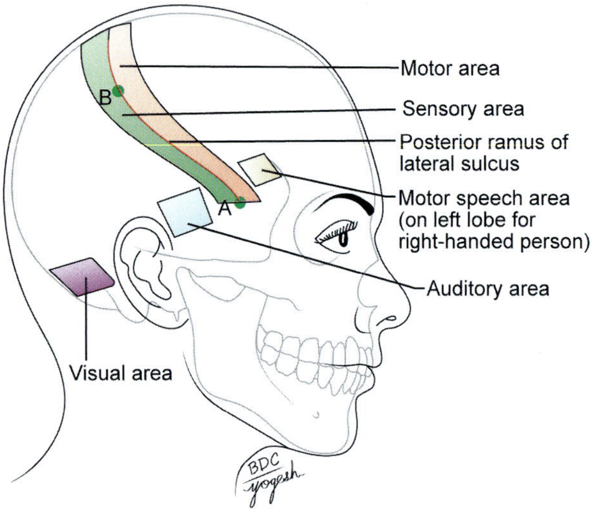

Fig. 15.4: Surface marking of the functional areas of the cerebral cortex (right lateral view)

3. *Motor speech area*: It is marked on the left (in right handed person) just above and anterior to the pterion.
4. *Auditory area*: It is marked little above and anterior to the auricle and below the posterior ramus of the lateral sulcus.
5. *Visual area*: It is marked on each side above the external occipital protuberance.

RADIOLOGICAL ANATOMY OF THE BRAIN

IMAGING OF CNS

The imaging of central nervous system is important for diagnosis and treatment of a patient with neurological disorders. Plain radiograph of skull and spine is still basic primary investigation, and they provide many important information in CNS disorders.

Computerised tomography (CT) scan and magnetic resonance imaging (MRI), positron emission tomography (PET scan) and single photon emission computed tomography (SPECT) are useful for neuroimaging.

Functional neuroimaging: It helps in assessing the metabolic and functional activities of brain. It includes EEG (electroencephalography), PET scan, functional MRI, SPECT scan and magnetic resonance spectrography (MRS).

The imaging modalities are useful for:

1. Diagnosis or detection of intracranial tumours, injuries, degenerative diseases, and infections.
2. For detection of activities and functioning of entire brain or a particular area of the brain.
3. To measure the level of different metabolites in the brain or detect metabolic disorders.
4. To determine the neurotransmitter activity in a specific part of brain.

Imaging with Plain X-ray

The anteroposterior (AP), lateral and Towne's (fronto-occipital) views give idea about (Fig. 15.5):

1. Skull bones, bone erosion, fractures, vascular markings
2. Aneurysm of vessels
3. Neurological tumours such as neurogliomas, meningiomas
4. Sites of calcifications – pineal gland, choroid plexus
5. Midline shift.

Imaging with X-ray Contrast Media

A *contrast media* containing *iodine* or *barium* is injected in the ventricles of brain or in subarachnoid space or blood vessels and radiograph is taken. These *contrast radiographs* are as follows:

1. *Myelography* – the contrast media is injected into spinal subarachnoid space.
2. Ventriculography – the contrast media is injected into ventricles of brain
3. Cerebral angiography (carotid or vertebral).

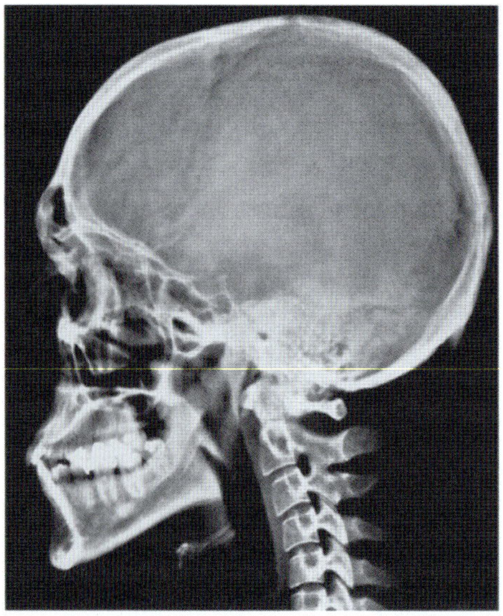

Fig. 15.5: Lateral view of skull and cervical vertebrae

Ultrasonography (USG)

It is noninvasive, painless and a safe imaging technique. *Contrast media* is a substance that is introduced into a part of body (blood vessels or ventricles of brain) to improve the visibility of internal structure during radiography.

Uses:

1. For assessing foetal CNS development
2. For detecting midline shift
3. Doppler effect is useful for assessing blood flow through carotid arteries
4. Postnatally, USG is useful before closure of fontanelle.

Computerised Tomography or CT Scan

It is noninvasive radiographic imaging. It provides more detailed information than plain radiographs. It gives sectional views of brain. These images can be assembled to produce three-dimensional images.

Scale in CT scan: The structures are seen ranging from back, grey to white in colour as follows:

Black colour → air → fat → water → CSF → white matter → grey matter → blood → bone → metal → white colour. Thus, the bones look white, ventricles and CSF look black, and soft tissue has variable shades of grey colour.

Cranial CT scan gives information about size and shape of ventricles of brain, size of brain tissue, injuries, hematoma, calcified tissues, tumours, infarction, abscess, and encephalitis (Fig. 15.6).

Spinal CT scan gives information of intervertebral disc, spinal cord injury, subarachnoid space (with injection of contrast media).

Magnetic Resonance Imaging (MRI)

In MRI, the body is exposed to high energy magnetic field and using radiowaves, the sectional images are captured. MRI gives higher details of soft tissues and less hazardous than CT scan (Fig. 15.7). It provides good contrast between grey and white matters. MRI takes 30 to 40 minutes for imaging whereas CT scan takes only 5 minutes. MRI cannot be done in patients with artificial joints, eye implants, intrauterine devices and pacemakers.

MRI is useful in detection of tumours of brain, developmental anomalies, vascular aneurysm, stroke, trauma, disease of pituitary gland, multiple sclerosis, and so on.

Positron Emission Tomography (PET)

In the PET scan, radioactively labeled, metabolically active chemical is injected in bloodstream. Then, the emission of *positron-emitting radioactive isotopes* is measured and images of brain created. Based on the tissue activity, the images show (Fig. 15.8): Black – rainbow colours – red colour.

Black or darkest violet indicates absence of activity and red indicates very high activity. The PET scan is useful in detection of *cancers*. It is useful in detection

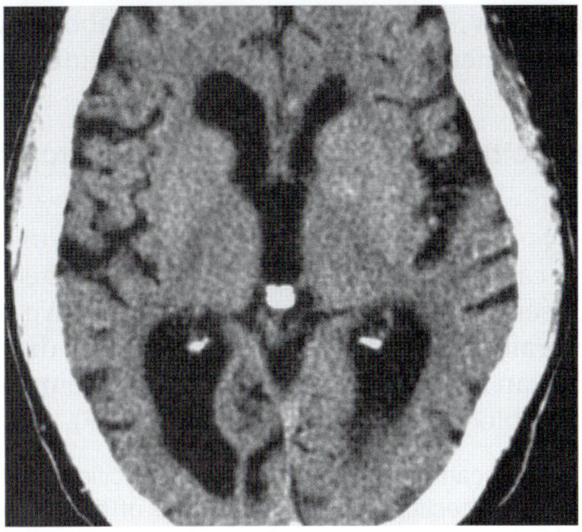

Fig. 15.6: Computerised tomography (CT) scan

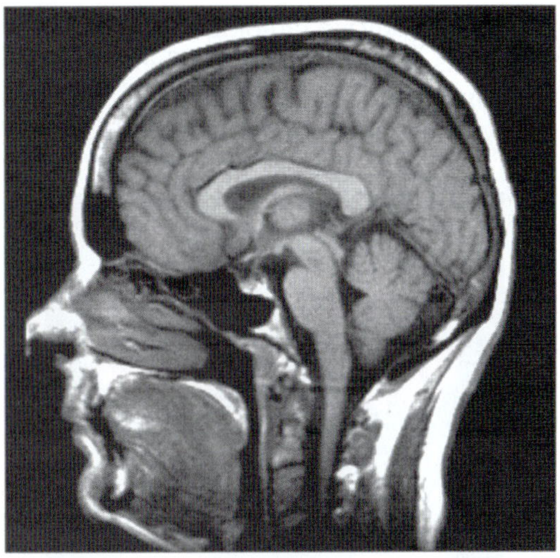

Fig. 15.7: Magnetic resonance imaging (MRI)

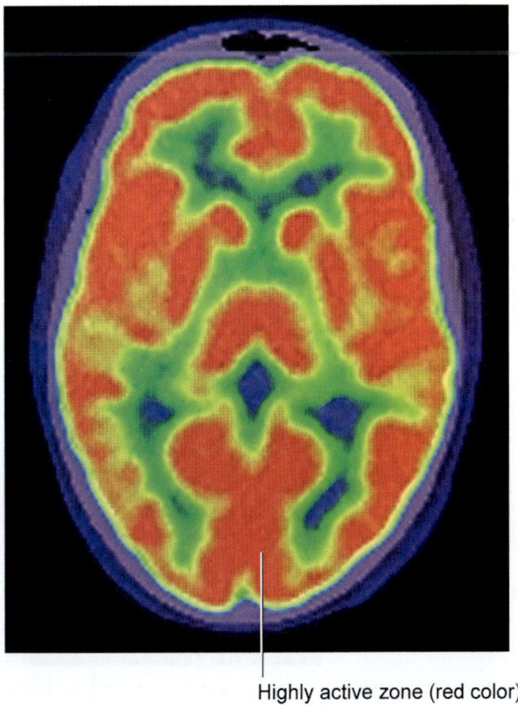

Fig. 15.8: Positron emission tomography (PET) scan (*Image courtesy*: Dr Abhijeet Taori)

of blood flow, oxygen and glucose metabolism, brain activity, dementia/Alzheimer's disease, and ischemic areas.

Single Photon Emission Computed Tomography (SPECT)

It uses *gamma-ray-emitting radioisotopes*. It is useful for *epilepsy* cases. The radioactive tracer is injected at the time of seizure, and it is taken-up by the active regions of the brain. The taken-up tracer does not distribute. Hence, scan is done after termination of seizure. SPECT measures blood flow to the brain (Fig. 15.9).

Note: The CT scan is useful for detection of calcified pineal gland and also for detection of dilated ventricle of brain in case of hydrocephalus (Figs 15.10 and 15.11).

Cerebral Angiography

Cerebral angiography is a radiological technique by which cerebral vessels can be visualised. The arterial system is visualised by carotid angiography (Fig. 15.12), and the vertebral system by vertebral angiography (Fig. 15.13).

Dye: About 10 to 12 ml of 30% pyelocil or diodone.

Technique: For carotid angiography, the common carotid artery is located at the carotid tubercle and the dye is injected percutaneously. A series of skiagrams are taken rapidly at intervals of 1 second. Within 2 seconds after the commencement of injection, the dye reaches the cerebral arteries, and after 2 seconds it is in the veins. After another two seconds or so, the dye passes into the intracranial venous sinuses. The skiagrams taken at different intervals provide arteriograms, venograms (or phlebograms) and sinograms.

Similarly for vertebral angiography, the dye is injected into the vertebral artery and skiagrams are taken as described above.

Indications: Cerebral angiography is helpful in diagnosis of intracranial tumours, haematomas, aneurysms and angiomas.

MR angiography: This technique employs modification so that blood vessels can be visualised without injecting the dye. The conventional angiography is still preferred.

Digital subtraction angiography (DSA): In this procedure, low concentrations of contrast media are used. Bones and

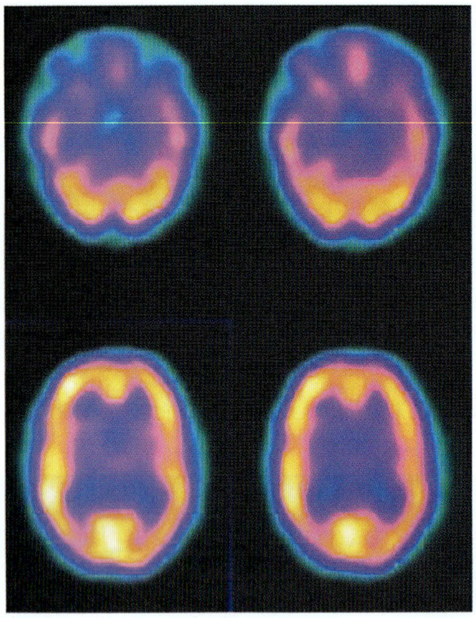

Fig. 15.9: Single photon emission computed tomography (SPECT) scan (*Image courtesy*: Dr Abhijeet Taori)

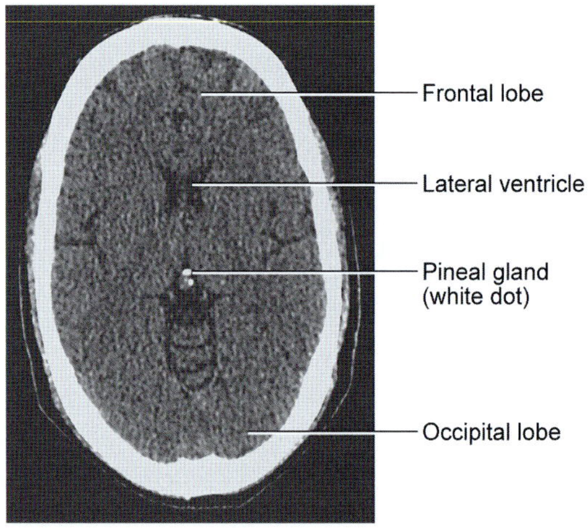

Fig. 15.10: Calcified pineal gland (due to aging) on CT scan (*Image courtesy*: Dr Abhijeet Taori)

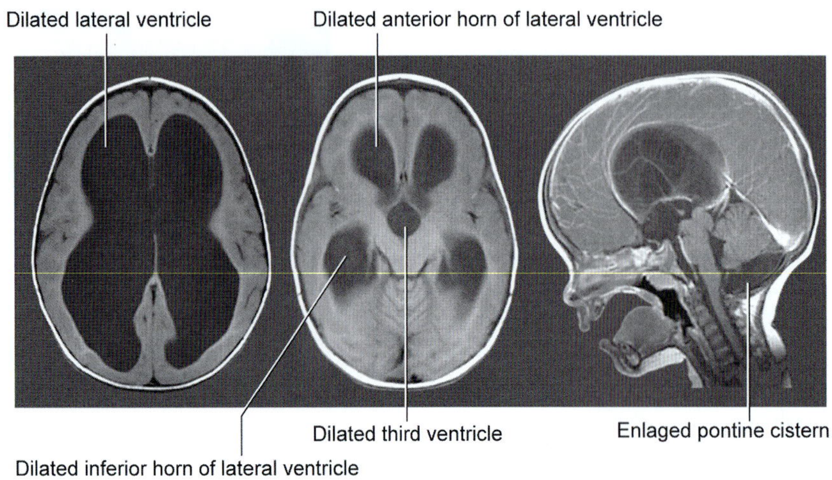

Fig. 15.11: Dilated ventricles (hydrocephalus) on CT scan (*Image courtesy*: Dr Abhijeet Taori)

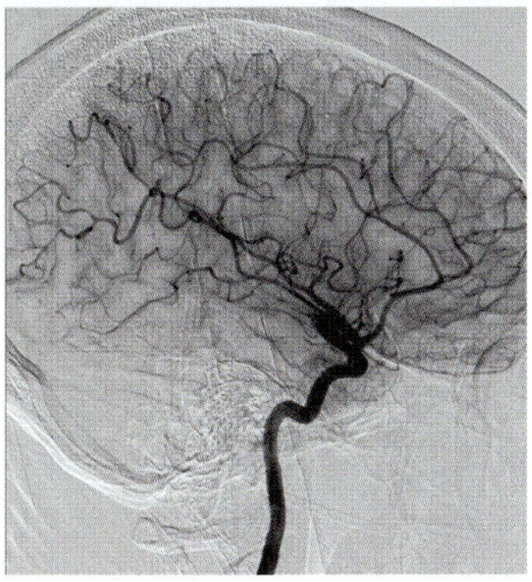

Fig. 15.12: Carotid angiography

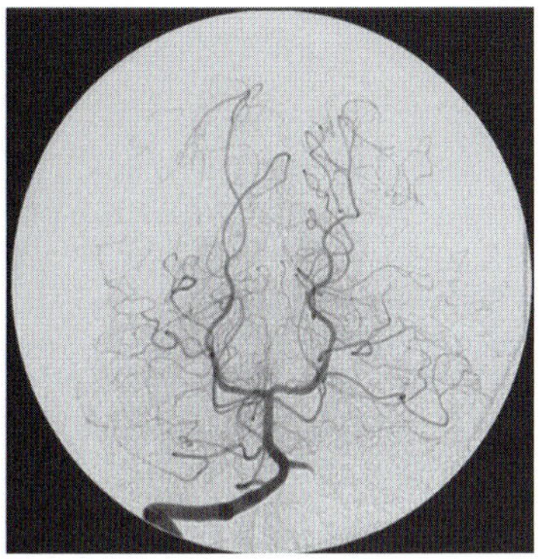

Fig. 15.13: Vertebral angiogram

muscles are removed with the help of the computer. Ideal method is arterial DSA wherein diluted contrast medium is injected into the artery to see its course, branches and their diseases.

Because of these modern and safe procedures, the older techniques—pneumoencephalography, ventriculography and myelography—have become obsolete.

Electrophysiological Methods

a. *Electromyography (EMG):* This is the study of electrical activity accompanying the muscle contraction. It is also used to study the action of various muscles.
b. *Electroencephalography (EEG):* The pattern of electrical activity of brain is analysed by putting electrodes in the scalp at different points and recording it in the machine.
c. *Nerve conduction studies* done to estimate the rate of conduction through the nerve fibres.

These procedures may be used according to the requirement of the patient.

BDC's Anatomy *e*-book

1. Evolution of the head
2. Further reading

Chapter

16

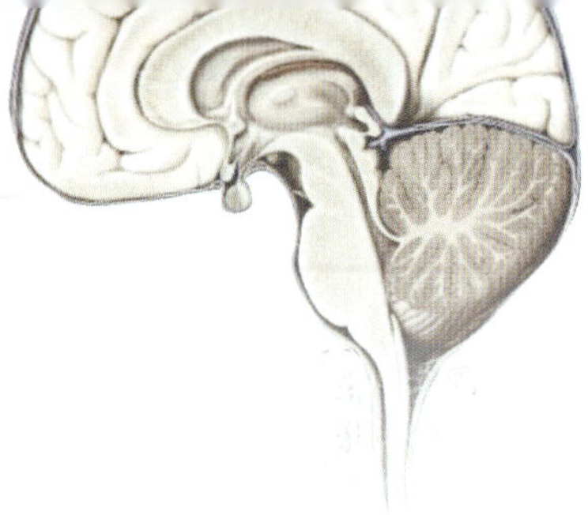

Autonomic Nervous System

Autonomic nervous system comprises sympathetic and parasympathetic components. It is also called *visceral nervous system* (Figs 16.1a and b).

Sympathetic system is active during fright, flight or fight. During any of these activities, the pupils dilate, skin gets pale, blood pressure rises, blood vessels of skeletal muscles, heart, lungs and brain dilate. There is hardly any activity in the digestive tract due to which the individual does not feel hungry. The person is tense and gets tired soon. This is the larger of the two components of autonomic nervous system.

Parasympathetic system has the opposite effects of sympathetic system. This component is sympathetic (kind) to the digestive tract. In its activity, digestion and metabolism of food occurs. Heart beats normally. Person is relaxed and can do creative work.

Autonomic nervous system is controlled by brainstem and cerebral hemispheres. These include reticular formation of brainstem, thalamic and hypothalamic nuclei, limbic lobe and prefrontal cortex including the ascending and descending tracts interconnecting these regions.

Comparison of parasympathetic and sympathetic nervous systems is given in Table 16.1.

SYMPATHETIC NERVOUS SYSTEM: THORACOLUMBAR OUTFLOW

It consists of two ganglionated trunks, their branches, prevertebral ganglia, and plexuses. It supplies all the viscera of thorax, abdomen and pelvis, including the blood vessels of head and neck, brain, limbs, skin and the sweat glands as well as arrector pilorum muscle of skin.

The preganglionic fibres are axons of neurons situated in the lateral horns of T1–L2 segments of spinal cord. They leave spinal cord through their respective ventral roots, to reach sympathetic ganglia and beginning of ventral rami via white rami communicantes (wrc) [singular: ramus communicans]. There are 14 wrc on each side. These fibres can have following alternative routes (Fig. 16.2):

- They relay in the ganglion of the sympathetic trunk, postganglionic fibres pass via the grey rami

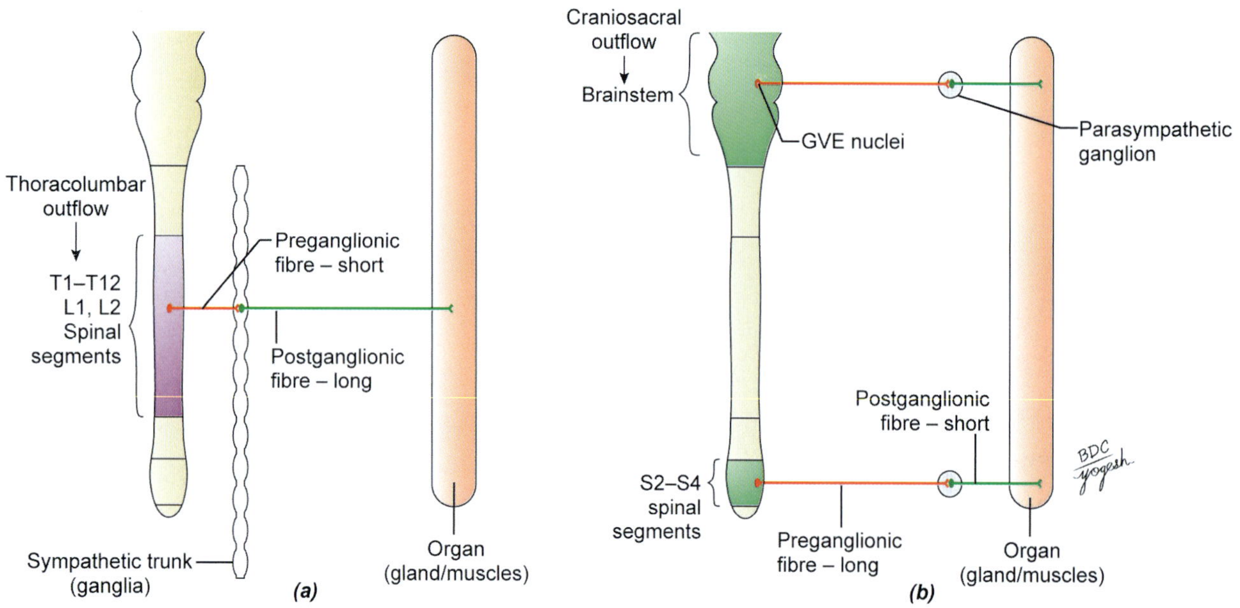

Figs 16.1a and b: (a) Sympathetic nervous system and (b) parasympathetic nervous system (GVE: General visceral efferent)

TABLE 16.1: Comparison of parasympathetic and sympathetic nervous systems

	Parasympathetic	*Sympathetic*
Outflow	Craniosacral outflow	Thoracolumbar outflow
Preganglionic neuron	Located in midbrain, pons and medulla oblongata and pass through III, VII, IX, X cranial nerves and also along S2–S4 segments of spinal cord	Located in lateral horn of spinal cord from T1–T12 and L1–L2 segments
Preganglionic fibres	Longer (Fig. 13.3b), myelinated	Shorter (Fig. 13.3a), myelinated
Relay of impulses	Occurs in neurons close to viscera	Occurs in neurons little away from the viscera they supply
Postganglionic fibres	Short, nonmyelinated	Long, nonmyelinated
Neurotransmitter	Both at preganglionic endings and postganglionic endings, acetylcholine is released	At preganglionic endings, acetylcholine is released. At postganglionic endings, adrenaline is released, except in cases of sweat glands where acetylcholine is released
Number of synapses	Preganglionic neuron makes synapses with much smaller number of neurons. Impulses are localised	Preganglionic neuron makes connection with large number of postganglionic nerve cells and impulses are widespread
Postganglionic supply	Only the viscera are supplied by postganglionic fibres. These do not supply blood vessels of skeletal muscles	All the viscera are supplied by post-ganglionic fibres. The only exception is suprarenal gland which is supplied by the preganglionic fibres
Functions	These activities are discrete as well as isolated and conserve the body energies	These activities are mass reactions, widely diffuse in their action. These reactions are catabolic in nature and are used in fright, flight or fight
Action of skin	Nil	Sudomotor, pilomotor and vasomotor
Effect on blood vessels	Blood vessels to the glands of gastrointestinal tract are dilated	Blood vessels to skeletal muscles (cholinergic), heart and brain are dilated
Effect of gastrointestinal system	Secretory to the glands, motor to the smooth muscles and inhibitory to the sphincters of gut	Decreases the secretory activity of glands, including the peristalsis of gut. It is motor to the sphincters
Effect on pupil	Pupil is constricted, lens curvature is increased as in reading	Dilates the pupil
Heart	Slows the pulse, maintains normal blood pressure	Tachycardia, rise in blood pressure. Dilates the coronaries
Lungs	Increase the secretions of glands of lungs and is bronchoconstrictor	Decrease the secretions, is bronchodilator. Adrenaline-like drugs are given in asthma
Urinary bladder	Both filling and emptying of urinary bladder are controlled by parasympathetic system	Supplies only blood vessels of bladder, sphincter vesicae is contracted by sympathetic action during ejaculation
Erectile tissue	Relaxes, causes erection	—
Action	Conserves energy	Prepares for emergency

communicantes (grc) and get distributed to the blood vessels of skin, sweat glands and to arrector pili muscles.

- These may pass through the corresponding ganglion and ascend to a ganglion higher before terminating in the above manner.
- These may pass through the corresponding ganglia and descend to a ganglion lower and then terminate in the above manner.
- Postganglionic fibres from upper thoracic ganglia supply the thoracic viscera.
- Some preganglionic fibres pass to corresponding ganglia and emerge from these (unrelayed) in the form of splanchnic nerves to supply the abdominal and pelvic viscera after synapsing in the ganglia situated in the abdominal cavity.
- A few fibres of splanchnic nerves reach the medulla of the suprarenal gland.

Sympathetic trunks on either side of the body extend from cervical region to the coccygeal region where both trunks fuse to form a single *ganglion impar.* Sympathetic trunk has cervical, thoracic, lumbar, sacral and coccygeal parts. The branches of each part are discussed below.

Cervical Part

It extends from base of skull to the neck of 1st rib. It has three ganglia—superior, middle and inferior cervical ganglia. Branches of these ganglia are tabulated in Table 16.2.

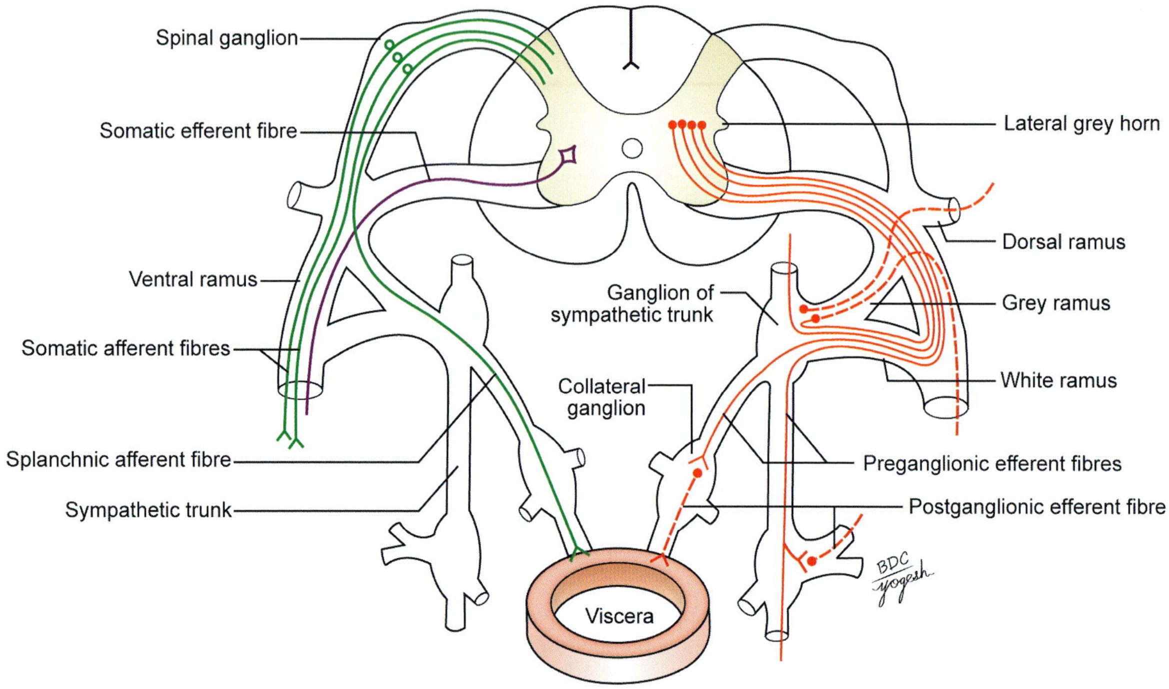

Fig. 16.2: Components of a typical spinal nerve

TABLE 16.2: Branches of superior, middle and inferior cervical ganglia

	Superior cervical ganglion	*Middle cervical ganglion*	*Inferior cervical ganglion*
Arterial branches	i. Along internal carotid artery as internal carotid nerve ii. Along common carotid and external carotid arteries	Along inferior thyroid artery —	Along subclavian and vertebral arteries —
Grey rami communicantes	Along cervical 1–4 nerves	Along 5 and 6 cervical nerves	Along 7 and 8 cervical nerves
Along cranial nerves	Along IX, X, XI, XII cranial nerves	—	—
Visceral branches	Pharynx, thyroid, cardiac	Cardiac	Cardiac

Thoracic Part

There are usually 11 ganglia on the sympathetic trunk of thoracic part. 1st ganglion lies on neck of 1st rib and is usually fused with inferior cervical ganglion and forms stellate ganglion. The lower ones lie on the head of the ribs. The sympathetic trunk continues with its abdominal part by passing behind the medial arcuate ligament.

The ganglia are connected with the respective spinal nerves via the white ramus communicans (from the spinal nerve to the ganglion) and the grey ramus communicans (from the ganglion to the spinal nerve, i.e. ganglion gives grey (ggg)).

Branches

1. Grey rami communicantes to all the spinal nerves of thorax, i.e. T1–T12. The postganglionic fibres pass along the spinal nerves to supply cutaneous blood vessels, sweat glands and arrector pili muscles.
2. White rami communicantes from upper 4–6 ganglia travel up the cervical part of sympathetic trunk to relay in the three cervical ganglia. Fibres from the lower thoracic ganglia T10–L2 pass down as preganglionic fibres to relay in the lumbar or sacral ganglia.
3. Second to fifth ganglia give postganglionic fibres to heart, lungs, aorta and oesophagus.
4. Lower eight ganglia give fibres which are preganglionic (unrelayed) for the supply of abdominal viscera. These are called splanchnic (visceral) nerves (*see* BD Chaurasia's Human Anatomy Vol 1, Fig. 14.15).
   - Ganglia T5–T9 give fibres which constitute greater splanchnic nerve.
   - Ganglia T10–T12 give fibres that constitute lesser splanchnic nerve.
   - Ganglia L1–L2 give fibres that constitute lowest splanchnic nerve.

Abdominal/Lumbar Part

It runs along the medial border of psoas major muscle. It is continuous with the pelvic part by passing behind the common iliac vessels. There are four ganglia in the lumbar or abdominal part. Only upper two ganglia receive white ramus communicans from the ventral primary rami of first and second lumbar nerves.

Branches

1. Grey rami communicantes to the L1–L5 spinal nerves. These pass along the spinal nerves to be distributed

to the sweat glands, cutaneous blood vessels and arrector pili muscles (sudomotor, vasomotor and pilomotor).
2. Postganglionic fibres pass medially to the aortic plexus.
3. Postganglionic fibres pass in front of common iliac vessels to form hypogastric plexus, which is also supplemented by branches of aortic plexus.

Aortic plexus: This plexus is formed by preganglionic sympathetic, postganglionic sympathetic, preganglionic parasympathetic and visceral afferent fibres around the abdominal aorta. This plexus is concentrated around the origin of ventral and lateral branches of abdominal aorta. These are known as coeliac plexus, superior mesenteric plexus, inferior mesenteric plexus and renal plexus.

Pelvic/Sacral and Coccygeal Parts of Sympathetic Trunk

Pelvic part runs in front of sacrum, medial to ventral sacral foramina. Caudally, the two trunks unite and fuse into a single ganglion impar in front of coccyx. There are four ganglia in this part of sympathetic trunk. Their branches are:

1. Grey rami communicantes to the sacral and coccygeal nerves.
2. Branches to the pelvic plexuses.

Collateral/Prevertebral Ganglia and Plexuses

Coeliac plexus is the largest of the three autonomic plexuses, coeliac, superior mesenteric and inferior mesenteric plexuses. It is a dense network of nerve fibres which unite the two coeliac ganglia. The ganglia receive the greater splanchnic nerves, lesser splanchnic nerves of both sides including some filaments of vagi and phrenic nerves.

Coeliac ganglia are two irregularly shaped ganglia. Each ganglion receives greater splanchnic nerve. The lower part of the ganglion receives lesser splanchnic nerve and is also called aorticorenal ganglion. The aorticorenal ganglion gives off the renal plexus which accompanies the renal vessels.

Secondary plexuses arising from coeliac and aorticorenal plexus are distributed along the branches of the aorta, namely phrenic, splenic, left gastric, hepatic, intermesenteric, suprarenal, renal, gonadal, superior and inferior mesenteric plexuses.

Superior Hypogastric Plexus

This plexus lies between the two common iliac arteries and is formed by: (i) aortic plexus, and (ii) branches from lumbar sympathetic ganglia. It divides into right and left inferior hypogastric plexuses (pelvic plexus); which runs on the medial side of internal iliac artery and is supplemented by pelvic splanchnic nerves (parasympathetic nerves). Thus, inferior hypogastric plexus contains both sympathetic and parasympathetic nerves. These are for the supply of the pelvic viscera along the branches of the arteries.

PARASYMPATHETIC NERVOUS SYSTEM

Craniosacral Outflow

Preganglionic parasympathetic fibres are present in four cranial nerves, e.g. III, VII, IX, and X cranial nerves and also along S2–S4 spinal nerves. Four ganglia namely ciliary, pterygopalatine, submandibular and otic, are concerned with efferent parasympathetic fibres of III, VII and IX nerves.

1. Oculomotor parasympathetic fibres arise in midbrain, from the Edinger-Westphal nucleus. Preganglionic fibres pass through the III nerve and leave as motor root along the nerve to inferior oblique muscle to enter the *ciliary ganglion*. These fibres are relayed in the ciliary ganglion, and the postganglionic fibres pass via the short ciliary nerves to be distributed to ciliaris and sphincter pupillae muscles.
2. Facial nerve contains efferent parasympathetic fibres. These are the axons of neurons of superior salivatory nucleus. These fibres leave the brain as nervus intermedius, and form part of the facial nerve and pass along its chorda tympani branch. Chorda tympani nerve joins the lingual nerve in the infratemporal fossa. These fibres travel with the lingual nerve to reach submandibular ganglion. Fibres of chorda tympani nerve relay in this ganglion from where postganglionic fibres supply the submandibular and sublingual salivary glands.

   Greater petrosal branch of facial nerve joins the deep petrosal (sympathetic fibres) to form the *nerve of pterygoid canal*. Only greater petrosal nerve fibres relay in the *pterygopalatine ganglion*. These postganglionic fibres supply lacrimal gland, glands of nose, pharynx and palate.
3. Glossopharyngeal nerve contains the axons of the inferior salivatory nucleus. They travel through IX nerve and are given off in its tympanic branch which forms tympanic plexus from where the lesser petrosal nerve starts. The lesser petrosal nerve relays in the otic ganglion. The postganglionic fibres are given to the auriculotemporal nerve to reach the parotid salivary gland.
4. Vagus or X cranial nerve contains efferent parasympathetic fibres. They have their origin in the dorsal nucleus of vagus and pass along its pulmonary, cardiac, oesophageal, gastric and intestinal branches.

Sacral Outflow

Pelvic Splanchnic Nerves

These are the preganglionic fibres constituting the sacral component of the craniosacral outflow of the parasympathetic nervous system. These arise from lateral horn cell of S2–S4 segments of spinal cord. The axons of these neurons pass along the ventral rami of S2–S4 nerves to join the inferior hypogastric plexus to be distributed to the pelvic viscera.

Some of the parasympathetic fibres ascend from inferior hypogastric plexus to reach superior hypogastric plexus and finally the inferior mesenteric plexus. Thereafter, these fibres are distributed along the branches of inferior mesenteric artery to supply left one-third of transverse colon, descending colon and pelvic colon. These preganglionic fibres relay in the neurons situated in the wall of the viscera.

Efferent Pathways of Cranial Part of Parasympathetic Nervous System

Preganglionic parasympathetic fibres are present in four cranial nerves, e.g. cranial nerves III, VII, IX, X and along spinal nerves S2–S4. Four ganglia, namely ciliary, pterygopalatine, submandibular and otic, are concerned with efferent parasympathetic fibres.

NERVE SUPPLY OF THE VISCERA

See BD Chaurasia's Human Anatomy Vol 1, Fig. 14.15.

Heart

Preganglionic sympathetic neurons are located in lateral horns T1–T5 segments of spinal cord. These fibres pass along the respective ventral roots of thoracic nerves to synapse with the respective ganglia of the sympathetic trunk. After relay, the postganglionic fibres form thoracic branches which intermingle with the vagal fibres, to form cardiac plexus.

Some fibres from T1–T5 segments of spinal cord reach their respective ganglia. These fibres then travel up the cervical part of the sympathetic chain and relay in superior, middle and inferior cervical ganglia. After relay, the postganglionic fibres form the three cervical cardiac nerves. Preganglionic parasympathetic neurons for the supply of heart are situated in the dorsal nucleus of vagus nerve.

Sympathetic activity increases the heart rate. Larger branches of coronary arteries are mainly supplied by sympathetic nerves. It causes vasodilation of coronary arteries. Impulses of pain travel along sympathetic fibres. These fibres pass through sympathetic trunk and reach the spinal cord via T1–T5 spinal nerves. Thus, the pain may be referred to the area of skin supplied by T1–T5 nerves, i.e. retrosternal and medial side of the left upper limb. Since one is more conscious of impulses coming from skin than the viscera, one feels as if the pain is in the skin. This is the basis of the referred pain.

Smaller branches of coronary arteries are supplied by parasympathetic nerves. These nerves are concerned with slowing of the cardiac cycle. The nerves reach the heart by two plexuses—superficial and deep cardiac.

Superficial Cardiac Plexus

- Superior cervical cardiac branch of left sympathetic trunk.
- Inferior cervical cardiac branch of left vagus nerve.

Deep Cardiac Plexus

It consists of two halves which are interconnected and lie anterior to bifurcation of trachea.

Right half	*Left half*
Superior, middle, and inferior cervical cardiac branches of right sympathetic trunk	Only middle and inferior branches of left sympathetic trunk
Cardiac branches of T2–T4 ganglia of right side	Same
Three cervical cardiac branches of right vagus	Two cervical cardiac branches of left vagus
Two branches of right recurrent laryngeal nerve arising from neck region	Same, but coming from thoracic region

Branches from the plexus give extensive branches to pulmonary and right and left coronary plexuses. Branches from the coronary plexuses supply both the atria and the ventricles. Left ventricle receives richer nerve supply because of its larger size.

Lungs

The lungs are supplied from the anterior and posterior pulmonary plexuses. The anterior plexus is an extension of deep cardiac plexus. The posterior plexus is formed from branches of vagus and T2–T5 sympathetic ganglia. Small ganglia are found on these nerves for the relay of parasympathetic (brought via vagus nerve) fibres. Parasympathetic system is bronchoconstrictor (motor) whereas sympathetic system is inhibitory. Sympathetic stimulation causes relaxation of smooth muscles of bronchial tubes (bronchodilator). The pressure of inspired air also causes bronchodilation.

Gastrointestinal Tract

Oesophagus

- Cervical part of oesophagus receives branches from recurrent laryngeal nerve and middle cervical ganglion of sympathetic trunk.
- Thoracic part gets branches from vagal trunks and oesophageal plexus as well as from sympathetic trunks and greater splanchnic nerves.
- Abdominal part receives fibres from vagal trunks (i.e. anterior and posterior gastric nerves), thoracic part of sympathetic trunks, greater splanchnic nerves and plexus around left gastric artery. The nerves form a plexus called myenteric plexus between two layers of the muscularis externa and another one in the submucous layer.

Stomach

Sympathetic supply reaches from coeliac plexus along gastric and gastroepiploic arteries. A few branches also reach from thoracic and lumbar sympathetic trunks. Parasympathetic supply is derived from vagus nerves. The left vagus forms anterior gastric, while right vagus comprises posterior gastric nerve. The anterior gastric nerve supplies cardiac orifice, anterior surface of body as well as fundus of stomach and pylorus.

Posterior gastric nerve supplies posterior surface of body and fundus till pyloric antrum. It gives number of coeliac branches which form part of the coeliac plexus.

Vagus is secretomotor to stomach. Its stimulation causes secretion which is rich in pepsin. Sympathetic system inhibits peristalsis and is motor to the pyloric sphincter. It also carries pain fibres from stomach.

Small Intestine

The nerves of this part of the gut are derived from coeliac ganglia formed by posterior gastric nerve (vagus) and splanchnic nerves (sympathetic) and the plexus around superior mesenteric artery. These nerves form myenteric plexus and submucous plexus. Parasympathetic fibres relay in the ganglion cells present in these plexuses. Parasympathetic system is secretomotor to the intestines and inhibits the sphincters. Sympathetic system inhibits the peristaltic movements of intestine but stimulates the sphincters. The autonomic nerves in the intestine form enteric nervous system.

Large Intestine

Large intestine, except the lower half of anal canal, is supplied by both components of autonomic nervous system. The derivatives of midgut, i.e. caecum, vermiform appendix, ascending colon and right two-thirds of transverse colon receive their sympathetic nerve supply from coeliac and superior mesenteric ganglia and parasympathetic from vagus nerve.

Left one-third of transverse colon, descending colon, sigmoid colon, rectum and upper half of anal canal (developed from hindgut) receive their sympathetic nerve supply from lumbar part of sympathetic trunk and superior hypogastric plexus through the plexuses on the branches of inferior mesenteric artery. Its effect is chiefly vasomotor. Parasympathetic supply of colon is received from pelvic splanchnic nerves S2–S4. Pelvic splanchnic nerves give fibres to inferior hypogastric plexuses to supply rectum and upper half of anal canal. Some of inferior hypogastric plexuses pass up through superior hypogastric plexus and get distributed along the branches of inferior mesenteric artery to the left third of transverse colon, descending and sigmoid colons.

Rectum and Anal Canal

Sympathetic fibres pass along inferior mesenteric and superior rectal arteries and also via superior and inferior hypogastric plexuses.

Parasympathetic supply is from pelvic splanchnic nerves, which join inferior hypogastric plexus. This supply is motor to muscles of rectum and inhibitory to internal sphincter.

The external anal sphincter is supplied by inferior rectal branch of pudendal nerve. Afferent impulses of physiological distension of rectum and sigmoid colon are carried by parasympathetic nerves, whereas pain impulses are conveyed both by the sympathetic and parasympathetic nerves.

Pancreas

Branches of coeliac plexus pass along the arteries. Effect of sympathetic nerve is vasomotor. The nerve fibres make synaptic contact with acinar cells before innervating the islets. The parasympathetic ganglia lie in sparse connective tissue of the gland and the islet cells.

Liver

Nerves of the liver are derived from hepatic plexus which is an offshoot of coeliac plexus. This contains both sympathetic and parasympathetic fibres. These accompany the blood vessels and bile duct. Both types of nerve fibres also reach the liver through various peritoneal folds.

Gallbladder

Parasympathetic and sympathetic nerves of gallbladder are derived from coeliac plexus, along the hepatic artery (hepatic plexus) and its branches. Fibres from the right phrenic nerve (C4) through the communication of coeliac and phrenic plexuses also reach gallbladder in the hepatic plexus. Thus, the reason of pain in the right shoulder (from where impulses are carried by lateral supraclavicular nerve C4) in cholecystitis is the stimulation of phrenic nerve fibres (C4) due to the communication between phrenic plexus and hepatic plexus via coeliac plexus. Coeliac plexus gets fibres from thoracic 7 ganglia. Thoracic 7 nerve supplies skin over inferior angle of scapula. Hepatic plexus, an offshoot of coeliac plexus, supplies gallbladder. So pain of gallbladder is also referred to inferior angle of right scapula.

Urinary System

The kidneys are supplied by renal plexus formed from coeliac ganglion, coeliac plexus, lowest thoracic splanchnic nerve, and first lumbar splanchnic nerve. The plexus runs along the branches of renal artery to supply the vessels, renal glomeruli and tubules. These are chiefly vasomotor in function.

Ureter is supplied in its upper part from renal and aortic plexus, middle part from superior hypogastric plexus and lower part from hypogastric nerve and inferior hypogastric plexus.

Vesical Plexus

Sympathetic fibres arise from T11–T12 segments and L1–L2 segments of spinal cord. Parasympathetic fibres arise from S2–S4 segments of spinal cord, which relay in the neurons present in and near the wall of urinary bladder. Parasympathetic system is motor to the muscular coat and inhibitory to the sphincter; sympathetic system is chiefly vasomotor. Emptying and filling of urinary bladder is normally controlled by parasympathetic system only.

Male Reproductive Organs

Testicular plexus accompanies the testicular artery to reach the testis. It is formed by renal and aortic plexus, and also from superior and inferior hypogastric plexuses. This plexus supplies the epididymis and ductus deferens.

Prostatic plexus is formed from inferior hypogastric plexus and branches are distributed to prostate, seminal vesicle, prostatic urethra, ejaculatory ducts, erectile tissue of penis, penile part of urethra and bulbourethral glands. Sympathetic nerves cause vasoconstriction, and parasympathetic nerves cause vasodilatation.

Comparison of parasympathetic and sympathetic nervous systems is tabulated in *see* Table 16.1.

Female Reproductive Organs

The ovary and uterine tube receive their nerve supply from plexus around the ovarian vessels. This plexus is derived from renal, aortic plexuses and also from superior and inferior hypogastric plexuses. Sympathetic fibres derived from T10–T11 segments of spinal cord are vasomotor in nature whereas parasympathetic fibres are probably vasodilator in function.

Uterus

It is supplied by uterovaginal plexus, formed from the inferior hypogastric plexus. The sympathetic fibres are derived from T12 to L1 segments of spinal cord. Parasympathetic fibres arise from S2–S4 segments of spinal cord. Sympathetic system causes uterine contraction and vasoconstriction, while parasympathetic nerves produce vasodilatation and uterine inhibition. Vagina is supplied by nerves arising from inferior hypogastric plexus to uterovaginal plexus. These supply wall of vagina including vestibular glands and clitoris. Parasympathetic fibres cause vasodilator effect on the erectile tissue.

AFFERENT AUTONOMIC FIBRES

Autonomic afferents are peripheral processes of pseudounipolar cells in some cranial and spinal nerve ganglia. The terminals of autonomic nerves may be loops, rings, tendril-like endings, a few encapsulated ones in the walls of viscera. Viscera are sensitive to stretch, ischaemia and distension. These sensations cause pain and reach up to the level of consciousness.

General visceral afferent fibres are in III, VII, IX, X cranial nerves, S2–S4 nerves and in T1–L2 spinal nerves.

Vagus nerves has a large general visceral afferent component. The superior ganglion is somatic and inferior ganglion is visceral in nature. Their central processes end in dorsal nucleus of vagus or tractus solitarius. Afferents are reached from pharynx and oesophagus via IX, X cranial nerves which are concerned with swallowing reflexes. In the thorax, afferent fibres arise from walls of great vessels, aortic and carotid bodies and bronchial musculature (for cough reflex). General visceral afferent fibres from stomach and intestine also terminate in the dorsal nucleus of vagus which may be responsible for nausea and hunger.

CLINICAL NEUROANATOMY

1. Removal of stellate ganglion improves the blood supply to the upper limb. But its removal causes ***Horner's syndrome*** which is comprised of:
   - Anhidrosis of the same side of face
   - Partial drooping of upper eyelid, i.e. ptosis
   - Enophthalmos
   - Constriction of the pupil
   - Loss of ciliospinal reflex
   - Flushing of face
2. Arteries of the upper limb are innervated by sympathetic fibres. Preganglionic fibres originate from the cell bodies of T2–T5 spinal segments. Fibres ascend in the sympathetic trunk and synapse with middle and inferior cervical ganglia. Postganglionic fibres join the nerves which constitute the brachial plexus, get distributed to the arteries of the upper limb in each region. These fibres may be cut to relieve the symptoms of ***Raynaud's disease***.
3. T2–T5 ganglia and stellate ganglia may be removed in cases of intractable angina pectoris.
4. Arteries of lower limb are supplied by lower three thoracic and upper two lumbar segments of the spinal cord. Femoral artery is supplied by sympathetic fibres from femoral and obturator nerves. Posterior tibial artery receives the postganglionic fibres from common peroneal and tibial nerves. ***Buerger's disease*** may be treated by lumbar sympathectomy.
5. ***Megacolon:*** There is absence of ganglion cells and failure of innervation of the smooth muscle layers of pelvic colon.
6. ***Referred pain:*** If the somatic nerves from skin and afferent fibres from viscera enter the same segment of the spinal cord, the phenomenon of referred pain occurs. Visceral pain in the appendix is produced due to either spasm of its muscle, or distension of its lumen. The afferent impulses ascend through the superior mesenteric plexus, lesser splanchnic nerve to reach the spinal cord at T10 level. Impulses from the skin around umbilicus are also carried by T10 segment.

   Brain is more conscious of impulses from skin. So in early case of appendicitis, though there is stimulation of sympathetic fibres of appendix, person thinks the impulses are arising from skin of umbilicus. So pain of early appendicitis is referred to the umbilicus. Later on when parietal peritoneum is inflamed, pain is localised in the right iliac fossa.
7. Pain fibres from the body of the uterus pass with sympathetic nerves through the hypogastric plexus and the lumbar splanchnic nerves to cells on the dorsal roots of the lower thoracic and upper lumbar nerves. Afferents from cervix pass in dorsal roots of upper sacral nerves. Cauterisation of cervix does not cause pain whereas stretch (dilatation) of cervix is painful.

BDC's Anatomy *e*-book

1. Viva voce questions

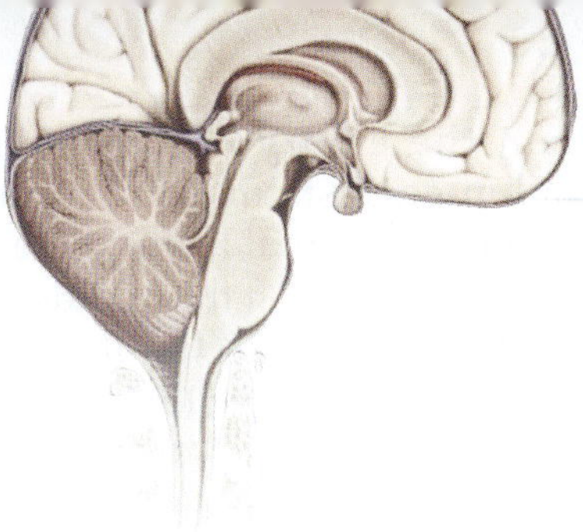

Chapter

17

Development of Nervous System

Competency:

AN64.2 Describe the development of neural tube, spinal cord, medulla oblongata, pons, midbrain, cerebral hemisphere and cerebellum.

DEVELOPMENT OF BRAIN

NEURAL TUBE

The whole of nervous system develops from ectoderm except the blood vessels and the microglia (neuroglial tissue) (Figs 17.1 and 17.2).

At the beginning of 3rd week of development, the ectodermal germ layer has the shape of a flat disc that is broader in cephalic region than in the caudal region. With the appearance of the notochord and its inductive influence, ectoderm overlying the notochord thickens to form a slipper-shaped plate, called neural plate. Cells of the plate make-up neuroectoderm and with induction, the process of neurulation starts. The plate is located in the mid-dorsal region in front of the primitive pit. Its lateral edges get raised to form the neural folds.

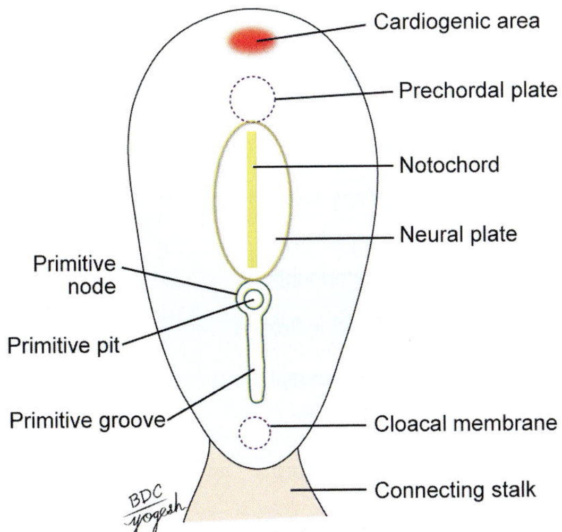

Fig. 17.1: Germ disc showing neural plate

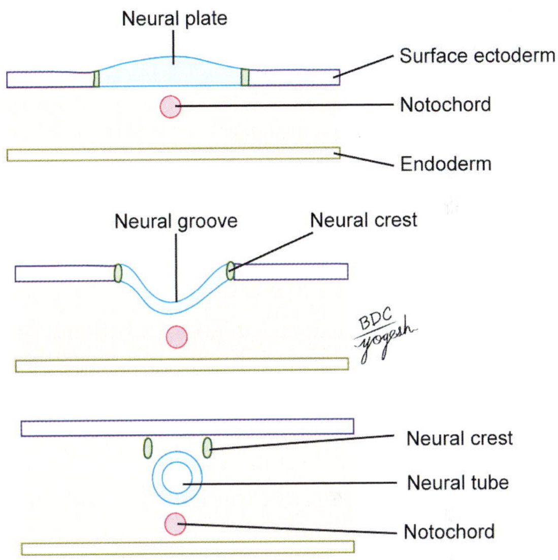

Fig. 17.2: Formation of neural plate and neural crest

With further development, the neural groove between the two folds on either side becomes deeper. Eventually, the neural folds approach each other in midline and finally fuse, thus forming the neural tube. Fusion begins in the cervical region and proceeds in cephalocaudal direction. At the most cranial and caudal ends of the embryo, fusion is delayed and the cranial and caudal neuropores temporarily form open connections between the base of neural tube and the amniotic cavity.

Final closure of cranial neuropore occurs on 25th day and caudal neuropore two days later of the embryonic life, and eventually neuropores disappear leading to a closed tube.

Before the neural tube is completely closed, it is divisible into an enlarged cranial part with three divisions which forms brain and a caudal tubular part which forms spinal cord.

The cephalic end of the neural tube shows three divisions (Fig. 17.3):

1. Prosencephalon or forebrain
2. Mesencephalon or midbrain
3. Rhombencephalon or hindbrain.

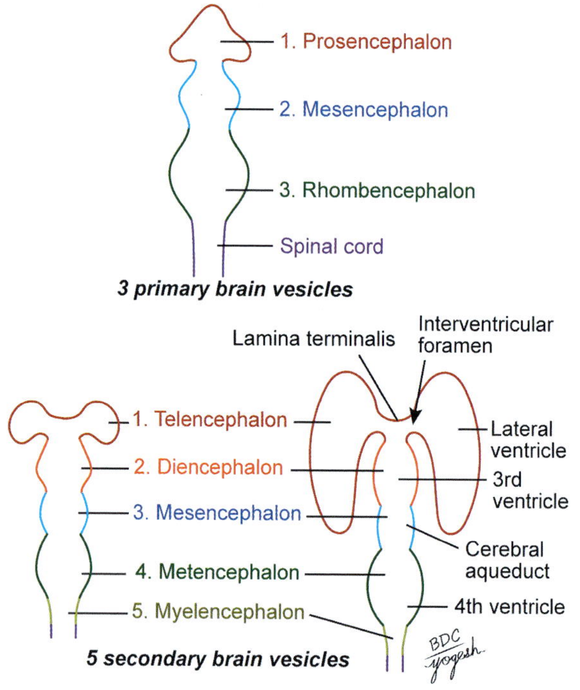

Fig. 17.3: Developing brain vesicles

Further Development of the Brain

Prosencephalon, mesencephalon and rhombencephalon are first arranged cephalocaudally. Soon it develops four flexures (Figs 17.4a and b). These are:

a. *Cervical flexure:* It appears at the junction of rhombencephalon and spinal cord.

b. *Cephalic or mesencephalic flexure:* This flexure is located in the region of midbrain.

c. *Rhombencephalic flexure:* The mesencephalon is separated from rhombencephalon by a furrow called rhombencephalic flexure.

d. *Pontine flexure:* When the embryo is 5 weeks old, the prosencephalon consists of two lateral outpocketings—the primitive cerebral hemispheres. At this stage, a deep furrow appears at the middle of rhombencephalon. This is called pontine flexure, and it divides rhombencephalon into metencephalon and myelencephalon.

The flexures change orientation of various parts of brain.

The lumen of the spinal cord, the central canal is continuous with that of primitive brain vesicles.

The cavity of rhombencephalon is known as fourth ventricle, those of cerebral hemisphere are lateral ventricles and cavity of diencephalon is third ventricle.

Cavity of lateral ventricles communicates with that of third ventricle through interventricular foramen of Monro. Cavity of third and fourth ventricles is connected through narrow cerebral aqueduct of Sylvius.

Neural Crest Cells and their Derivatives

During folding of the neural tube, a group of cells are formed along each side of neural groove and after the formation of neural tube, lie between the surface ectoderm and neural tube. These cells (ectodermal in origin) migrate laterally, and are called neural crest cells. They extend from prosencephalon at the cranial end of the tube to the level of caudal somites (Fig. 17.5).

Derivatives of the neural crest cells are as follows:

Dorsal mass of cells

A. Neuroblast cells
- Dorsal root ganglia
- Sensory ganglia of V, VII, IX and X cranial nerves
- Skeletal elements of pharyngeal arches
- Odontoblast of teeth
- Parafollicular cells of thyroid gland.

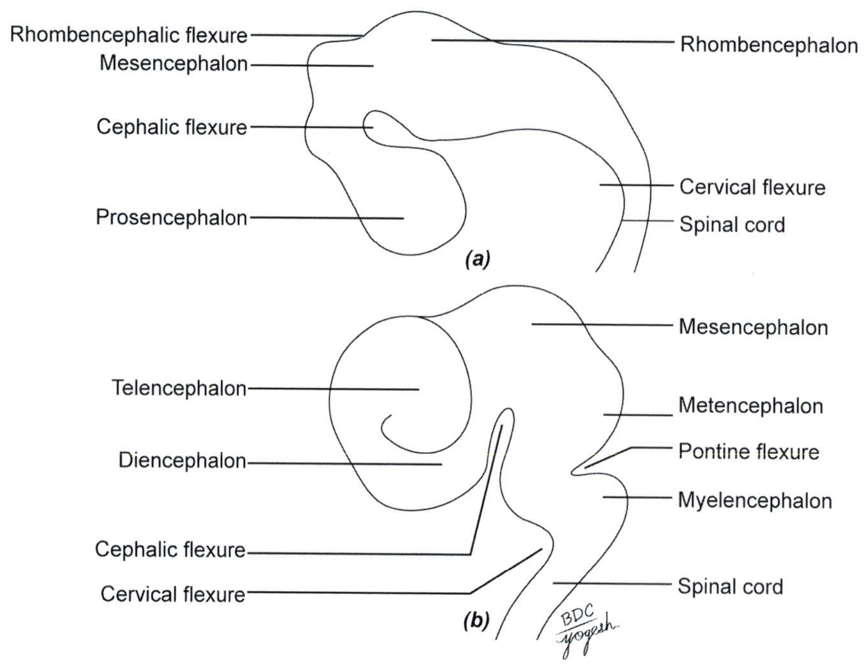

Figs 17.4a and b: Development of the various flexures of the brain

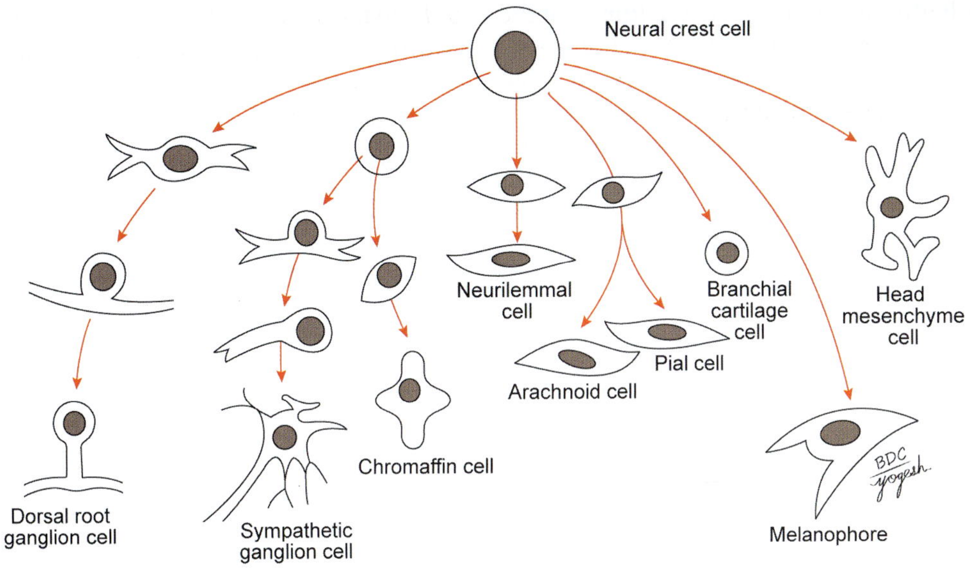

Fig. 17.5: Development of neural crest cells

B. Spongioblast cells
   - Satellite cells in ganglion
   - Schwann cells.

C. Pluripotent cells
   Melanocytes.

Ventral mass

A. Sympatho-chromaffin organ

B. Sympathoblasts
   - Sympathetic ganglionic neurons
   - Parasympathetic ganglionic neurons (ciliary, pterygopalatine, submandibular and otic).

C. Chromaffin cells
   - Chromaffin cells of medulla of adrenal gland
   - Para-aortic body
   - Argentaffin cells in respiratory system
   - Enterochromaffin cells in gut.

Other derivatives

- Facial bones and vault of skull
- Dermis of face and neck
- Muscles of ciliary body
- Sclera and choroids of eyeball
- Substantia propria and posterior epithelium of cornea
- Pharyngeal arch cartilages
- Semilunar valves in heart
- Spiral and bulbar septum in heart.

Diencephalon

The median part of prosencephalon forms diencephalon. It comprises a roof plate and two alar plates. The choroid plexus of third ventricle is formed from ependymal cells of roof plate and the vascular mesenchyme.

After the formation of the telencephalon, the lateral wall of diencephalon becomes thickened and gets divided into three regions, by appearance of two sulci.

These are called epithalamic and hyothalamic sulci, and the central part between the two sulci is called thalamus. The part above the epithalamic groove is a small region represented by habenular nuclei and pineal body. The part below the hypothalamic groove forms hypothalamus.

Pineal body or epiphysis develops from the most caudal part of roof plate. The pineal body initially appears as an epithelial lining in the midline, but by the 7th week of intrauterine life, it begins to evaginate. Eventually, it becomes a solid organ located on the roof of the mesencephalon. It serves as a channel through which light and darkness affect endocrine and behavioural rhythms, i.e. circadian rhythm. In the adult, calcium is frequently deposited in the epiphysis and it even serves as a landmark on an X-ray skull.

As a result of proliferative activity; the various nuclei of thalamus are formed by multiplication of cells in the mantle layer of the wall of diencephalon.

Hypothalamus forming lower portion of the alar plate differentiates into a number of nuclear areas which serve as regulation centre of the visceral functions, i.e. sleep, digestion, body temperature and emotional behaviour.

The prominent group of these nuclei is mammillary body, which forms distinct protuberance on the ventral surface of the hypothalamus on each side of the midline.

Telencephalon

The telencephalon consists of two lateral outpocketings, the cerebral (right and left) hemispheres and a median portion, the lamina terminalis. The cavities of hemispheres, the lateral ventricles, communicate with the lumen of diencephalon, through the interventricular foramen of Monro.

Cerebral Hemispheres

Cerebral hemispheres arise as bilateral (right and left) evaginations at the beginning of 5th week of development from the lateral wall of prosencephalon. By the middle of 2nd month of development, the basal part of hemisphere, i.e. the part which is initially formed by the forward extension of thalamus, begins to increase in size. As a result, this area bulges into the lumen of the lateral ventricle as well as into the foramen of Monro.

In the region where the wall of hemisphere is attached to the roof of diencephalon, the neuroblasts fail to develop and it remains very thin. Here the hemispheric wall consists of a single layer of ependymal cells covered by vascular mesenchyme and together they form choroid plexus. Due to disproportionate growth of various parts of hemisphere, the choroid plexus protrudes into lateral ventricle along a line known as choroid fissure.

Above the choroid fissure, the wall of hemisphere is thickened, thus forming the hippocampus which mainly has an olfactory function and this part bulges into lateral ventricle.

With further growth and expansion, the hemispheres cover the lateral aspect of diencephalon, mesencephalon and cranial portion of metencephalon.

Corpus Striatum

Some of the cells of the mantle layer in thick basal part of lateral wall of hemisphere form corpus striatum. It expands posteriorly and gets divided into two parts:

a. A dorsomedial portion—the caudate nucleus
b. A ventrolateral portion—the lentiform nucleus.

This division occurs by axons passing to and from the cortex of the hemisphere. The fibre bundle thus formed is known as internal capsule (Fig. 17.6).

Lobes of Brain

Continuous growth of cerebral hemispheres in anterior, dorsal, posterior and inferior directions results in formation of frontal, parietal, occipital and temporal lobes. As the growth in the region of corpus striatum slows down, the area between temporal and frontal lobes becomes depressed and forms the insula. The area is later overgrown by adjacent lobes and at the time of birth is almost completely covered. In later part of fetal life due to growth in a limited area, the sulci and gyri make their appearance. This is to accommodate more neurons in a limited area.

Cerebral Cortex

From development point of view, the cerebral cortex consists of:

a. The hippocampal cortex
b. Pyriform cortex
c. The neocortex.

The developing telencephalon has a medial wall, apposed to the counterpart of the opposite side, a superolateral wall and a basal wall. The hippocampal cortex develops in medial wall, pyriform cortex in the marginal layer—superficial to corpus striatum, and neocortex in the superolateral region. Earlier formed cells are neuroblasts. Motor areas of the cortex are rich in pyramidal cells, while the sensory areas have abundance of granular cells (Fig. 17.7).

Cerebral Commissures

In the adult, the right and left halves of the cerebral hemispheres are connected by a number of fibre bundles called commissures, which cross midline.

- The most important is lamina terminalis. It is part of the wall of the neural tube that closes the cranial end of the prosencephalon. After the appearance of telencephalic vesicles, lamina terminalis lies in the anterior wall of third ventricle. Neurons growing from one hemisphere pass to the other through the lamina terminalis. So, it becomes thickened to form commissured plate.
- *Anterior commissure*: The first of the crossing bundles to appear is anterior commissure. It consists of fibres connecting the olfactory bulb and related brain areas of one hemisphere to those of opposite side.
- Hippocampal or fornix commissure is the second to appear.
- *Corpus callosum*: It is the most important commissure. It appears in the 10th week of development and connects non-olfactory areas of the right and left sides.
- *Optic chiasma*: It appears in the anterior wall of diencephalon and contains fibres from medial halves of two retinas.

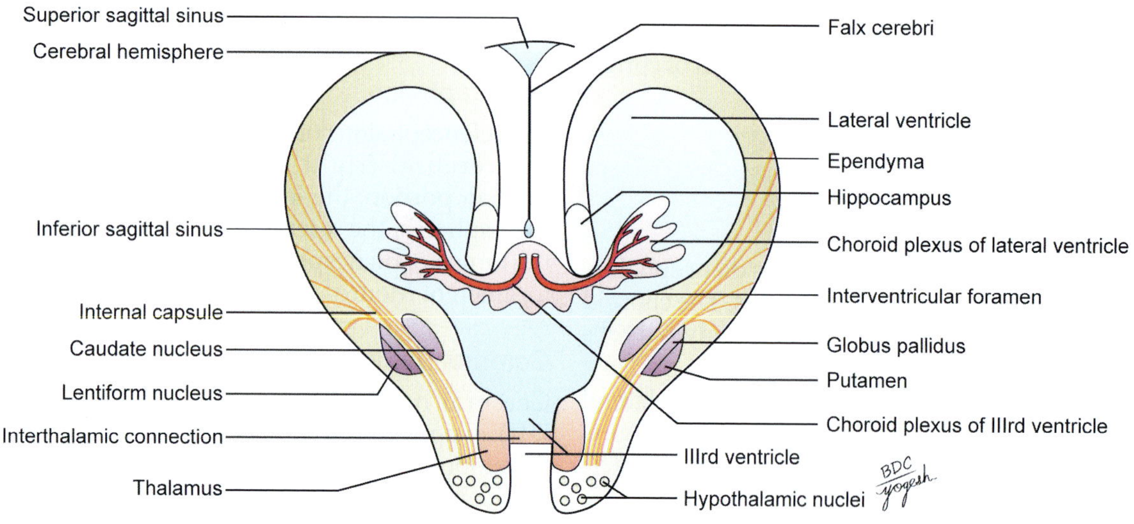

Fig. 17.6: Development of caudate and lentiform nuclei. Between these two nuclei, the fibres of internal capsule are seen

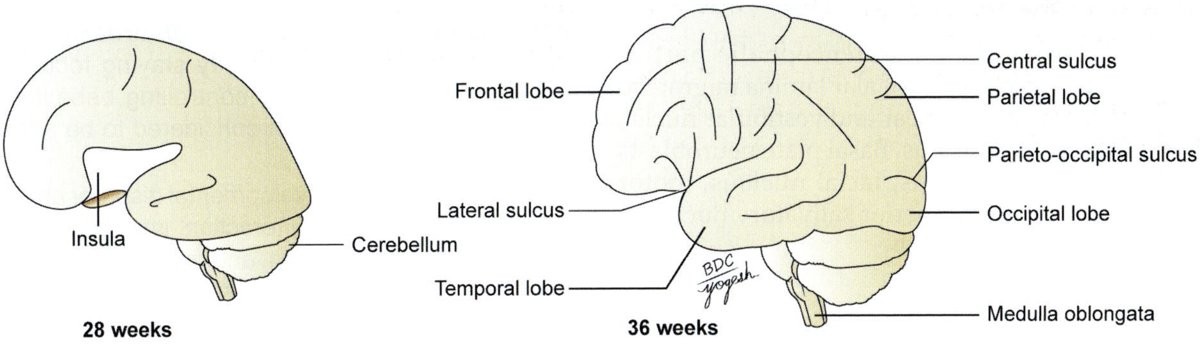

Fig. 17.7: Developmental stages of cerebral cortex

Development of Spinal Nerve Roots

Motor nerve begins to appear during the 4th week of development, arising from nerve cells located in the basal lamina (ventral horn) of spinal cord. Dorsal nerve roots form the collection of fibres arising from the cells of the dorsal root ganglia (spinal ganglion). Central processes from these ganglia form bundles that grow into spinal cord opposite the dorsal horns. Almost immediately, spinal nerve divides into dorsal and ventral rami. Dorsal primary rami supply dorsal axial musculature and skin of back. Ventral primary rami supply limbs, ventral body wall and form major nerve plexuses, i.e. cervical, brachial and lumbosacral plexuses (Figs 17.8a and b).

The peripheral processes of the dorsal nerve root ganglia grow upwards to form sensory component of the spinal nerve. Axons of neurons in the dorsal grey column enter marginal layer to form ascending tracts of the spinal cord, and the axons of cells of neurons developing in various parts of brain enter the marginal layer to form descending tracts.

As the mantle layer forms the dorsal and ventral columns, the white matter becomes subdivided into dorsal, ventral and lateral white columns.

Positional Changes of Spinal Cord

During the third month of intrauterine life, the spinal cord extends the entire length of embryo. Due to rapid growth of dura mater and vertebral column as relative to the neural tube, the terminal end of spinal cord is located, at birth, at the level of 3rd lumbar vertebra. This process of recession continues after birth, as a result of which, in the adult, spinal cord usually ends at the upper border of 2nd lumbar or at lower border of 1st lumbar vertebra.

Below this level, a thread-like extension of pia mater forms filum terminale and is attached to the periosteum of coccyx. Nerve fibres below the level of cord are called cauda equina (horse's tail).

Because of this recession of spinal cord, the intervertebral foramen no longer lie at the level at which corresponding nerves emerge from the spinal cord. The nerves run obliquely to reach their respective foramen. The obliquity is least in lower cervical region, gradually increases and is more in lumbar, sacral and coccygeal regions.

One advantage of this recession of spinal cord is when cerebrospinal fluid is tapped for diagnostic purposes. During a lumbar puncture, the needle is inserted at the lower lumbar level, avoiding the lower end of the cord.

DEVELOPMENT OF BRAINSTEM

Development of Medulla Oblongata

Medulla oblongata develops from caudal myelencephalic part of the rhombencephalic vesicle. Neuroblasts from the alar plate of the neural tube at this level will develop into the sensory nuclei of the medulla. The neuroblasts of basal plate will give rise to the motor nuclei.

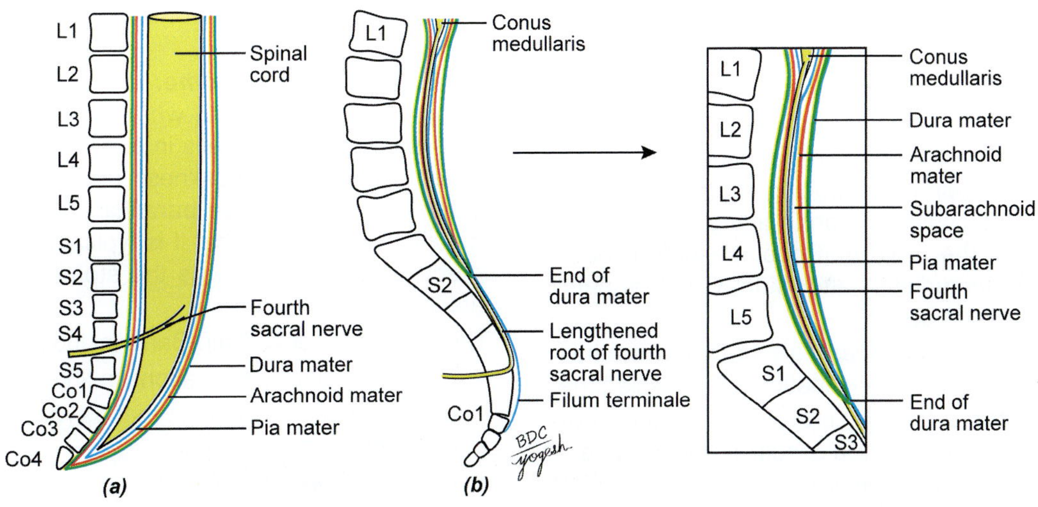

Figs 17.8a and b: Ascent of the spinal cord: (a) In intrauterine life and (b) in adult; and inset

Development of Pons

Pons develops from cranial metencephalic part of rhombencephalic vesicle. Cells of alar lamina migrate to form the pontine nuclei, cochlear and vestibular nuclei, and trigeminal sensory nucleus. Basal plate neuroblasts give rise to abducens nucleus, facial nucleus, motor nucleus of trigeminal and superior salivatory nucleus.

Development of Midbrain

Midbrain develops from middle vesicle or the mesencephalon. Alar lamina cells multiply and fuse to form 4 colliculi. These cells also migrate ventrally to form red nucleus and substantia nigra. The basal lamina forms the crus cerebri.

DEVELOPMENT OF CEREBELLUM

Cerebellum develops from the neurons of alar lamina of metencephalic part of the rhombencephalic vesicle. These neurons migrate dorsally and form the rhombic lip which forms the cerebellum. The earliest part to develop is the archicerebellum. In its centre, the paleocerebellum develops, splitting the archicerebellar parts into two parts—the lingula and flocculonodular lobe. Lastly, the paleocerebellar part is also split by the development of neocerebellum in its centre into two parts—the anterior lobe except lingula and pyramid with uvula.

Competency:
AN64.3 Describe various types of open neural tube defects with its embryological basis.

CLINICAL NEUROANATOMY

Down syndrome: Down syndrome (DS) is a set of physical and mental traits caused by a gene problem which happens before birth. The affected persons may have some degree of intellectual disability. Normally, a person has 46 chromosomes. But, a person with DS has 47 chromosomes having extra or abnormal chromosomes changes the way the brain and body develops.

Clinical features: Flat face, small ears, slanting eyes, small mouth, short neck, short arms and legs, low muscles tone, loose joints, and below average intelligence.

Cerebral palsy: It is a neurological disorder by a nonprogressive brain injury or malformation that occurs while the child's brain is undergoing development. The brain damage is caused by brain injury or abnormal development of the brain that occurs—before birth, during birth or immediately after birth. Cerebral palsy may be of different types.

Clinical features: Affected parts are body movements, muscles control, muscle coordination and muscle tone.

Craniosynostosis (*cranio*, cranium; *syn*, together; *ostosis,* relating to bone): It is a condition in which one or more of the fibrous sutures in an infant (very young) skull prematurely fuses by turning into bone (ossification).

Attention deficit hyperactive disorder (ADHD): A disorder that includes difficulty staying focused and paying attention, difficulty controlling behaviour and hyperactivity. ADHD is not considered to be a learning disability.

Autism: It is a neurodevelopmental disorder characterised by impaired social interaction, impaired verbal and non-verbal communication, and restricted and repetitive behaviour. Autism affects information processing in the brain by altering how nerve cells and their synapses connect and organise. How this occurs is not well understood.

Symptoms: Impaired social interaction, impaired verbal and non-verbal communication, restricted and repetitive behaviour.

Causes: Genetic and environmental factors.

Convulsion: A sudden, violent, irregular movement of the body, caused by involuntary contraction of muscles and associated especially with brain disorders such as epilepsy, the presence of certain toxins or other agents in the blood or fever in children.

Epilepsy: It is a chronic disorder, the hallmark of which is recurrent, unprovoked seizures or convulsions. A person is diagnosed with epilepsy, if they have two unprovoked seizures (or one unprovoked seizure with the likelihood of more) that were not caused by some known and reversible medical condition like alcohol withdrawal or extremely low blood sugar.

Spinal stenosis: It is narrowing of the spinal canal. The narrowing of the spinal canal limits the amount of space for the spinal cord and nerves. Pressure on the spinal cord and nerves due to limited space can cause symptoms such as pain, numbness, and tingling.

Spina bifida: It is a birth defect where there is incomplete closing of the backbone and membranes around the spinal cord. There are three main types: Spina bifida occulta, meningocele, and myelomeningocele. The most common location is the lower back, but in rare cases it may be the middle back or neck. Occulta has no or only mild signs. Signs of occulta may include a hairy patch, simple, dark spot, or swelling on the back at the site of the gap in the spine. The meningocele typically causes mild problems with a sac of fluid present at the gap in the spine.

Guillain-Barre syndrome: It is a rare but serious autoimmune disorder in which the immune system attacks healthy nerve cells in one's peripheral nervous system. This leads to weakness, numbness and tingling. It can eventually cause paralysis. The cause of this condition is unknown, but it is typically triggered by an infectious illness, such as the stomach flu or a lung infection.

The symptoms of Guillain-Barre include:

- Tingling or prickly sensations in fingers and toes
- Muscle weakness in legs that travels to upper body and gets worse over time
- Difficulty in walking steadily
- Difficulty moving eyes or face, chewing or swallowing

- Severe lower back pain
- Loss of bladder control
- Fast heart rate
- Difficulty breathing
- Paralysis

Stroke: It occurs when the supply of blood to the brain is either interrupted or reduced. When this happens, the brain does not get enough oxygen or nutrients, and brain cells start to die. Ischemic strokes are caused by arteries being blocked or narrowed, and so treatment focuses on restoring an adequate flow of blood to the brain.

Hemorrhagic strokes are caused by blood leaking into the brain, so treatment focuses on controlling the bleeding and reducing the pressure on the brain.

Chiari malformation: It is a condition in which brain tissue extends into the spinal canal. It occurs when part of the skull is abnormally small or misshapen, pressing on the brain and forcing it downward. Chiari malformation is categorised into three types, depending on the anatomy of the brain tissue that is displayed into the spinal canal. Chiari malformation type I develops as the skull and brain are growing. As a result, signs and symptoms may not occur until late childhood or adulthood. The paediatric forms, Chiari malformation type II and type III, are present at birth (congenital).

Spina bifida: In spina bifida, the vertebral arches and spines of a few vertebrae do not develop. Underneath the bony defect, the spinal cord and meninges may also be affected due to failure of mesenchyme forming the vertebral arches. Types of spina bifida (Fig. 17.9) are:

a. *Spina bifida occulta:* The defect is only bony.
b. *Meningocele:* Meninges protrude through the bony defect.
c. *Meningomyelocele:* Meninges and spinal cord protrude through the bony defect.
d. *Rachischisis:* The spinal cord and meninges do not develop.

DEVELOPMENT OF AUTONOMIC NERVOUS SYSTEM

Sympathetic Portion

Sympathetic pathways consist of two neurons, i.e. preganglionic and postganglionic. The preganglionic neurons develop in the mantle layer of thoracolumbar segments of spinal cord—T1–L2 segments. These neurons are located in the general visceral efferent column or intermediate zone and form the lateral horn of the spinal cord. The axons arising from these neurons are myelinated and pass into ventral nerve roots to enter spinal nerves. After a short course, they leave the spinal nerve and pass towards postganglionic neurons.

Postganglionic neurons develop in the 5th week of intrauterine life; cells originating in the neural crest of the thoracic region migrate on each side of spinal cord towards the region immediately behind the dorsal aorta. Here they form a bilateral chain of segmentally arranged sympathetic ganglia interconnected by longitudinal nerve fibres. Together they form the sympathetic chains located on each side of vertebral column. From positions in the thorax, neuroblasts migrate towards cervical and lumbosacral regions, thus extending sympathetic chain to their full length. The arrangement is obscured in the cervical region by fusion of the ganglia.

Some neuroblasts migrate in front of aorta to form preaortic ganglia like coeliac, and mesenteric ganglia.

The nerve fibres originating in the visceroefferent column (lateral horn) of thoracolumbar segments of spinal cord synapse with neurons of sympathetic ganglion at the same level in sympathetic chain or pass through the chain to preaortic or collateral ganglion. The preganglionic fibres have myelin sheath and stimulate sympathetic ganglion cells. Passing from spinal nerves to sympathetic ganglion, they form the white ramus communicans. Since the visceroefferent column extends from T1–L2 segments of spinal cord, white rami communicantes are found only at T1–L2 levels.

Axons of sympathetic ganglion cells are called postganglionic fibres and have no myelin sheath. They pass either to other levels of sympathetic chain or extend to heart, lungs and intestinal tract.

Other fibres known as grey rami communicantes pass from sympathetic chain to spinal nerves and from there to peripheral blood vessels, arrector pilorum muscles and sweat glands. Grey rami communicantes are found at all levels of spinal cord.

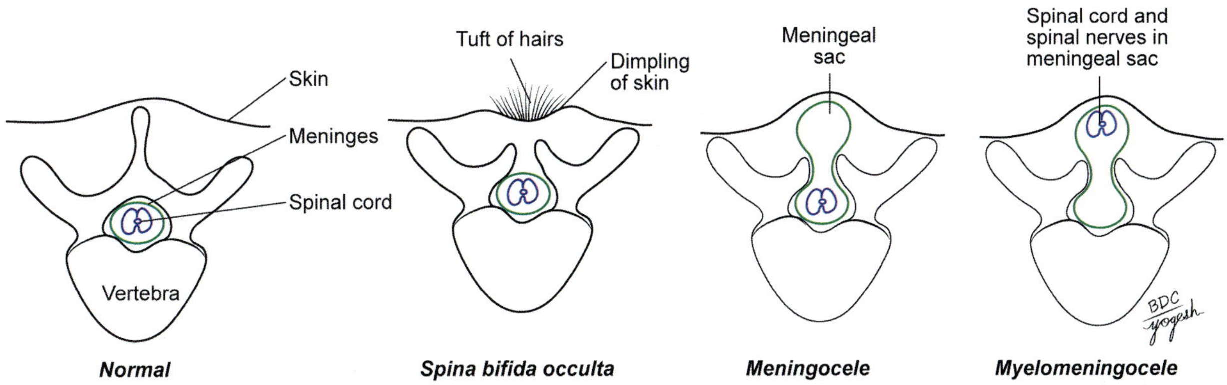

Fig. 17.9: Types of spina bifida

Parasympathetic Portion

Preganglionic neurons are formed in the brainstem and sacral region of spinal cord.

These neurons in the brainstem are located in general visceral efferent column. These give rise to Edinger-Westphal nucleus, lacrimatory, superior salivatory and inferior salivatory nuclei and dorsal nucleus of vagus. Their axons constitute the cranial parasympathetic outflow.

The sacral preganglionic neurons are derived from the mantle layer of sacral part of the spinal cord, their axons constitute the sacral parasympathetic outflow.

Postganglionic neurons of cranial region are derived from neural crest cells. These neurons form ciliary, otic, sphenopalatine and submandibular ganglia and also the ganglia associated with various viscera supplied by vagus nerve. Postganglionic axons arise from these neurons in the ganglia and supply constrictor pupillae, lacrimal gland, salivary gland and various viscera.

According to some investigators, postganglionic neurons of the brain arise from same region as the preganglionic neurons and migrate along the path followed by postganglionic fibres.

In the sacral region, the postganglionic neurons migrating from the sacral part of the spinal cord supply pelvic viscera and distal one-third of transverse colon, descending colon, pelvic colon, and rectum.

BDC's Anatomy *e*-book

1. Molecular regulation of development of spinal cord and brain
2. Viva voce questions

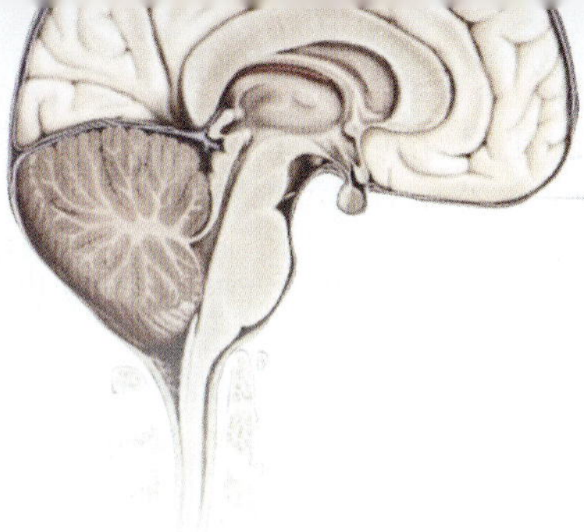

Appendix

Ventricles, Cranial Nerves and Arteries

SUMMARY OF THE VENTRICLES OF THE BRAIN

LATERAL VENTRICLE

The lateral ventricle comprises a central body and three horns—anterior, posterior and inferior. Their walls are enumerated.

Body or Central Part

Roof: Trunk of corpus callosum.

Floor: Superior surface of thalamus, thalamostriate vein, stria terminalis, body of caudate nucleus.

Medial: Septum pellucidum, body of fornix.

Anterior Horn

Roof: Anterior part of trunk of corpus callosum.

Anterior: Genu and rostrum of corpus callosum.

Floor: Head of caudate nucleus.

Medial wall: Septum pellucidum and column of fornix.

Posterior Horn

Roof and lateral wall: Tapetum of corpus callosum.

Medial wall: Bulb of posterior horn above and calcar avis below.

Inferior Horn

Roof and lateral wall: Tapetum, tail of caudate nucleus, stria terminalis and amygdaloid nucleus.

Floor: Pes hippocampus, hippocampus, alveus, fimbria, dentate gyrus and collateral eminence.

THIRD VENTRICLE

The third ventricle lies between the two thalami. The components of its boundaries and recesses are enumerated:

Anterior wall: Lamina terminalis, anterior commissure, anterior column of fornix (*see* Fig. 9.1).

Posterior wall: Pineal body and cerebral aqueduct.

Floor: Optic chiasma, tubercinerium, infundibulum, mammillary body, posterior perforated substance and tegmentum of midbrain.

Roof: Ependyma, tela choroidea.

Lateral wall: Medial surface of thalamus, medial aspect of hypothalamus, epithalamus and interventricular foramen.

Recesses: Infundibular recess, optic recess, pineal recess, suprapineal recess (*see* Fig. 9.1).

FOURTH VENTRICLE

The cavity of fourth ventricle is situated dorsal to pons and upper part of medulla oblongata and ventral to the cerebellum. Its boundaries, recesses, apertures and continuations are mentioned here:

Lateral boundaries: Gracile tubercle, cuneate tubercle inferior cerebellar peduncles and superior cerebellar peduncles.

Upper part: Facial colliculus on the dorsal surface of pons.

Intermediate part: Vestibular nuclei, medullary striae.

Lower part: Upper part of medulla oblongata containing hypoglossal and vagal triangles.

Roof: Superior medullary velum, thin sheet of pia mater and ependyma with median aperture, inferior medullary velum (*see* Fig. 7.2).

Recesses in roof: One median dorsal, two lateral dorsal and two lateral.

Apertures: One median—foramen of Magendie, two lateral—foramina of Luschka (left and right).

Continuity: Above with cerebral aqueduct. Below with central canal of spinal cord.

NUCLEAR COMPONENTS OF CRANIAL NERVES

The cranial nerve nuclei, their locations and functions are listed in Table A.1.

ARTERIES OF BRAIN

Vertebral Artery

Vertebral artery, a branch of 1st part of subclavian artery, is divided into four parts:

1. *First part:* Lies deep in the neck in the vertebral triangle; gives no branches.

TABLE A.1: Cranial nerve nuclei

Component	*Nucleus*	*Location*	*Function*
General somatic efferent (GSE) (supply skeletal muscle of somatic origin)	Oculomotor nucleus	Midbrain at the level of the superior colliculus	Supply 4½ extrinsic muscles of the eyeball except the lateral rectus and the superior oblique
	Trochlear nucleus	Midbrain at the level of the inferior colliculus	Superior oblique muscle through the trochlear nerve
	Abducent nucleus	Lower part of the pons	Lateral rectus muscle through the abducent nerve
	Hypoglossal nucleus	Extends into both the open and closed parts of the medulla	Seven out of eight muscles of the tongue through the hypoglossal nerve
Special visceral efferent (SVE) (supply striated muscle derived from the branchial arches)	Motor nucleus of the trigeminal nerve	Upper part of the pons	Muscles of mastication through the mandibular nerve
	Nucleus of the facial nerve	Lower part of the pons	Various muscles innervated by the facial nerve
	Nucleus ambiguus	In both the open and closed parts of the medulla	Stylopharyngeus muscle through the glossopharyngeal nerve; and Muscles of the soft palate, the pharynx and the larynx through the vagus nerve and the cranial part of the accessory nerve
General visceral efferent (give origin to preganglionic neurons that relay in a peripheral autonomic ganglion. Postganglionic fibres arising in the ganglion supply smooth muscles or glands)	Edinger-Westphal nucleus	In the midbrain in close relation to the oculomotor nucleus	Through the oculomotor nerve to the ciliary ganglion to supply the sphincter pupillae and the ciliaris muscles
	Lacrimatory nucleus	In the lower pons	Fibres that pass through the facial nerve and its branch, the greater petrosal nerve to relay in the pterygopalatine ganglion and supply the lacrimal, nasal, palatal and pharyngeal glands
	Superior salivatory nucleus	In the lower part of the pons	Through the facial nerve and its chorda tympani branch to the submandibular ganglion for supply of the submandibular, sublingual salivary glands and glands in the oral cavity
	Inferior salivatory nucleus	In the lower part of the pons just below the superior nucleus	Through the glossopharyngeal nerve to the otic ganglion for supply of the parotid gland
	Dorsal nucleus of the vagus	Open and closed parts of the medulla	Fibres that pass through the vagus nerve to be distributed to thoracic and abdominal viscera (the ganglia concerned are present in the walls of the viscera supplied)
General visceral afferent (GVA) and special visceral afferent (SVA)	Nucleus of solitary tract	In the medulla and extends into both its closed and open parts	Its lower part receives general visceral sensations as follows: a. Through the glossopharyngeal nerve from the tonsil, pharynx, posterior part of the tongue, carotid body and carotid sinus b. Through the vagus nerve from the pharynx, larynx, trachea, oesophagus and other thoracic and abdominal viscera Its upper part also receives sensations of taste (special visceral afferent) as follows: a. From the anterior two-thirds of the tongue, and the palate except circumvallate papillae through the facial (VII) nerve in its superior part b. From the posterior one-third of the tongue through the glossopharyngeal nerve (IX) including the circumvallate papillae in its middle part c. From the posteriormost part of the tongue and from the epiglottis through the vagus (X) nerve in its inferior part

(Contd.)

TABLE A.1: Cranial nerve nuclei *(Contd.)*

Component	*Nucleus*	*Location*	*Function*
General somatic afferent (GSA)	Main or superior sensory nucleus of the trigeminal nerve	Upper part of the pons	Fine and discriminatory touch, pressure sensation from head and neck
	Spinal nucleus of the trigeminal nerve	Medulla	Pain, temperature from forehead, cheek, from around mouth
	Mesencephalic nucleus of the trigeminal nerve	Midbrain	Exteroceptive sensations (touch, pain, temperature) from the skin of the face, through the trigeminal nerve; and from a part of the skin of the auricle through the vagus (auricular branch) and through the facial nerve. Proprioceptive sensations from muscles of mastication reach the mesencephalic nucleus through the trigeminal nerve. The nucleus is also believed to receive proprioceptive fibres from the ocular, facial and lingual muscles, teeth and temporomandibular joint
Special somatic afferent (SSA)	Cochlear nuclei (dorsal and ventral)	Pons	Impulses of hearing through the cochlear nerve
	Vestibular nuclei (superior, spinal, medial and lateral)	Pons	Receive fibres from the semicircular canals, the utricle and the saccule through the vestibular nerves

2. *Second part:* Passes in the foramen transversaria of C6–C1 vertebrae; gives spinal branches for supply of meninges and spinal cord.
3. *Third part:* Lies in the suboccipital triangle, on the posterior arch of atlas vertebra and gives branches to muscles of suboccipital triangle.
4. *Fourth part:* Enters the cranial cavity through foramen magnum. Joins with the same artery of opposite side to form basilar artery at the lower border of pons.
   The fourth part gives:
   a. Meningeal branches
   b. Posterior spinal artery
   c. Anterior spinal artery
   d. Posterior inferior cerebellar artery
   e. Medullary branches.

Basilar Artery

Right and left vertebral arteries unite at the lower border of the pons to form a median basilar artery, which gives following branches:

1. Anterior inferior cerebellar
2. Pontine branches
3. Labyrinthine branches
4. Superior cerebellar
5. Posterior cerebral.

Internal Carotid Artery (ICA)

1. Cervical part gives no branches.
2. Petrous part gives: (i) caroticotympanic for the middle ear, and (ii) pterygoid branches.
3. Cavernous part gives branches to: (i) trigeminal ganglion, and (ii) superior and inferior hypophyseal branches.
4. Cerebral part gives following branches:
   a. Ophthalmic artery which supplies outer layers of eyeball and retina through central artery of retina which is an end artery
   b. Anterior cerebral artery
   c. Middle cerebral artery continuation of ICA
   d. Posterior communicating artery
   e. Anterior choroidal artery.

Circle of Willis

Circle of Willis is formed by union of (i) anterior cerebral, (ii) terminal part of internal carotid, (iii) posterior communicating branch of internal carotid, (iv) joining the posterior cerebral branch of vertebral artery on each side. The two anterior cerebral arteries are joined by anterior communicating artery.

Branches of Circle of Willis

Central branches: These are long, thin, numerus end arteries which supply deeper structures like internal capsule and basal ganglia.

Choroidal branches: Choroidal branches of internal carotid and posterior cerebral arteries supply choroid plexuses of the ventricles.

Cortical branches: These are:

a. *Anterior cerebral:* Chief artery on the medial surface of cerebral hemisphere till parieto-occipital sulcus. It also supplies 1 cm wide area on the superolateral surface, along the superomedial border. The area includes motor and sensory areas of lower limb and perineum.
b. *Middle cerebral:* Main artery of the superolateral surface supplying major parts of motor and sensory areas. It also supplies motor speech, auditory and vestibular areas.
c. *Posterior cerebral:* Chief artery of the tentorial surface and occipital lobe. This is the artery of visual cortex.

BDC's Anatomy *e*-book

1. Clinical terms
2. Viva voce questions

RIGHT THALAMUS

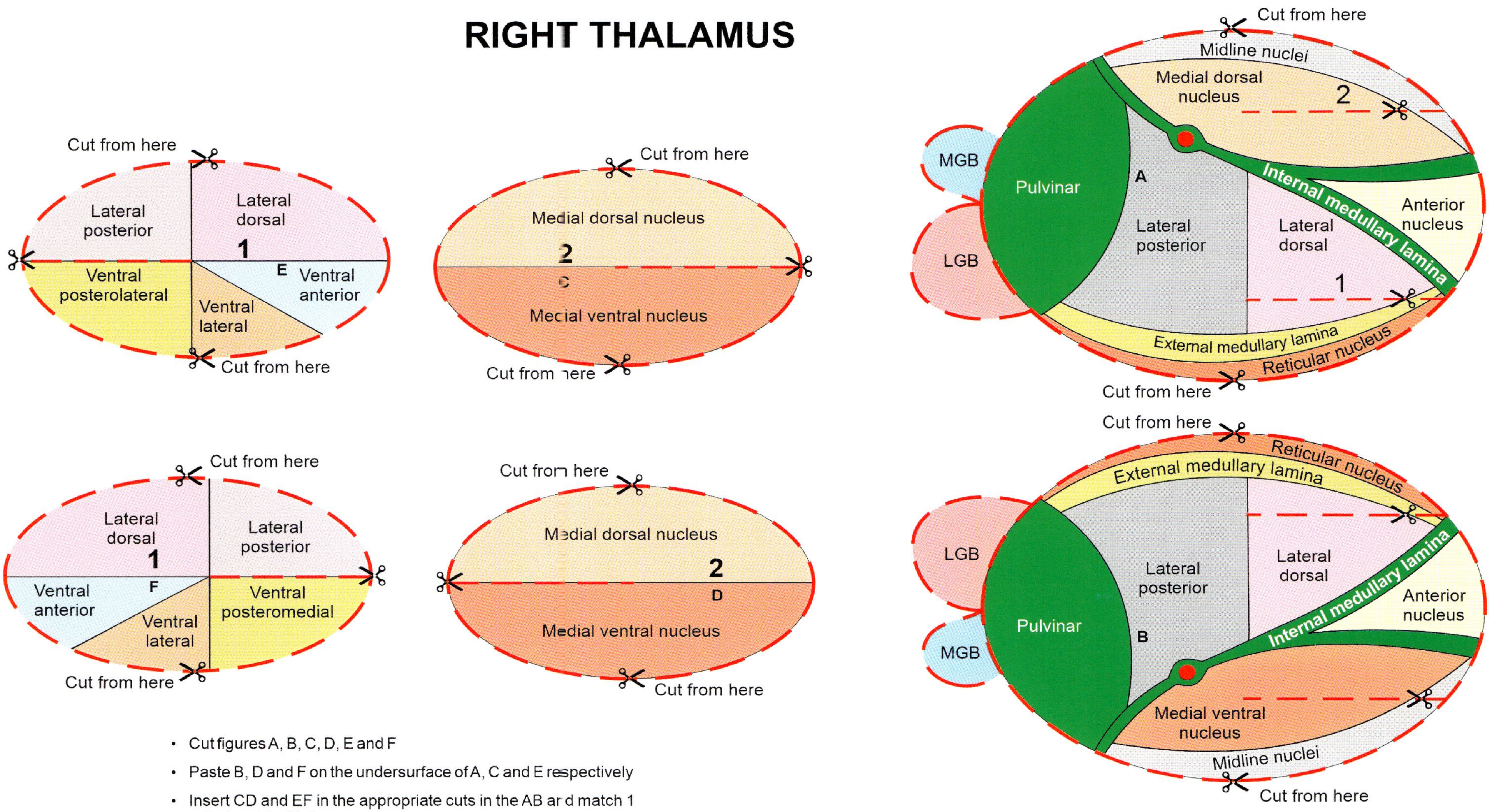

- Cut figures A, B, C, D, E and F
- Paste B, D and F on the undersurface of A, C and E respectively
- Insert CD and EF in the appropriate cuts in the AB ar d match 1 with 1 and 2 with 2

Index

A

Agnosia 135
Agraphia 134
Allergic rhinitis 53
Alzheimer's disease 176
Amyotrophic lateral sclerosis 46
Anosmia 53, 156
Aphasia 136
Apraxia and akinesia 134
Argyll Robertson pupil 56, 98
Arteries of brain 162, 193
  basilar artery 195
  circle of Willis 195
    anterior cerebral 195
    central branches 195
    choroidal branches 195
    cortical branches 195
    middle cerebral 195
    posterior cerebral 195
  internal carotid artery 164, 195
  vertebral artery 162, 193
Ascending tracts 41
  exteroceptive sensations 52
    anterior spinothalamic 42
    lateral spinothalamic 41
  neurons of 43
Astereognosis 135
Athetosis 140
Attention deficit hyperactive disorder 190
Autism 190
Autonomic nervous system 178

B

Babinski's sign 7
Ballismus 140
Basal nuclei 137
    amygdaloid body 140
    claustrum 139
  corpus striatum 138
    caudate nucleus 138
    functions of 139
    lentiform nucleus 138
Bell's palsy 69
Benedikt's syndrome 98
Binasal hemianopia 55
Bitemporal hemianopia 55
Blood supply of brain 162
Blood supply of spinal cord 47
Blood supply of the brainstem 171
Blood–brain barrier 167
Brainstem 8, 84, 171
Brown-Séquard syndrome 46
Bulbar palsy 90

C

Caseous lymph nodes 80
Cauda equina syndrome 34
Cellular architecture 1
  grey matter and white matter 7
  neuroglial cells 5
  neuron 1
  reflex arc 7
Cerebellopontine angle 93
Cerebellum 99
  blood supply 106
  connections of 104
  external features 99
  functions of 106
  grey matter of 126
  histological structure 103
  morphological divisions 102
Cerebral hemisphere 8, 126
Cerebral palsy 190
Cerebral vascular disease 171
Cerebrospinal fluid (CSF) 28
Cerebrum 126
  histology 136
Charcot's artery of cerebral haemorrhage 145, 169
Chiari malformation 191
Chorea 140
Circulus arteriosus or circle of Willis 195
Cisternal puncture 28
Complete transaction of spinal cord 46
Compression of III nerve 59
Conus medullaris syndrome 34
Convulsion 190
Cranial nerves 49, 193
Craniosynostosis 190
Crocodile tears syndrome 69

D

Deafness 72
Descending tracts 38
  extrapyramidal tracts 39
    comparison of pyramidal and extrapyramidal tracts 41
    lateral reticulospinal 40
    medial reticulospinal 40
    rubrospinal 40
    vestibulospinal 40
  pyramidal or corticospinal tracts 38
    anterior 42
    lateral 41
Destructive lesion of primary motor area 134
Diabetes insipidus 122
Diencephalon 114
  connections and functions of 118
  epithalamus 119
  hypothalamus 120
  metathalamus 117
    lateral geniculate body 119
    medial geniculate body 117
  subthalamus 122
  thalamus 114
Disturbance of sleep 124
Divisions of nervous system 1
  anatomical 1
  functional 1
Down syndrome 190

E

Eighth cranial nerve 71
  pathway of hearing 71
  vestibular pathway 72
Eleventh cranial nerve 79
  course and distribution 79
    cranial root 80
    spinal root 80
  functional components 79
Embolism 171
Epilepsy 190

F

Facial nerve palsy in newborn 69
Fifth cranial nerve 62
  branches of 63
    mandibular nerve 64
    maxillary nerve 63
    ophthalmic nerve 63
  nuclear columns 50
    motor component 49
    sensory components 49
First cranial nerve 52
Foster Kennedy syndrome 56
Fourth cranial nerve 60
Fourth ventricle 109
  angles 112
  cavity and recesses of 112
  communication 109
  floor 109
  lateral boundaries 109
  openings in the roof 112
  roof 111
  tela choroidea of 112
Frey's syndrome 66
Froin's syndrome or loculation syndrome 29

Functional areas of cerebral cortex 133
areas of special sensations 135
hearing 135
smell 136
taste 136
vestibular area 136
vision 136
motor areas 132
frontal eye field 134
motor speech area of Broca 134
prefrontal cortex 134
premotor 133
primary 134
supplementary 134
sensory areas 134
first somesthetic area 134
receptive speech area of Wernicke 135
second somesthetic area 135
somesthetic association cortex 135

G

Glossopharyngeal neuralgia 75

H

Haemorrhage—cortical or subcortical 171
Hemianopia 55
Hemiballismus 122
Hemiplegia 169
Hippocampal-amygdala complex 156
Homonymous hemianopia 55
Horner's syndrome 184
Hydrocephalus 112
Hydrocephalus in infants 124
Hyperglycaemia 124
Hypertensive encephalopathy 171

I

Injury to lower part of medulla oblongata 90
Injury to pharyngeal branch 79
Injury to right recurrent laryngeal nerve 79
Internal carotid artery 164, 195
branches 164
anterior cerebral artery 164
anterior choroidal artery 164
middle cerebral artery 164
ophthalmic artery 164
posterior communicating artery 164
Intersegmental tracts 45
Investigations required in a neurological case 176
angiography 176
computerised tomography 175
electrophysiological methods 177
lumbar puncture 28, 31
magnetic resonance imaging 175
positron emission tomography 175
X-ray skull 174
Irritation of the auricular branch of the vagus 78
Irritation of the recurrent laryngeal nerve 78

J

Jacksonian epilepsy 134
Jugular foramen syndrome 75

L

Laminar organisation in spinal cord 36
Lateral ventricle 148
anterior horn 150
central part 150
inferior horn 150
boundaries 150
posterior horn 150
boundaries 150
Lesion of the pyramidal tract 157
Lesions of spinal root of accessory nerve 80
Limbic system 151
Papez circuit 155
rhinencephalon 151
Loss of corneal blink reflex 65
Loss of jaw jerk reflex 65
Loss of sneeze reflex 65
Lumbar epidural space 28
Lumbar puncture 31
Lumbar puncture in a child 31

M

Medial medullary/Dejerine syndrome 89
Medulla oblongata 84
blood supply 89
external features 84
internal structure 87
Meniere's syndrome 73
Meninges 22
arachnoid mater 23
cisterns 26
cerebellomedullary 26
cisterna pontis 26
interpeduncular 26
lumbar 26
of great cerebral vein 26
of lateral sulcus 26
dura mater 22
folds of 23
extradural spaces 25
pia mater 25
subarachnoid space 25
subdural spaces 25
Midbrain 94
external features 95
internal structure 95
subdivisions 96
Millard-Gubler syndrome 94
Myasthenia gravis 21

N

Nerve supply of the viscera 182
Ninth cranial nerve 73
Nuclear components of cranial nerves 193
abducent 194
facial 194
glossopharyngeal 194
hypoglossal 194
oculomotor 194
olfactory 194
optic 194
trigeminal 194
trochlear 194
vagus and cranial part of CN XI 194
vestibulocochlear 194
Nuclei of spinal cord 36
in anterior grey column 36
in lateral grey column 36
in posterior grey column 36

O

Occlusion of anterior cerebral artery 169
Optic neuritis 55

P

Papilloedema 28
Paralysis of both vocal cords 79
Paralysis of the vagus nerve 78
Parasympathetic nervous system 181
craniosacral outflow 181
efferent pathways of cranial part 182
sacral outflow 181
Parinaud's syndrome 98
Parkinsonism 140
Parts of the nervous system 7
central nervous system 7
peripheral nervous system 8
Pathway of pain and temperature 157
Pathway of proprioceptive (kinaesthetic) impulses 158
Pathway of touch 158
crude touch 158
fine touch 158
Perivascular spaces 169
Pharyngitis 75
Poliomyelitis 35
Pons 90
basilar part 92
blood supply 93
external features 91

internal structure 91
tegmentum in the lower part of 92
tegmentum in the upper part of 93
Pontine haemorrhage 93
Pseudobulbar palsy 90
Pyramidal tract 157

R

Ramsay-Hunt syndrome 69
Receptors 18
functional classification 18
exteroceptors 18
interoceptors/enteroceptors 18
proprioceptors 18
motor efferent endings 20
skeletal muscle 20
sensory afferent 18
free nerve endings 19
Krause's end bulb 19
lamellated (pacinian) corpuscles 19
Merkel endings 19
neuromuscular spindles 20
neurotendinous spindle of Golgi 19
Ruffini's corpuscles 19
tactile corpuscles of Meissner 19
Referred pain 184
Reticular formation 159
connections 160
functions 159
location and identify 159

S

Scotoma 55
Second cranial nerve 53
optic pathways 54
Seventh cranial nerve 66
Sixth cranial nerve 61
Sixth nerve paralysis 62
Spasmodic torticollis 80
Spina bifida 190
Spinal cord 30
Spinal nerves 33
Spinal stenosis 190
Stroke 191
Subarachnoid haemorrhage 31
Summary of the ventricles of the brain 193
fourth ventricle 193
lateral ventricle 193
third ventricle 193
Surface anatomy 173
borders of cerebral hemisphere 173
central sulcus 173
functional areas of cerebral cortex 173
lateral sulcus 173
Sympathetic nervous system, thoracolumbar outflow 178
abdominal/lumbar part 180
branches 179
cervical part 179
pelvic/sacral and coccygeal parts 181
prevertebral ganglia and plexuses 181
superior hypogastric plexus 181
thoracic part 180
Syringomyelia 42

T

Tabes dorsalis 35
Thalamic syndrome 117
Taste pathway 159
Tenth cranial nerve 75
Third cranial nerve 58
Third ventricle 123
Thrombosis 164
of posterior cerebral artery 164
of posterior inferior cerebellar artery 164
of superior cerebellar artery 164
of the paracentral artery 192
Tracts of the spinal cord 37
Trigeminal neuralgia 65
Tumours of pons 94
Twelfth cranial nerve 80

U

Uncinate fits 156

V

Veins of the brain 170
characteristics of 170
groups of 170
external cerebral 170
internal cerebral 170
terminal 170
Ventricular puncture 28
Vertebral arteries 162
basilar artery 163, 195
anterior inferior cerebellar artery 163
labyrinthine artery 163
pontine branches 164
superior cerebellar artery 164
two terminal posterior cerebral branches 164
branches of posterior cerebral arteries 185
intracranial branches 162
anterior spinal artery 163
medullary branches 163
meningeal branches 163
posterior inferior cerebellar artery 162
posterior spinal artery 162
Vertigo 72

W

Weber's syndrome 59, 98
White matter of cerebrum 141
association fibres 141
long 141
short 141
commissural fibres 142
corpus callosum 142
internal capsule 143
blood supply 145
fibres of 145
projection fibres 142